T0358187

Pain and Pleasure in Classical Times

Columbia Studies in the Classical Tradition

The titles published in this series are listed at *brill.com/csct*

Pain and Pleasure in Classical Times

Edited by

W. V. Harris

BRILL

LEIDEN | BOSTON

The Library of Congress Cataloging-in-Publication Data is available online at http://catalog.loc.gov

Typeface for the Latin, Greek, and Cyrillic scripts: "Brill". See and download: brill.com/brill-typeface.

ISSN 0166-1302
ISBN 978-90-04-37949-7 (hardback)
ISBN 978-90-04-37950-3 (e-book)

This book is printed on acid-free paper and produced in a sustainable manner.

Nam neque nos agere hoc patriai tempore iniquo possumus aequo animo

LUCRETIUS I, 41–42

∵

Contents

Preface

Pain and Pleasure in Classical Times is the fruit of a conference that took place at Columbia's Center for the Ancient Mediterranean on April 17th and 18th, 2015. The idea that brought the conference into being was that the analysis of pain and pleasure as they were experienced and as they were thought about in classical antiquity had been too segmented. Literature scholars, ancient historians, archaeologists and philosophers all had plenty to learn from each other in this area. From an ancient historian's point of view, certainly, there were and are many intriguing lines of enquiry (I describe some of them in the Introduction).

'Best laid schemes'. A distinguished cast and lively discussions did not produce anything remotely like a comprehensive view of the subject, and it is to be hoped and expected that further studies will proliferate. A conference about classical pain is currently being organized at the University of Exeter. Some of the papers given at our conference were too peripheral, some papers were promised for publication but not delivered—the usual difficulties of publishing conference proceedings. Such difficulties made me especially grateful to three distinguished scholars who did not attend the conference, Véronique Boudon-Millot, James Davidson and David Konstan, for agreeing to publish highly relevant articles here.

It is my pleasure to thank all the contributors for their hard work and co-operation, and all the numerous scholars whose names do not appear in the table of contents but who took part in the conference and/or provided advice subsequently. But most of all I wish to thank two Columbia graduate students, Ursula Poole, who co-organized the conference with me, and Evan Jewell, who as the Coordinator of the Center at the time laboured unflaggingly to make it a success.

W. V. Harris
Berlin, November 2017

Abbreviations

Not listed are the various abbreviations which the contributors have used to refer to the works of classical authors. In case of obscurity see Liddell-Scott-Jones, *Greek-English Lexicon* or Glare, *Oxford Latin Dictionary*.

AJPh	*American Journal of Philology*
ANRW	H. Temporini (ed.), *Aufstieg und Niedergang der römischen Welt*
BA	*Beazley Archive* (www.beazley.ox.ac.uk/pottery/)
CAG	Commentaria in Aristotelem Graeca
CMG	*Corpus Medicorum Graecorum*
CPh	*Classical Philology*
CQ	*Classical Quarterly*
CUF	Collection des Universités de France
FGrHist	F. Jacoby (ed.), *Die Fragmente der griechischen Historiker*
IG	*Inscriptiones Graecae*
IGUR	*Inscriptiones Graecae Urbis Romae*
Kühn	C. G. Kühn (ed.), *Claudii Galeni Opera Omnia* (Leipzig, 1821–1833), 20 v.
Littré	É. Littré (ed.), *Hippocrates, Oeuvres complètes* (Paris, 1839–1861), 10 v.
LS	A. A. Long and D. Sedley (eds.), *The Hellenistic Philosophers* (Cambridge, 1987), 2 v.
LSJ	H. Liddell, R. Scott and H. S. Jones, *Greek-English Lexicon* (ninth edition).
OSAPh	*Oxford Studies in Ancient Philosophy*
PBACAPh	*Proceedings of the Boston Area Colloquium on Ancient Philosophy*
RE	A. Pauly, G. Wissowa, etc. (eds.), *Realencyclopädie der classischen Altertumswissenschaft*
SJPh	*Southern Journal of Philosophy*
SVF	H. von Arnim (ed.), *Stoicorum Veterum Fragmenta*
TAPhA	*Transactions of the American Philological Association*
TLG	Thesaurus Linguae Graecae
ZPE	*Zeitschrift für Papyrologie und Epigraphik*

Notes on Contributors

Elizabeth Asmis
is Professor of Classics at the University of Chicago. She is the author of *Epicurus' Scientific Method* and numerous articles on Plato, Philodemus, Lucretius, Seneca, Epictetus, Marcus Aurelius, and others. Her most recent articles are: 'Seneca's Originality' (*The Cambridge Companion to Seneca*, eds. Bartsch and Schiesaro, [Cambridge, 2015], 224–38); 'Art and Morality' (*A Companion to Ancient Aesthetics*. eds. Destrée and Murray [Blackwell, 2015], 486–504); and 'Lucretius' Reception of Epicurus: *De Rerum Natura* as a Conversion Narrative', *Hermes* 144 (2016), 239–61. Her current research focuses on Epicurean social philosophy, Hellenistic aesthetics, and the reception of Lucretius.

Véronique Boudon-Millot
is the Director of the Research Centre on Ancient Medicine at the CNRS (French National Centre for Scientific Research) at the Sorbonne in Paris. She leads the programme for the publication of Galen's works in the CUF (Collection des Universités de France, also known as collection Budé). She has published widely on ancient medicine, philosophy and science. Her publications include over 100 articles written in French, English and Italian. She has edited and translated seven Galenic treatises, with introduction and commentary, in the CUF (in 2000, 2007, 2010 and 2016) and she has published a biography of Galen (2012).

Wei Cheng
(PhD, Humboldt-Universtität zu Berlin, 2015) is Assistant Professor of Classics at the University of Peking (Beijing). His thesis examined Aristotle's understanding of pleasure and pain in historical context. His research focuses on Plato, Aristotle, and the Old Academy. At the moment he is working on several articles related to the study of ancient concepts of mental life.

James Davidson
is Professor of Ancient History at the University of Warwick. He is the author of *Courtesans and Fishcakes* and *The Greeks and Greek Love*, which won the Mark Lynton History Prize, the Randy Shilts Award for Gay non-fiction and the Lambda Literary Award for Lesbian Gay Bisexual and Transgender non-fiction.

Vanessa de Harven
is Assistant Professor of Philosophy at the University of Massachusetts, Amherst. In addition to research interests in Plato's moral psychology and

Socratic intellectualism that are reflected in her contribution to this volume, de Harven specializes in Stoic metaphysics. In particular, she has work on Stoic *corporealism*, the nature of their *incorporeals* (including especially their novel semantic entities, the *lekta*, roughly, the meanings of our words), and the status of pure products of thought, like creatures of fiction and mathematical entities, which are *neither corporeal nor incorporeal*.

Marcus Folch

is an Associate Professor of Classics at Columbia University. His work focuses on ancient Greek literature and philosophy, performance in antiquity, and incarceration in the ancient world. He is the author of *The City and the Stage: Performance, Genre, and Gender in Plato's Laws*, as well as articles and chapters on ancient literary criticism, the dialogue between ancient Greek philosophy and the poetic tradition, classical reception in the 20th century. He is currently at work on a book entitled *Bondage, Incarceration, and the Prison in Ancient Greece and Rome: A Cultural and Literary History*.

W. V. Harris

is Shepherd Professor of History at Columbia University and was Director of the Center for the Ancient Mediterranean there for seventeen years. His most recent book is *Roman Power: a Thousand Years of Empire* (Cambridge, 2016). In 2016–2017 he was a fellow of the Wissenschaftskolleg zu Berlin, working principally on the environmental history of the ancient Mediterranean. He is a Corresponding Fellow of the British Academy.

David Konstan

is Professor of Classics at New York University and Professor Emeritus of Classics and Comparative Literature at Brown University. Among his publications are *"A Life Worthy of the Gods": The Materialist Psychology of Epicurus; Greek Comedy and Ideology; Friendship in the Classical World; The Emotions of the Ancient Greeks; Before Forgiveness: The Origins of a Moral Idea; Beauty: The Fortunes of an Ancient Greek Idea*; and *In the Orbit of Love: Affection in Ancient Greece and Rome*. Konstan is a fellow of the American Academy of Arts and Sciences and an honorary fellow of the Australian Academy of the Humanities.

Wolfgang-Rainer Mann

is Professor of Philosophy at Columbia University. He is the author of *The Discovery of Things: Aristotle's* Categories *and Their Context* (Princeton, 2000). More recently, he has written several papers on the reception of Greek philosophy by various Roman authors.

Samuel D. McVane
earned his PhD in the Classical Studies program at Columbia University (2018). His dissertation explores the relationship between paradox and ignorance in the philosophy and style of Seneca's *Letters on Ethics*. He currently teaches Latin at Doane Academy in Burlington, New Jersey.

Katja Maria Vogt
is Professor of Philosophy at Columbia University. She specializes in ancient philosophy, ethics, and normative epistemology. Her publications include *Skepsis und Lebenspraxis* (Freiburg, 1998, paperback with new material 2015), *Law, Reason, and the Cosmic City: Political Philosophy in the Early Stoa* (Oxford, 2008), *Belief and Truth: A Skeptic Reading of Plato* (Oxford, 2012), *Desiring the Good: Ancient Proposals and Contemporary Theory* (Oxford, 2017) and numerous articles. She is the editor of *Pyrrhonian Skepticism in Diogenes Laertius* (Tübingen, 2015), and is currently co-authoring with Jens Haas a series of papers on *Ignorance and Action*.

Caroline Wazer
completed her PhD in Ancient History at Columbia University in 2017. Her thesis was entitled *Salus Patriae: Public Health in the Early Roman Empire*.

CHAPTER 1

Introduction: Pain and Pleasure as a Field of Historical Study

W. V. Harris

Pain and pleasure may not be neat opposites, like heat and cold; so at least Ryle argued.[1] Nonetheless it is unsurprising that they should be thought of in that way, and at least since Empedocles[2] they have constantly been paired together throughout the western philosophical and literary tradition. And if we study their manifestations in a given culture—such as classical antiquity—together, we may hope to gain some psychological insight into its diverse peoples and their cultural productions.[3]

The relevant bibliography about pain and pleasure in past cultures is by no means scanty, and the history of pain has begun to receive wide-ranging treatments.[4] But we lack a satisfactory history of pain in antiquity, and as for the ancient history of pleasure, it has been fragmented into the history of sex and the history of extravagances and luxuries, to the neglect of the many other pleasures that life offers. Meanwhile the experts on ancient philosophy have often seemed to operate as if we knew what tastes and what presuppositions about pain and pleasure Greeks and Romans brought with them when they philosophized. In short, there is still much more territory to explore, and in particular there is a gorgeously rich cultural history to be written—a history to which this book is no more than a prolegomenon.

---

1 Ryle 1954, 49–50 (and elsewhere). 'Most of the questions which can be asked about aches, tickles and other sensations or feelings cannot be asked about our likings and dislikings, our enjoyings and detestings. In a word, pleasure is not a sensation at all' (49). But—in the best tradition of philosophy—he loads the dice against physical pleasures, and pleasure is not in any case synonymous with liking or enjoying. The most interesting reaction to Ryle's views that is known to me is Puccetti 1969; for other views see Wolfsdorf 2013, 221–65.

2 31 A 86 and A 95 D-K = D 235 and D 236 Laks-Most. The terms he uses for (feeling) pain are *lupeisthai* and *algêdôn*.

3 In his essay *Über den Schmerz* that deplorable figure Ernst Jünger wrote 'Tell me your relation to pain, and I will tell you who you are!' (Jünger 2008 [1934], 1). That is the particular claim of a militarist, but if we add pleasure—'Tell me your relation to pain and pleasure, and I will tell you who you are!'—the assertion makes some sense.

4 Note especially Moscoso 2012, Bourke 2014.

DOI:10.1163/9789004379503_002

A linguistic observation is necessary here, although it is rather obvious. The very words for pain and pleasure, for feeling pain and feeling pleasure, are, in both classical and modern languages, deeply complicated. Simply consider the terminology in Greek, Latin, English and German. It is obvious, though often in practice forgotten, that *odunê, dolor, pain* and *Schmerz* are not exactly synonymous (certainly not when it comes to psychic or emotional pain).[5] The same applies to *hêdonê, voluptas, pleasure* and *Vergnügen* (the inventor of psychoanalysis wrote *Jenseits des Lustprinzips*—was that really 'the *pleasure* principle', as the standard translation has it?). It would be a very worthwhile undertaking to describe the semantic fields of the four Greek and Latin terms just mentioned, and of a dozen or so other relevant Greek and Latin terms, all of which evolved over time (see especially the chapters contributed to this book by Boudon-Millot and McVane, but others as well). It may even be possible to explain these developments.

This is not simple pedantry: these terms overlap but they are seldom or never synonymous. Euripides has Phaidra give as examples of pleasure (*hêdonê*) long talks, leisure—and shame (*aidôs*) (*Hipp.* 383–5), a passage that has worried commentators a good deal.[6] They would have had to worry much more if a Latin writer had classified *pudor* as a *voluptas*. Or again: Plato assures us that the philosopher-ruler would live 729 (3^6) times 'more pleasurably' (or should we say 'pleasantly'?)—*hêdion*—than the tyrant (*Rep.* IX.587e); a Latin counterpart could hardly have said, without causing puzzlement, that the philosopher-ruler had 729 times as much *voluptas*.

It can indeed be argued that we should put the terms 'pain' and 'pleasure' on one side if we are going to understand the *roughly* equivalent phenomena in the ancient world (and also that the Greeks and Romans should be dealt with quite separately). We cannot empathize with the *odunai, lupai, ponoi, algêmata*, and so on, of the Greeks unless we attend very closely to the contours of these concepts (though I have argued elsewhere that for historians empathy in any precise sense is in any case fool's gold).[7] This is not a matter of philologist's purism, but of understanding the psychology of the people we are attempting to study. And not only of the individuals but of their collectivities as well. In his excellent book *The Lure of the Arena: Social Psychology and the Crowd at the Roman Games* (2011) the late Garrett Fagan showed how an ancient historian

---

5 On the looseness—or is it richness?—of the Greek terminology of pain see for example below pp. 39–40, 59 n.20, etc.

6 Kovacs 1980, etc.

7 Harris 2010.

widely read in social psychology can do this; and James Davidson's paper in this collection take us further in that direction.

∴

Later I will suggest some of the open questions that a cultural historian of classical pain and pleasure might profitably try to answer. But first I will give a brief account of what I think the authors of this volume have achieved. Such a procedure unavoidably over-simplifies—no summary can do justice to a richly argued scholarly article—, but it may help readers to relate the papers to each other and to map out the whole territory.

James Davidson—whose book *Courtesans and Fishcakes* (1997) was a major contribution to the cultural history of classical Greece—at once raises very large questions. Do the near-universal pleasures of eating, drinking and fornicating have a history? Yes. Fish-consumption, avoided by the Greeks at Troy, even though they lived ten years by the sea, and roast-meat consumption, had cultural flavours, both for Homer and his audience, and still later for Plato. Modern (i.e. fourth-century BC) love, often disreputable, contrasts with the Homeric love of Achilles and Patroclus. But a most extraordinary aspect of Greek thinking about the pleasures of sex and of wine-drinking is that ample myths told who *invented* them, just as Greeks loved to tell who invented almost any social practice, from marriage to the cultivation of olives and figs. It was Laius (the father of Oedipus) who invented homosexuality—unless it was the Cretans, or Poseidon. Then there was the question who was first taught by Dionysus the art of making wine and the art of drinking it properly.

Such stories were not merely learned lucubrations, they were widely present in the culture, especially in the cult of Dionysus and depictions of that god's epiphany. The Hippocratic *On Ancient Medicine* meanwhile asserts that the diet of the Greeks had been 'discovered and developed during a long period of time'. What do all these contrasts between the more or less remote past and the present mean? Davidson offers a multi-layered answer, emphasizing 'the centrality of Eros in Greek thinking and the overwhelming power of *erôs* in Greek experience'. Carnal pleasures are fresh, we discover them. But they also need to be managed—and different Greeks, and of course the barbarians, do that differently.

Véronique Boudon-Millot transports us into the world of medicine, or rather of physiological theory, mainly in Galen. After a careful consideration of some of the common Greek words for pleasure and pain, she examines how these concepts functioned in medical thinking. If pain and pleasure are taken to be simply sensations, that leads to the supposition that they can both be distributed among all the senses. It then came easily, in fact naturally, to a Greek philosopher to suppose that pain arises from what in sensory experience does not accord with 'nature', and that pleasure arises from a return to 'nature' (Galen quotes Plato's *Timaeus* and 'Hippocrates'). The intensity of the pain or pleasure is proportional to the brusqueness or otherwise of the change perceived by the sense in question.

From this theorizing Galen draws some practical conclusions. Pleasure and pain are not only symptoms, they are also among the 'small causes' of illness, so he claims (xv.903K). This turns into an argument in favour of sexual moderation: not too much pleasure but not too little. (None of this has any basis in what we would count as observed physiological fact—but Galen was still doctor enough to recommend specifics to heighten and to lower sexual desire). Lastly, there is a role of pain and pleasure in therapeutics, a disputed matter in antiquity; what is most fascinating is the frequent emphasis in medical writers on making treatments as pleasant as possible ('ancient medical thought expressed gentleness as its deepest originality').

My contribution also concerns medicine. Clearly the author of the Hippocratic *On Breaths* was telling the most frightful lie when he advertised the medical art of his time by claiming (1.2) that it rid the sick of the greatest evils, 'illnesses, suffering (*lupês*), pains (*ponôn*), and death. For all these things medicine (*iatrikê*) provides a manifest cure'. And such claims won an astonishing degree of acceptance in classical Greece.[8] In reality, both popular medicine and doctors were still largely helpless in the face of pain. Hippocratic doctors were expected to be able to allay pain, but most of their ideas about how to do it were themselves painful or dangerous or both, although they could very occasionally help. Scholars are often much too optimistic about this. The obstacles in the way of discovering effective analgesics were admittedly formidable. But I argue in my chapter that there was some definite progress, though it was very slow.

Who was most responsible for some small later advances it is impossible to say, given our ignorance about Hellenistic medicine, but by the time of Celsus and Dioscorides doctors and others had realized more clearly what opium and mandragora might do. Relief was still hard to come by, however, especially if your doctor happened to belong to the 'Methodist' sect.[9] By Galen's time there had been some further progress, though it remains unknown how much lower-level physicians knew and were able to put into practice. Anesthesia for

---

8   To name two texts out of many, consider [Aeschylus], *Prometheus Vinctus* 478–83, and the passage in *Nicomachean Ethics* 10.4 quoted below by Wei Cheng (p. 175).

9   On the medical sects see most recently Leith 2016.

surgery also became more possible, though it always remained very dangerous. I then briefly raise the questions whether Greeks and Romans behaved
differently from us in the face of physical pain (yes, sometimes at least), and
whether they actually felt pain differently (debatable).

Continuing with medicine and the 'Methodists', *Caroline Wazer* asks what
their claim to treat patients 'pleasurably' really amounted to. Was it a false
promise? Roman laypeople were well aware that medical treatment was very
often painful. A contrary tradition also appears, maintaining that sexual pleasure was good for a woman's health, and that a doctor might prescribe things
that were pleasant to eat (evidence of Martial). But the Methodist Antonius
Musa prescribed cold baths in winter (and was considered to have saved
Augustus' life), and this and other evidence shows that members of that sect
sometimes forgot about pleasurable treatments.[10]

I started this introduction with the philosophers, and all readers of the Greek
philosophers meet the hedonism of the Epicureans and the anti-hedonism of
many of the others. But what do we in fact mean by hedonism? *Katja Vogt*
sets out to answer this question, classifying philosophers as hedonists, anti-
hedonists and also, crucially, as 'non-hedonists', that is to say those who 'reject
hedonism while admitting that there are good pleasures'. She distinguishes
between psychological hedonism—Epicurus' claim that all humans do in fact
pursue pleasure—and normative hedonism, which is of course rejected by
Plato and Aristotle. But Epicurus' hedonism is sophisticated, distinguishing
carefully between different kinds of pleasures and pains.

Plato and Aristotle are to be qualified as non-hedonists not anti-hedonists,
since 'they never seem to call into question that pleasure is a positive experience'. The good human life in the *Philebus* (the Platonic dialogue especially
concerned with pleasure) contains pleasures, and Aristotle also ascribes value
to pleasure. It is the Stoics (though they were not the first) who are the anti-
hedonists who claim that pleasure is in every instance irredeemably bad,
whatever that may mean. Plato and Aristotle had made claims about *which*
pleasures were bad, tending of course to select the least intellectual ones. Vogt
ends with a discussion of what Aristotle has to say about the variety of pleasure
at the beginning of *Nicomachean Ethics* Book 10.

Wolfgang Mann and *Vanessa de Harven* in their turn concentrate on the
other Platonic dialogue besides the *Philebus* that is most important in this
context, the *Protagoras*, and on the dispute among its modern interpreters as
to whether Socrates is represented there as a theorist of hedonism. In the last

---

10   But one might say that cold baths, whatever the season, were a very mild remedy by the
      standards of the bleeding, purging and cauterization that other doctors favoured.

part of this disjointed dialogue he has seemed to some readers to endorse a kind of hedonism, and he does indeed introduce a calculus of pleasure (an antecedent of utilitarianism). Contrary to the views of some scholars, however, Mann and de Harven argue that a close reading of the dialogue shows that Socrates is never represented as having committed himself to any form of philosophical hedonism. A careful and contextualized reading of the crucial passage in *Protagoras* 358ab reveals that Socrates is never represented by Plato as having endorsed hedonism *himself*, but merely as having used that position as a dialectical strategy. The Socrates of the *Protagoras* is not therefore anomalous.

But what of the Epicureans? *Elizabeth Asmis* takes the case of Lucretius, starting from the notorious passage at the beginning of Book II where the poet, in a priamel, may seem to endorse gloating over the sufferings of others in storms and battles.[11] She holds that Lucretius can be at least partially defended from this reading if we put the passage in its pedagogical, and specifically Epicurean-pedagogical, context. In Book I Lucretius has been 'cajoling and pressing the student to keep going, like a hound, ... who must seek out the truth for himself'. The poet needs to urge the student on to persevere with the study of the complex reasoning that he/she is about to meet. Escape from misery is the goal of Epicurean teaching, and it is freedom from misery (the misery of shipwreck and of battle) that provides the steps in the priamel. There is no reason to think Lucretius deficient in pity, certainly not (I would add) by Roman standards.

At the beginning of Book II, Lucretius has not told us what life will be like when we are free of religion. The reward is 'to hold the serene temple of wisdom', in short to experience Epicurean *ataraxia*, freedom from disturbance. The poet's message is a message of encouragement, free of any feeling of contempt. This paper shows in short how the priamel fits into the structure of the poem as a whole.

On to the Stoics. Taking Seneca seriously as a philosopher, *Sam McVane* analyses his thinking about pleasure, which does not adhere strictly to previous Stoic doctrines, as far as we can tell. In a paper that pays careful attention to language, McVane argues that the kinds of *gaudium* (joy) discussed in Seneca's *De vita beata* are to be identified with the 'joys' that are 'accompaniments' or

---

11 'It is sweet, when the winds are buffeting the water on the great sea, to gaze from the land on the great toil of another; not because it is a sweet pleasure that anyone should be distressed, but because it is sweet to perceive from what evils you yourself are free. Sweet it is, too, to behold great contests of war marshaled over the plains, when you have no part in the danger. But nothing is more pleasant than to occupy the serene temples, well fortified, that have been erected by the teachings of the wise', I, 1–8.

epigennêmata of virtue. These are 'the affective side of the sage's thinking and actions in so far as they are virtuous'. They are not emotions but 'moods or generalized states of mind' that are part of the Stoic account of a good life. He works hard to get around the difficult Stoic view that the sage 'never takes pleasure in anything', not even discovery or conversation, let alone love or a fine wine.

McVane further addresses the paradox that, according to Seneca, while the Stoic sage is always in this state of joy, he may at the same time be in physical pain and even undergoing torture. He ingeniously attempts to resolve the paradox by analysing 'joy' and invoking the psychological state baptized by the psychologist Mihaly Csikszentmihalyi as 'flow'.

We return to Aristotle, via his great Severan-age commentator Alexander of Aphrodisias. There are two separate treatments of pleasure in the *Nicomachean Ethics*, in Books VII and X, which seem to describe the way in which pleasure is connected with activity (*energeia*)—the crucial concept in Aristotle's analysis of pleasure—somewhat differently. His claim in Book X that pleasure stands in a 'supervenient' (*epiginomenon*) relationship to activity has been understood in different ways. *Wei Cheng*, in an especially rich paper which is correspondingly difficult to summarize adequately, divides these interpretations into what he calls the 'extrinsic' reading and the 'intrinsic' reading. The one supposes that pleasure is a by-product of an activity, while the other understands Aristotle to be saying that pleasure is the *perfection* of the activity upon which it supervenes. Cheng argues that Alexander based his anti-hedonistic argument on the 'extrinsic reading', and that the 'hedonists' whom Alexander criticizes appealed to the 'intrinsic reading'.

Alexander's hostility towards hedonism was commonplace by his time, and it led him to perform somersaults in order to 'purify' Aristotle's thought of even the slightest hedonistic taint. His position is that 'pleasures supervene *no less* on shameful activities [than on noble ones]' (*PE* 145.20–21); pleasure is therefore 'neither immanent in perfect activities nor does it (even partly) constitute these activities. Accordingly, there is no intrinsic relation between pain and bad activities'.[12] Cheng argues that Alexander here makes the analysis of pleasure in *Nicomachean Ethics* X more a matter of ethics than Aristotle intended. In short, he sounds somewhat like a Stoic, and must have seemed so to other Aristotelians of his time.

David Konstan remarks on the fact that Aristotle's *Rhetoric* did not include *lupê*, grief or distress, among the *pathê*, a term which we distort somewhat when we translate it by 'emotions'. Aristotle's view follows from the fact that

---

12   Cheng, p. 196.

lupê also includes physical pain, and from his opinion that *pathê* always involve judgement of some kind, whereas *lupê*, even in the sense of distress, was a more 'elementary' response. Indeed *pathê*, for Aristotle, involve not simply judgements but moral judgements about other humans. When the Stoics invented the concept of *propatheiai*, 'pre-emotions',[13] grief could be fitted into that category. But there is a difficulty: humans, unlike animals, can experience *prolonged* grief, as a result for example of bereavement; the Stoics of course disapproved. 'Nevertheless', Konstan argues, 'there are fundamental differences between inveterate grief and the kind of sentiments that Aristotle included under the term *pathos*'. Prolonged grief, he suggests, was too immune to reason to be admitted as a *pathos*; and all the *pathê* listed in Aristotle's *Rhetoric* to one degree or another 'involved a concern for justice' as well as a responsiveness to reasoning.

Finally *Marcus Folch*, in an extraordinarily rich and suggestive essay, approaches the history of pain and pleasure through an analysis of Plutarch's essay on the lateness of divine punishment, *De sera numinis vindicta*. It is important to Plutarch's anti-Epicurean position to show that god really does punish the evil-doer, and he even claims that there are no real delays. Sometimes god reserves punishment for the evil-doer's descendants, and that according to Plutarch is right and proper. In the dialogue's concluding myth, with which Plutarch attempts to bolster his case, he tells of one Aridaeus, who toured the afterlife and saw the evil-doers being punished, culminating in Nero, who was about to be reincarnated as a swan or a frog.

But much more is going on in this text. Folch contends that Plutarch's essay 'presents its reader with a meditation on the emotions of pain and pleasure that human suffering and vice engender', and he explains the philosophical and literary underpinnings of Plutarch's ideas. Yet Nero's appearance in the final scene of the Aridaeus story also complicates matters, and Folch invites us to think that Plutarch's essay finally amounts to 'a sophisticated act of double-speak and authorial deflection, in which its philosophical defense of divine providence is rewritten as censure of the Roman emperor', an emperor, it will remembered, who had favoured the Greeks and been favoured by them.

∴

Amid the great range of possibilities that a cultural history of ancient pain and pleasure offers to us, the following themes seem especially promising (I will

---

13   As to when that happened cf. Harris 2001, 110.

limit myself to seven). Some of them are adumbrated elsewhere in this book, others not. All need to be discussed diachronically.

(1) An initial imperative concerns terminology, and language more generally (see above, p. 2).[14] Ample material for several Ph.D. dissertations.

(2) What was the cause and the character of each kind of *psychological pain* that ancient people commonly experienced? We might take such experiences as terror, shame and bereavement and ask, on the one hand, whether ancient people experienced them as pains, and on the other hand (and this has been done quite a lot) what their specific manifestations were in different places and periods. For Plato, anger (*orgê*), fear, yearning, mourning, love, jealousy, envy 'and all such things' are *lupai* (*Philebus* 47d), i.e. pains or at least distressful experiences. But he is of course trying to make a point, namely that all pleasures are mixed with pain except the pleasure of knowing, as well as exploiting the (from our point of view) vagueness of the term *lupê*.[15] This 'vagueness', incidentally, allows trivial discomforts to be counted as *lupai*: Aristotle, who is arguably as precise in his use of language as any other Greek writer, considers that writing, for instance, and calculating can be *epilupos* (*EN* 10.5.1175b18), a cause of *lupê*.

Merely to take a handful of questions, should we think that the rise of consolation literature—commonly traced to the Hellenistic philosopher Crantor—reflects a greater intensity of feeling about the deaths of individuals? Was bereavement different in a society characterized by short and highly variable life-expectation?[16] When Euripides has Orestes remark that the perception of other people's sufferings 'gnaws' human beings (*Electra* 290–1), we wonder how true this was of his Athenian audience—whose members had been complicit in their share of collective brutality. And it depends which 'other people': it is assumed in the *Philebus* that there is nothing wrong with rejoicing in the misfortunes of one's enemies (49d).[17] How much, to take another case, were people painfully haunted by fear of death, or by fear of an existence after death? Or by fear of the death, wounds and destruction of warfare?

---

14   As far as pain is concerned note the important contribution of Roby 2016.

15   On the semantic range of *lupê* see now Thumiger 2017, 363.

16   See especially Kotsifou 2012.

17   'Socrates: But it is neither unjust nor envious to rejoice (*chairein*) in the misfortunes of our enemies, is it? Protarchus: No, of course not'. Whether this is consistent with what Plato wrote elsewhere need not be decided here. For the background see Dover 1974, 182. Dover maintained that enmity was much more characteristic of classical Athens than of the world in which he lived ('few of us expect to be involved for long in a relationship deserving the name of enmity', 181).

Such questions can obviously be multiplied, and they lead us into the grey area between psychic and physical pain. What the historian wants to know is how far such feelings extended, and, ideally, how and why they waxed and waned from one epoch to another. And as noted earlier, individual and group feelings will need to be distinguished from each other.

(3) The history of *physical pain* is less simple than might be supposed, as I suggest in Chapter 4. A number of intriguing historical questions suggest themselves.[18] Did people generally believe, at any period, that they could obtain relief from physical pain, either from doctors or from the variety of other sources that I have discussed elsewhere under the heading 'popular medicine'?[19] In the absence of effective analgesics, at least for most of their history, were the Greeks and Romans so accustomed and resistant to pain that they often did not count as pains that would be considered rather serious by modern people, as is suggested, for instance, by Scribonius Largus' comments on a certain dental procedure (*Compositiones* 53)?[20] To what extent did the comfortably-off adult males discount the pains of other kinds or classes of people?[21]

(4) While psychic and physical pains may sometimes be hard to tell apart, *psychic and intellectual pleasures* are even more commonly difficult to distinguish from sensory pleasures.[22] It might be a good idea to discard the traditional distinction entirely. The person who takes pleasure in looking at a work of art or a fine building or who takes pleasure in music is commonly considered to be experiencing a sensory pleasure, but since that pleasure may depend on ratiocination and knowledge, it seems misleading to put it in the same box with the pleasures of eating, drinking and fornicating, even though these too

---

18   Here I should most warmly thank Daniel King (Exeter) for sending me in advance of publication the text of his book *Experiencing Pain in Imperial Greek Culture* (Oxford, 2018). In his highly critical introduction, he appears to state his aim as 'a subtle understanding of the way in which pain might be managed in medical contexts, [and] how it is shaped by different relationships or different visions of the body's biology' (8–9). But it is only in the halls of literature departments that a scholar can write that 'the body's reality is debatable' (10). Another key claim, that 'embodied pain experience was underpinned by the emergence of a particular understanding of the physical *sōma* in this period [the first three centuries AD]' (12), warns us that 'discourse', not ordinary humanity, is going to be the focus in what follows. But further criticism would be out of place here.

19   Harris 2016.

20   See below, p. 68.

21   For this aspect of the early history of modern anesthesia see Bourke 2014, chapter 9.

22   For the neurology of pleasure see in general Kringelbach and Berridge 2010, where the editors list and elicit answers to seventeen 'fundamental pleasure questions' (7–22).

may be the subject of refined discrimination. Psychic pleasures, in any case, like psychic pains, are perhaps highly culture-specific.

That is indeed a claim that deserves a detailed investigation. We have been accustomed to think, for instance, that the evident pleasure that many Romans, including many members of the elite, experienced while they watched gladiatorial fighting and the slaughter of large wild animals was a hallmark of their culture. Garrett Fagan, however, argued forcefully that taking pleasure in painful spectacles is a commonplace of human history—so what made the Roman case special?[23] (The answer is perhaps not far to seek: institutionalization, and what that demonstrates about Roman society as a whole). The papers of Asmis and Folch in this collection touch on the question of what we may generically call gloating or *Schadenfreude*, but there is clearly more to do. And this is of course a Greek problem as well as a Roman one. A famous story in *Republic* Book IV (439e–440a) tells of Leontion son of Aglaion, who as he walked by the Long Walls of Athens could not resist the pleasure of looking at the corpses of those whom the public executioner had done to death (evidence, according to Plato, of the divided nat ure of the soul). Most Greeks, presumably, had no difficulty in understanding Leontion's voyeurism.[24] The question arises in any case whether ancient cultures gloated and felt *Schadenfreude* with fewer inhibitions than modern cultures do (if we can identify anything that can be called a modern culture). The same question applies to the literary and artistic taste for portrayals of violence and suffering that are so widespread in the ancient world from the *Iliad* to Ammianus Marcellinus and beyond.

As with psychic pains, so with psychic pleasures there is a vast territory for a historian to explore. We have been mesmerized by Greek philosophers into speaking as if such pleasures will have consisted of the intellectual pleasures to which they themselves gave preference. Meanwhile ordinary Greeks and Romans took personal or vicarious pleasure in victories (military, athletic and personal),[25] took pleasure in the growth and flourishing of their children (if they were fortunate in this respect), took pleasure in safely completed sea-voyages and harvests, and took pleasure in conversation, friends—and (*pace* Aristotle) in doing nothing. And notoriously—a much-discussed theme—they took pleasure in dramatic performances. For all this it is necessary to

---

23 Fagan 2011, chapter 2.

24 But Plato uses no word for pleasure here.

25 Cf. *EN* 7.4.1147b30: 'victory, honour, wealth'.

go far beyond the usual philosophical sources,[26] which tend to divide pleasures into the highly cerebral and the sensory, ignoring a vast range of human
experience.[27]

(5) There could also be a history of Graeco-Roman *physical pleasures*. As
I remarked earlier, modern writing on the subject has tended to dissolve
into the history of sex (which has concentrated heavily, in the United States at
least, on the unpleasurable aspects) and on extravagances and luxuries. The
study of ancient sexuality has nonetheless suffered, surprisingly perhaps, from
a neglect of the complexities of erotic pleasure, which are clearly enough
attested in a variety of Greek and Latin authors.

We need a much wider view, and a more democratic one. Admittedly one
important chapter in the history of pleasure concerns refinement: how, when
and why did it come about that some sensory pleasures—those connected in
particular with the senses of taste (gastronomy), sight and hearing—came to
be preferred by connoisseurs? We lack a history of taste—in the wider sense—
in the classical world. But an account of preferences for foodstuffs (*garum!*)
and other sensory experiences needs to go far beyond connoisseurs in any
strict sense, indeed it needs to consider as wide a range of people as possible. Such a history would also require some understanding of evolutionary
biology.[28] But it is a cultural history that is required.

(6) Two broadly negative attitudes towards pleasure recur in ancient texts,
philosophical and otherwise. One of them, which we might consider moderate, hierarchized pleasures, relegating sensuality of all kinds and promoting in-
tellectuality. The other amounted to a blanket condemnation of all pleasures.
But it would probably be a mistake to discuss these two attitudes separately,
simply because some of the greatest and most influential minds of antiquity,
including Plato and Aristotle, maintained divergent attitudes towards pleasure, sometimes within the same work.[29]

Students of Greek philosophy have devoted a great deal of energy to the
explication of both of these attitudes or positions (see in this volume the
papers of Vogt and Cheng in particular). But the history of philosophy has an
external aspect as well as an internal one;[30] in other words, no philosopher,

---

26   Cf. Chaniotis 2012, 25.

27   Even *EN* 10.3.1173b15–19 seems to head in that direction, while allowing space for pleasur-
     able memories and hopes.

28   Cf. especially Dickinson and Balleine 2010, Loonen and Ivanova 2015.

29   This is not the place to enter into details. See especially Harte 2014. For Antisthenes see
     below.

30   Cf. Herman 2006, 129–30.

not even Aristotle, is immune to contemporary society.[31] And the same applies even more obviously to the 'ordinary' writers of antiquity, those who picked up ideas rather than initiating them. For the cultural historian, meanwhile, both the moderate and the absolute anti-pleasure attitude offer a fascinating challenge.

Prudential advice to observe moderation in pursuing pleasures was no doubt as old as the hills. But with the first philosopher whose absolute-seeming condemnation of pleasure is well authenticated—Antisthenes, the follower of Socrates[32]—we are already faced with a quite different phenomenon. According to Antisthenes, he would rather have gone mad than feel pleasure, a famous saying (fr. 108 Caizzi = fr. 122 Prince).[33] Was he reacting against some of the features of the imperial Athens of his youth, or attempting perhaps to stake out a distinctive territory for a newly distinctive group, the students of the *phrontisterion*?[34] Such questions arise again and again throughout the history of the classical world, becoming all the more pressing when Stoicism gains wide influence under the Roman Empire.

This group of questions has wide relevance for the history of classical culture. How far example do pleasures of various kinds fit into ancient rhetoric or the ancient novel?

(7) Finally: pain, pleasure, and the state. Hitherto I have spoken about individuals or about crowds of individuals, or at most about individuals or crowds in their political manifestations. But what of the state, Greek or Roman? Most directly concerned are sumptuary legislation and norms, the role of the state in social welfare (including the provision of such amenities as baths) and euergetism, punishments and penological thinking, and state-sponsored spectacles. Even now, there is I think more to say about, for example, the contribution of ideas about austerity and the limitation of pleasure to sumptuary restrictions and legislation; about the contribution of callousness and gloating to the atrocious severity of punishments in not a few ancient states; and about the diverse pleasures provided by religious festivals. The interplay between ideas about pain and pleasure (and I mean ordinary people's ideas, not only those

---

31   As of course many students of Greek philosophy recognize: '[Plato's] concern with hedonism, and indeed philosophy generally, arose from his analysis of the ills of society in his time and his view of the sources of those ills in human nature' (Gosling and Taylor 1982, 3; but on the following page they shy away from following up on this observation).

32   Newly re-edited by S. H. Prince (2015).

33   As to how strongly anti-pleasure the views of Antisthenes really were see Prince 2015, 369.

34   It is intriguing that in *EN* 10.1.1172a29–33 Aristotle says of those who maintain that pleasure is wholly bad that some of them may not really believe it but wish to have an effect on people who are slaves of self-indulgence.

expressed by philosophers), social practices, and the state, deserves further investigation.

Less studied perhaps have been the disasters of war, in Goya's sense—which take us back to questions about sympathy and *Schadenfreude*.[35] The civilian victims of warfare—hard to study, admittedly—have received little attention.[36] And though we know considerably more about the mentalities of military personnel in both Greece and Rome than we did a generation ago, it might be revealing to consider what their expectations were with respect to pain and pleasure—and indeed whether disciplined soldiers are not commonly exceptions to facile ancient and modern assertions of the doctrine of 'psychological hedonism'.[37]

∴

The conspicuous absence in this collection is the iconographic evidence (though it is extensively used by James Davidson). No one can deplore this more than I do. My best efforts to elicit publishable papers from archaeologists have come to nothing; one hopes that others will be more fortunate. The relevant material is vast and very challenging, which may be part of the trouble. All sorts of questions come flooding in from other disciplines, as these pages strongly suggest. To what extent, for example, do gloating, sadistic voyeurism and in misogyny emerge as standard elements in classical art? (From Cassandra to the 'Punishment of Dirce'). Is it only the heroes who receive sympathetic treatment? What might the answers to these questions suggest to us about artists, patrons, or the general public? Visual pleasure has sometimes made its appearance in these pages, but there is much more to say. And what of the relationship between pleasure as it appears in the visual arts and the anti-hedonistic views that appear so often in this book? A project for the future.

---

35   But see very notably Dillon 2006.
36   But see now Raaflaub 2014.
37   For the meaning of this phrase see Katja Vogt's contribution to this volume.

CHAPTER 2

Post-primordial Pleasures: The Pleasures of the Flesh and the Question of Origins

James Davidson

What I want to examine in this paper are the links between pleasure and the origins of pleasure in ancient Greece—births of pleasure, discoveries of pleasure, first pleasures. This is part of a larger project looking at how time constructs pleasure and how pleasure constructs time: the degree to which the History of Pleasure—the presence in a community of a sense of pleasure's history, of a sense that pleasure has a history—can give a particular flavouring or colouring to a sense of the past and the present, and on the other hand, the degree to which pleasures themselves gain something or lose something from being plotted on to a timeline.

I will be confining myself to the pleasures of the flesh—eating, drinking and fornicating—and largely taking their status as pleasures for granted. I by no means wish to suggest these are the only pleasures worth talking about, but the carnal pleasures contest the boundaries of the definition of pleasure less strenuously than, say, the pleasures of train-spotting, stamp-collecting, or even the *goût de l'archive*, all of which have, apparently, given pleasure to millions. At the same time we must acknowledge the apparently universal character of these kinds of pleasures, which makes their cultural contextualization, and in particular their being mapped onto the field of time, more intriguing.

1   The Pleasures of Today

One of the ways in which pleasure and time are intertwined in Greek culture has now become something close to a commonplace in the scholarship of the pleasures of the flesh: the passion for or even obsession with fish in classical Athens and the ancient mystery of the 'fish missing from Homer'.[1] For, as Plato (and his comic poet contemporaries) noticed, the heroes of the *Iliad* don't eat fish even though they are encamped on the coast for a decade:

---

1   Davidson 1996, 57–64.

DOI:10.1163/9789004379503_003

You know that when his heroes are campaigning he doesn't give them fish to feast on, even though they are by the sea in the Hellespont, nor boiled meat either. Instead he gives them only roasted meat, which is the kind most easily available to soldiers, for it's easier nearly everywhere to use fire alone than to carry pots and pans ... Nor, I believe, does Homer mention sauces anywhere. Indeed, aren't even the other athletes aware that if one's body is to be kept in good condition, one must abstain from all such things?' 'Yes and they do well to be aware of it and to abstain from them'.

'If you think that', Socrates continues, 'then it seems you don't approve of Syracusan cuisine, or Sicilian-style dishes'. 'I do not'. 'Then you also object to Corinthian girls for men who are to be in good physical condition.... and Attic pastries ... I believe that we would be right to compare this diet ... to the kinds of lyric odes and songs that are composed in all sorts of modes and rhythms....

PLATO, *Republic* 404be[2]

It has not been too difficult to put these two odd features of Greek culture—classical fishmania (*opsomania*) and epic fishlessness (*anopsia*)—together. Fish was very strongly associated with the marketplace of the modern thalassocratic city of classical Athens—something you went shopping for, something you traded for money—while the selection, preparation, and consumption of meat was securely attached to central symbolic collective rituals, i.e. blood sacrifice. In this way fish-consumption was one large section of the category of food that was open to preference, connoisseurship, greed, and self-indulgence, thus allowing for the development or even overdevelopment of a particular kind of subjectivity: *opsophagia*.

But, as Plato points out so graphically, this consuming subject, this wish-listing, market-scanning, haggling, purchasing, and wolfing-down subject, the *opsophagos*, was at the same time a *contemporary* consuming subject, inseparable from the marketplace and money economy of Athens in the classical period. The pleasure of fish-consumption was very much a pleasure of today, like the pleasure of Corinthian courtesans and modern music.

Writers could play games with that strong contemporary flavouring of fish-consumption by transposing it onto the epic past or writing treatises on it, such as Archestratus's *Hēdupatheia*, in inappropriately Homeric hexameters, thus emphasizing the essential post-heroic temporality of fish-consumption through the effects of incongruity.

A whole genre of comedy, the mythological burlesque, depended for a lot of its comedy on the jarring juxtaposition of ancient heroic characters and plots

---

2   Cf. Eubulus 118.

with the trivial trappings of modern day life, which may be one reason why so many of the very many comic fragments mentioning fish come from the period when mythological burlesque was at its height in the fourth century BCE: fish was a topic rich in epochal bathos.[5]

This association of the pleasures of modern-market-bought fish with the life of the present day fell alongside other aspects of evanescence in the cultural construction of fish—its naturally early sell-by date, its fast disappearance from the market-stall, its disappearance from the plate or even from the pan—to give a sense of desperate urgency to the pleasure of consuming fish so that ancient descriptions of fish-lovers often bear a strong resemblance, strangely, to modern discourses about drug-addicts, desperate for their next fix. *Opsophagia* was not just of the present, as Plato implies, i.e. a quintessentially contemporary vice, it was also of the immediate present, the passing present, the *dies carpendus*, of the soon-to-go-off.[3]

Sex too could develop a flavouring of contemporaneity. The prominence of paid professional cithara-boys, often of slave status, for instance, in the defensive and combative fourth-century literature on Greek Homosexuality was not just a side-effect of the increasing complexity of modern music 'in all sorts of modes and rhythms' and the need for professional training in order to perform it. But inasmuch as the male and female *mousourgoi* hired to provide song and dance at classical *symposia* were often thought to have compromised their virtue by such intimate performances, the slave, ex-slave or simply low-status cithara-boys became associated with a less virtuous, more commoditized version of same-sex *erōs*.

In this way the handsome musicians were used to mark out more clearly the particular sexual subjectivity of men such as Misgolas, who was often seen in their company, with an implicit and sometimes explicit contrast with the subjectivities associated with the noble same-sex relationships of men in the heroic past like Achilles and Patroclus. For the cithara-boys, selected for their looks as much as their skill, seemed to foreground the element of sexual gratification over more traditional motivations and modalities in same-sex love such as, e.g., loyalty, honour, self-sacrifice, devotion and freedom.[4]

As for Plato's vaguely generalised 'Corinthian' courtesans, they too accumulated specific marks of contemporaneity, simply because they had become specific celebrities of a specific time-anchored cultural scene, not at all generalized but named and indeed (in)famous.[5] And comic poets were not so

---

3 Davidson 1997, ch. 1.

4 Davidson 2007, 451, 453, 455.

5 Davidson 2006, 29–51, cf. for instance *ta'pi Charixenes*, 'the age of Charixene', Aristophanes *Ecc.* 943.

chivalrous as to fail to note the passage of time in the lives of these named celebrities and the specific effects this passage of time had on their beauty, their availability and their price.[6]

Finally there is the whole question of morality. As is clear from Plato's brief list of modern pleasures, by emphasizing the novelty of pleasures and by drawing contrasts with the world of epic, in other words by *contemporizing* pleasures, he links pleasures to the debility of modern men in contrast to the heroes of Homer and provides some rhetorical assistance in a moral campaign to reduce or eliminate those pleasures of today, as if they were merely spoonfuls of froth on the surface of time, in order to regain the vigour of the past.

My first conclusion is very straightforward, even banal: For modern students of the ancient world, understanding the strangeness of ancient pleasure means understanding ancient pleasure in its ancient context, and an important part of that ancient context is the ancient temporal context. To understand how the Greeks thought about and even experienced pleasures of the flesh, it is helpful, or maybe even necessary, to think about how they had been plotted onto a timeline. We might even say that this temporal aspect of pleasure—the sense that pleasure has a history, a present and a past—is a central feature of how the Greeks understood pleasure.

2   Inventions of Love

But now I want to explore the other end of pleasure's timeline—not the ends in the fashionable contemporary scene, but the beginnings in the distant past—how the construction, the understanding and maybe even the experience of the pleasures of the flesh are affected by a concern with births, discoveries and origins in general. For one of the most startling features of the imagined past of the Greeks and one of the most peculiar features of its structuring of time is the obsession with 'firsts'. Jacob Burckhardt noted with some mischievous amusement that the Athenians alone boasted of having invented competition, law and justice, the cultivation of olives and figs, how to drink from wells, how to harness horses to carts and even 'how to walk upright'.[7] Other cities were no less proud of their own innovations. Halicarnassus, we now know, disputed the claim of the Athenian Cecrops to have invented marriage, insisting it was their own local hero Hermaphroditos who deserved the

---

6 E.g. Epicrates fr. 3.

7 Burckhardt 1998 [1898–1902], 219, with note 21, citing Aelian *VH* 3.38, Philochorus *FGrHist* 328 F 5b *ap.* Athenaeus 2.38cd cf. 5.179e, Burckhardt misses the qualification "upright after drinking".

credit.[8] In the Hellenistic world especially these firsts became almost a genre of literature, heurematology or protography, traces of which can be found even in the greatest monuments of Hellenistic literature—Callimachus's *Aitiai* for instance, or Apollonius's *Argonautika*. By the first century of our era Pliny the Elder and Hyginus were able to draw up long lists of first inventors—*quis quid invenit*—of a very wide range of things: fire, houses, sacrifice, taming animals, agriculture, pottery, dyeing cloth.[9]

These myths have the effect of presenting the world we see around us today as a world that has become, as a world that stands at the end of a long process not of evolution but of addition, as each accumulating innovation gradually makes the world look more like the one we are familiar with, stocking it with the things, the artefacts and institutions we see around us. By the same token such myths empty the past of such artefacts and institutions, turning the early epoch into a potentially dark, chaotic void. More important, they raise some pointed John-Lennon-like questions about the present, undermining its seeming normality and inevitability—imagine there's no marriage, imagine there's no houses, imagine there's no fire, imagine a world without slavery, a world without sacrifice, cloth, crops, pots, the disenfranchisement of women—provoking us into a game of historical Jenga or jackstraws to see what we can remove before the whole pile collapses and the past falls apart into something uselessly unrecognisable.[10]

Among these stories of firsts and origins are stories about the beginnings of the pleasures of the flesh. As has long been noted, one of the reasons that Eros—'fairest among the deathless gods, who unnerves the limbs and overcomes the mind and wise counsels of all gods and all men'—appears so early in Hesiod's *Theogony*, fourth thing in existence, by my count, is that a force of attraction is needed to get the primordial gods together.[11] After the theogonic hiatus caused by Uranus' pushing her progeny back into Earth's womb, sexual attraction was born again from the froth that surrounded his severed genitals in the form of Aphrodite, whose *moira* is 'sweet delight (*terpsis*) and gentle intimacy (*philotēs*)', who, indeed, gave her name, uniquely, to a particular sphere of human experience, to sexual pleasures, *ta aphrodisia*, 'the things of Aphrodite'.[12]

---

8   Lloyd-Jones, 1999, 1–14, esp. 2 ll. 19–20: *hos gamon heuren andrasi kai lechea prōtos edēse nomōi*, cf. Isager and Pedersen 2004.

9   Hyginus 274 and 277, Pliny *NH* 191–215, Kleingünther 1933, Thraede 1962.

10   For the story of how the women of Athens lost the vote, see Varro *ap.* Augustine, *City of God* 18.9.

11   Hesiod, *Theog.* 120–22, Vernant 1990, 465–78.

12   *Theog.* 206, cf. Pirenne-Delforge 1994, 419–33.

It has long been suspected, not unreasonably, that the reason the Greeks needed a boy-god of Love as well as an Aphrodite had something to do with the social institution of the love of boys, but according to their own mythology, the pleasures of homosexuality and/or the institution of Greek Love had a starting date rather later than Hesiod's Eros. According to a widespread Greek tradition, homosexuality even had a pioneer (an inventor, a discoverer, a sexual revolutionary, or a popularizer) in the form of Laius, father of Oedipus, who carried off Chrysippus, the handsome young son of his host, Pelops. So Plato in *Laws* can talk of 'following in nature's steps and enacting that law which held good before the days of Laius, declaring that it is right to refrain from indulging in the same kind of sexual intercourse with men and boys as with women'.[13] Elsewhere in the same dialogue he blames the invention of homosexuality—and here it is clear he is talking of sexual pleasure—*tas peri aphrodisia hēdonas*—on the Cretans and the Spartans, thanks to their all-male spaces of the gymnasium and the common mess.[14] Interestingly he accuses the Cretans of inventing both an inventor and a moment of invention in the form of Zeus's rape of Ganymede, as a false foundation-myth by which to justify their indulgence: 'Since they believe their laws and institutions come from Zeus, they added this slander against Zeus to mythology, so that it would be as the god's disciples, if you can believe it, that they would be enjoying this pleasure too'.[15] Pindar, however, put the date of the invention of homosexual *erōs* back a generation or two by making Poseidon besotted with Pelops in a time before either his younger brother, Zeus, became besotted with Ganymede or a young Laius became besotted with Pelops' son Chrysippus.[16]

The invention of love, especially same-sex *erōs*, could be considered something of a favourite topic of Plato. In *Phaedrus*, a divinely inspired Socrates gives a kind of allegorical reading of the myth of Ganymede, as if, this time, it was a true story misread or misheard by mortal poets. The eagle-rapt boy is used as a mythical model for the soul of the beloved, which is carried aloft on wings of love and produces a love-stream that drenches the admirer, i.e. Zeus, and splashes back on the beloved himself. This is Plato's myth of the invention

---

13   *Laws* 8. 836c. The example is very pertinent to Plato's argument inasmuch as later in the dialogue he suggests using myths and stories to create a cultural taboo against homosexuality in the same way that myths of e.g. Oedipus have created a taboo about incest, *Laws* 8.838b–839d.

14   *Ibid.* 1. 636bc.

15   *Ibid.* 636cd.

16   According to Pindar, Poseidon fell in love with Pelops and abducted him to serve the gods on Olympia, "where Ganymede would come on a second occasion". *Ol.* 1.43–4; cf. Davidson 2007, 221–7, and, on Laius and Chrysippus, 231–4.

of *himeros*—'imminent desire'—a name bestowed on this love-stream by Zeus himself, here probably allegorizing the stream of nectar and ambrosia that Ganymede was thought to pour for Zeus.[17] In the *Symposium* he has Pausanias allegorize the Hesiodic versus the Homeric versions of the birth of Aphrodite; the former, born from Ouranos's genitals, is the more ancient, purely masculine Heavenly 'Uranian' form of love, to be seen in the noble and restrained love of boys, while her younger alter-ego, 'Vulgar' Aphrodite Pandemos, the daughter of Zeus and Dione, is half female and represents the kind of hubristic love that is seen in love for women and the ignoble pursuit of boys.[18] In the same dialogue, Aristophanes proposes a very different myth of the origins of human sexual desire; each person is merely a slice of an original four-legged creature that ever longs to reconnect with its lost other half, with genitals moved to the front in order to assist in the act of temporary bodily re-joining, turning coition into the pleasure of (recreating) the past.[19]

Moreover, the vaunting on the part of the Cretans of Zeus's abduction of Ganymede as a model for their own homosexual practices, 'since they believe' comments Plato sarcastically 'that their laws and institutions come from Zeus', connects to a major theme of Plato's *Laws*: the story that Minos, king of Crete, Moses-like, received laws directly from Zeus in the cave to which the participants in the dialogue are walking. Indeed Aristotle states straightforwardly of Crete that 'the law-giver/Minos made intercourse to be directed towards males' to prevent overpopulation. It is hardly surprising therefore that the practices of Cretan homosexuality are described as part of 'the Cretan Constitution' both in Ephorus' account of Cretan customs and in the Aristotelian *Constitution of Crete*.[20] Indeed one of the most striking features of Greek discussion of Greek homosexuality is the constant reference to law and law-givers.[21] Plato's comment about the invention of the myth of Ganymede anticipates a debate later in the dialogue about what place should be given to homosexual sex in the laws and constitution of the new city. It was not Laius but the Theban lawgivers who institutionalized same-sex *erōs* in Thebes, according to Plutarch, and

---

17   Plato, *Phdr.* 255bc; cf. Davidson 13–14.

18   Plato, *Symp.* 180c–181e.

19   Plato, *Symp.* 191bc.

20   Plato, *Laws* 1.636bd, Aristotle, *Pol.* 1272a. Ephorus, *FGrHist* 70 F149 *ap.* Strabo 10.4,21, Aristotle fragment 611 (Rose). This explains why some ancient authors made Minos himself the abductor of Ganymede/ inventor of homosexuality, Suda, Mu 1092, s.v. 'Minos', Echemenes, *FGrHist* 459 F 1, Dosiadas, *FGrHist* 458 F 5, with Jacoby's notes ad loc.

21   On the importance of *nomos*, 'law/custom', *nomothesia* 'legislation' and *nomothetai* 'lawgivers' in the Greek discourse on Greek Homosexuality, see Davidson, 2007, 469–70.

it was Lycurgus, the Spartan lawgiver, according to Xenophon, who laid down how *paidikos erōs* was supposed to proceed in Sparta.[22]

3   First Tastings of Wine

Some of the most famous and pervasive myths of the origin of pleasure, of course, concerned epiphanies of Dionysus and the invention of wine. The most famous of these epiphanies happened in Thebes a generation or so before Laius invented homosexuality. 'Two things are primary for mortals', Tiresias claims in Euripides's *Bacchae*: the gifts of Demeter and the grief-ceasing, troubles-oblivionizing potion that Dionysus 'discovered' (*hēure*).[23] It took too long for Pentheus, the king of Thebes, to realise this truth and so he was plucked from the tree where he was spying on his Bacchant aunts and ripped limb from limb by his own mother.

In Attica priority was claimed by the mountain village of Icarion, which won authentication for its claim from the oracle at Delphi, and which already by the second half of the sixth century had an unusual colossal marble cult-statue of Dionysus seated with a kantharos cup, and by the fifth century was wealthy enough to offer loans, showing all the signs of being a major cult site.[24] According to the Icarians' myth of epiphany, which linked the invention of wine with the invention of tragedy and of processions of images of the phallus, Dionysus first taught the art of the vine to their hero Icarius, identified at some point with the constellation Boötes, the Wagoner. The shepherds who first tasted this new pleasure ended up in a drunken stupor that their bucolic colleagues misinterpreted as the deadly effects of a poison. They therefore murdered Icarius. When their drunken friends woke up with what can properly be called the mother of all hangovers they realised their mistake and fled, but the murder of Icarius did not go unpunished. Dionysus took on the form of a beautiful youth, a divine vengeful prick-tease, and having aroused in them the urge for intercourse he disappeared, leaving them with unresolvable erections. In agony they went to Delphi to ask how they might be relieved. The answer was that they should make images of their erections and offer them to the god. And this is why phalluses are carried in honour of Dionysus.[25]

---

22   Plutarch, *Pel.* 19.1, Xenophon, *Lac.* 2.12–14.

23   Euripides, *Bacchae* 279.

24   Pausanias 1.2,5, Romano 1982, 398–409, Whitehead 1986, 215–18.

25   Lucian scholia ed. Rabe pp. 211.14–212.8, 280. 4–12, scholiast ad Hom. *Il.* 22.29, cf. Luppe 1996, 29–33, Hyginus, *Fab.* 130, *Astr.* 2.4, Nonnus, *Dion.* 47.34–264, Burkert 1972, 223 n. 37, cf. Eratosthenes, *Erigone* frr. 22–6 (Powell).The myth is the subject of a famous mosaic

Dionysus is also in danger of violation in accounts of another epiphany on board the boat of the Tyrrhenian pirates, a tale told most famously in the *Homeric Hymn to Dionysus*, the criminals only realising the godhead of the handsome youth they had kidnapped when the mast starts sprouting tendrils and bunches of grapes, and terrifying visions of wild animals cause them to abandon ship, at which point they are turned into dolphins.[26] But it was not enough simply to know this god and this new pleasure of wine, you also had to know how to use it properly by mixing wine with water. This knowledge also had a founding hero in the form of the Attic king Amphictyon—'first man to blend'—, something he learnt from Dionysus himself, which is why, as Burckhardt observed, he was credited with teaching the world how to stand up, or rather, as Burckhardt failed to explain, to remain standing.[27]

4 Origins of Love and Wine in Images and Practices

Such myths are not merely obscure local fairy tales dug out of libraries by Hellenistic mythographers, they had a much wider presence in the culture and were celebrated in popular images and/or reflected in ritual practices. The Hesiodic early hatching of (winged) Eros, for instance, is invoked in Aristophanes' *Birds* as proof of the priority of winged creatures before whose appearance no sexual intercourse and therefore no *genesis* of gods could take place.[28] Eros was celebrated on the fourth day of every month, a reflection of or a provocation for, I have suggested elsewhere, the fact that he was born fourth in Hesiod's sequence of epiphanies in *Theogony*.[29] So we may even be able to discover a reflection of Hesiod's Theogonic sequence, a celebration of the birth of Eros, in the fact that the festival of Eros at his shrine on the slopes of the Acropolis in Athens was celebrated on the fourth day of the month

---

from the House of Dionysus in Nea Paphos, Cyprus, of the late second cent. CE; Icarius, named, is shown as an old man with his ox-cart; on the right are two figures labelled *hoi prōtoi oinon piontes*, cf. Dunbabin 1999, 227–9. Apollodorus 3.14.7 places the reception of Dionysus by Icarius, and that of Demeter by Celeus, in the reign of the second king of Athens, Pandion.

26   Homeric Hymns 7 *To Dionysus*, Apollodorus 3.37–8, Hyginus, *Astr.* 2.17. In Ovid's account, *Met.* 3.572–689, one of the pirates survives to join the *thiasos* and be interrogated by Pentheus. The threat of violation by the pirates is implicit in all the accounts that emphasize Dionysus's youthful beauty but explicit in Hyginus, *Fabulae* 134. and Servius on *Aeneid* 1.67.

27   Philochorus, *FGrHist* 328 F 5b *ap.* Athenaeus 2.38cd, cf. 5.179e.

28   Aristophanes, *Birds* 696–700.

29   Davidson 2007, 17 and 22–3.

Mounychion. The birth of Aphrodite, meanwhile, was the subject of a famous painting by Apelles in the temple of Asclepius in Cos, later even more famously re-imagined by Botticelli.[30] Apelles was said to have taken as his model the image of the courtesan Phryne, emerging from the waves during the festival of Aphrodite on Aegina—the courtesan, described as Aphrodite's 'interpreter and temple-keeper' (hypophētin kai zakoron), here clearly re-enacting as a form of pageant the goddess's birth rising from the waves.[31] The same pageant, it was believed, provided a model for Praxiteles' famous statue of the goddess for the temple of Aphrodite Euploia, Successful Sailing, in Cnidus.[32]

From the third century onwards poets celebrated the two works of art for their seductiveness but also for their realism—or rather for the sense they produced of witnessing the goddess's arrival on earth: 'Apelles saw Aphrodite herself brought forth naked from the wet-nurse sea, and that is how he drew her...', 'Apelles saw the Cyprian as she was escaping her mother's loins, still murmuring with foam ... not painted but alive', 'Apelles watched Aphrodite as she came up from the sea'.[33] 'This must be the work of Praxiteles' hands, or perhaps Olympus is bereft, the Paphian having come to Cnidus'. 'Where did Praxiteles see me naked?'[34]

It is more difficult to gauge the cultural impact of stories of the origins of homosexuality, especially the myths of Laius and of the rape of Ganymede, in Greek culture, short of noting that Plato thought them worth alluding to in his attack on the practice in Laws and in his allegorical re-interpretations in Phaedrus. But from the archaic to the Hellenistic period, poets compared their love for boys with that of Zeus, and their beloveds with Ganymede, while images of the pair often allude to a contemporary real world context, with indications of traditional courting-gifts like cockerels that might seem unnecessary for a prospective victim of abduction, bringing the myth into the world of late archaic Athens.[35] And it would have been a particularly unimaginative Cretan who did not anticipate Plato's conjecture and think of the abduction of Ganymede when he participated in the Cretan boy-abduction ceremony described by Ephorus, concluding as it did with a public sacrifice to Zeus.[36] There was at least one fifth-century tragedy on the subject of Laius's

---

30   Strabo 14.2,19.

31   Athenaeus 13.590de, Hyperides On Behalf of Phryne fr. 171 Jensen.

32   Athenaeus 13.590f–591a.

33   Anthologia Palatina 5.179 (Archias), 182 (Leonidas of Tarentum), P. Berol. 9812.6–9.

34   Anthologia Palatina 5. 159, 160, 162.

35   Theognis 1345–1350, Anthologia Palatina 12.68 (Meleager), 67 (Anon.) 65 (Meleager) 101 (Meleager).

36   Ephorus, FGrHist 70 F 149 ap. Strabo 10.4,21.

passion for Chrysippus—'the very first originator of love of males among the Greeks'—by Euripides, and other dramatic versions probably inspired the Italian vase-painters in their depictions.[37]

Dionysus's arrival is such a central feature of his myth and cult that he has sometimes been called the god of epiphany.[38] So the first appearance (of the god) of wine was commemorated in a number of cults with the arrival of his image. In Sicyon two red-faced and otherwise gold-covered images of the god were kept in secret and brought to the temple of Dionysus next to the theatre only one night a year, accompanied by a torch procession and hymns.[39] The statues were said to have been carved from the very tree that Pentheus fatefully climbed to spy on Dionysus's early converts. Delphi had told the Sicyonians to find the tree and to worship it equally with the god himself.[40]

Similarly in Athens the legendary arrival of (the cult of) Dionysus from Eleutherae on the Boeotian border was recreated every year on the eve of the City Dionysia with a procession of (the image of) Dionysus coming on the road from Eleutherae, a myth not about the introduction of one cult among many, but about *'the first introduction of the cult of Dionysos in Athens'*, as Christiane Sourvinou-Inwood has emphasised, reconstructing the entire festival with all its eventual performances as a kind of welcoming entertainment for a distinguished foreign visitor.[41] Appropriately a figure representing Pegasus of Eleutherae, who, after the inevitable initial opposition and punishment—another erection-affliction assuaged by the honouring of the god with phalluses—had introduced the Eleutheraean cult, was to be found alongside Dionysus, on the threshold of the city, just inside the Dipylon gate next to a shrine of Dionysus.[42]

There was, of course, another big festival in honour of Dionysus, the Anthesteria, which Thucydides calls 'more ancient'.[43] The festival was one of the most important and central in the lives of those who hailed from cities of an Ionian cultural allegiance—the closest thing they had to Christmas, it has been said, in terms of emotional appeal.[44] Appropriately this prior festival

---

37 Davidson 2007, 231–4. Aelian *NA* 6.15 on Euripides's presentation of Laius: *tou tōn arrhenōn erōtos ... Hellēnōn prōtistos arxas*. Rape of Chrysippus: Berlin Antikensammlung 1968.12.

38 Detienne 1986, 13–14: "le dieu le plus épidémique du panthéon c'est assurément Dionysos, qui fait de la parousie un mode d'action privilégié".

39 Pausanias 2.7.5–6.

40 Pausanias 2.2.7.

41 Sourvinou-Inwood 1994, 269–90, 274 [her italics].

42 Pausanias 1.2.5.

43 Thucydides 2.15. 4.

44 Parker 2007, 290.

was linked to the myth of Icarius, who as a wine-missionary was given priority over Pegasus.[45] In particular the death of Icarius's daughter Erigone, who
had hanged herself after finding her father's corpse, was commemorated in
the swinging festival called the *Aiora*, which is generally assigned to the third
day of the Anthesteria. And there were other potential reminders of the myth
in the festival, not just in the carrying of phalluses and the arrival of Dionysus
on a ship/wagon, and the excessive drinking followed by rituals for the hung
over 'survivors', but in the strange now-you-see-him-now-you-don't opening
and closing of the temple of Dionysus-in-the-marshes, opened only one day
a year, Day 2 of the festival (although processions are recorded only for Days 1
and 3, reflecting the brief arousing epiphany and disappearance of the longed-
for Dionysus to the satyriasic shepherds).[46] Finally, of course, the first taste
of wine is commemorated in the festival by the competitive drinking of neat
wine straight from a pouring jug on Day 2, Choes, and also by the custom of
offering on this occasion a first taste of wine to children, a cultural practice
that has resulted in the unearthing of large numbers of souvenir child-sized
wine-jugs.[47]

The invention of the practice of mixing wine with water also had a reflection in cult if one knew where to look for it, for Philochorus the local historian of Attica associates it with an altar of Upright Dionysus in the sanctuary
of the Seasons, adjacent to an altar of the Nymphs (i.e. water). He adds that
Amphictyon also established the custom that each symposium should begin

---

45   We should not exaggerate the degree to which the myth of Icarius dominated the
      Anthesteria. As Robert Parker has pointed out (2007, 375–6), the myths that were attached
      to the festival, or at least those that were thought worth mentioning by scholiasts, relate
      to a wide range of myths, the entertainment of a polluted Orestes in Athens, Deucalion's
      flood, a nice example of making do or *bricolage*, while the origin myths attached to myths
      of Pegasus or Icarius seem to relate to institutions of Dionysiac worship in general, e.g.
      Dionysus's wagon and the carrying of phalluses, rather than some specific practices of
      the Anthesteria/City Dionysia. On the other hand the evidence for an old important cult
      of Dionysus at Icarion is powerful, albeit strictly circumstantial, evidence that the myth
      of Icarius was not a late invention, Whitehead 1986, 215–18, Lewis 1956, 172. And if the
      myths seem to relate to Dionysiac practices in general, it is clear that those practices and
      indeed other peculiarities of the Anthesteria harken back to the epiphany of Dionysus,
      the origins of wine and/or the post-primordial period of the flood.

46   [Demosthenes] 59. 76, Thucydides 2.15.4. As Parker notes, there were processions to the
      temple on days 1, Pithoigia, and 3, Chutroi, but not, apparently, on day 2, Choes, the only
      day when the temple was open (Parker 2007, 291).

47   Parker 2007, 293, Hamilton 1992. Strictly speaking the first taste of wine is only an
      inference from the fact that children in their third year were crowned with flowers at the
      festival and, apparently, given a miniature *chous*, but it is as safe an inference as the one
      that allows us to infer a bridal bath from a *loutrophoros*.

with drinking a toast of neat wine to the *Agathos Daimon* as a 'demonstration of the power of the good divinity.... Moreover, he established the custom of repeating the name of Zeus the Saviour (*Sotēr*) over the mixed wine as a warning and reminder to drinkers that only when they drank in this way would they be safe and sound'.[48]

These introductions of wine to humankind are normally placed in the earliest strata of mortal mythology, soon after the autochthonous founders emerged from the earth, but the first taste of wine by those too primitive or remote from civilisation to have become used to it is a popular trope in Greek myth and legend. Milk-fed Polyphemus in the *Odyssey* is delighted with the wine Odysseus brings, comparing it to nectar and ambrosia. Uneducated in the dangers of the liquid he is soon sound asleep and vulnerable to blinding.[49] Another myth concerns Heracles's visit to the cave of the centaur Pholus. With him Dionysus had left a quantity of wine to be left untouched until Heracles should appear. When Heracles appeared, and perhaps at his insistence, the wine was opened. The bouquet attracted centaurs from miles around who, once they had tasted of the new kind of liquor, became somewhat aggressive to the point that Heracles was obliged to kill them with arrows dipped in the blood of the Hydra.[50] An even more famous centauromachy was the one at the wedding of the Lapith Pirithous. The story is already hinted at by Homer in the *Odyssey* when Antinous uses the example of the centaur Eurytion in the halls of Pirithous as an example of drunken insolence and its punishment; and Pindar vividly described the moment when the centaurs, intoxicated by the smell of wine, thrust their beakers of milk off the table and reached uninvited for the silver drinking-horns.[51]

Images of these introductions of wine/cult of Dionysus were among the most popular themes for Greek artists, whether decorating temples or cups. There is not much definite evidence for early representations of the epiphany of Dionysus in Icarion or of the introduction of his cult from Eleutherae.[52] But

---

48 Philochorus, *FGrHist* 328 F 5b *ap.* Athenaeus 2.38cd, On *Agathos Daimon* see Ogden, 2013, 298–9.

49 Homer, *Od.* 9.354–365.

50 Attached to this tale are the famous tales of the immortal centaur Chiron who was shot accidentally and swapped his immortality for Heracles's mortality to relieve the pain, and of the host Pholus himself who picked up one of the arrows, wondering that something so small could destroy a beast so magnificent, and, distracted in his wonderment, dropped it, fatally, on his own foot.

51 *Od.* 21.295–8, Pindar fr. 166 *ap.* Athenaeus 11.476bc.

52 Robertson 1986, 71–90, suggests that the figure on the reverse of a fragmentary *pelike* in the Getty—*Beazley Archive* 28880; Getty 81AE.62—is actually Ikarios, but identifications of the Attic hero, overwhelmingly in the work of 'The Affecter', e.g. *BA* 301311, 301322,

one of the most famous of all ancient vases is the borderless red-flooded tondo of Exekias' kylix in Munich showing the epiphany of Dionysus on the ship of the Tyrrhenians, as told in the Homeric Hymn.[53] The arrival of Dionysus at the head of a *thiasos* of satyrs and maenads was a popular theme on Attic drinking-cups and mixing-bowls from the sixth century to the end of the fifth, and his role as the bringer of wine or even as the proselytizer of the cult of wine is sometimes emphasized by his being paired on the same vase with scenes of the so-called 'mission' of Triptolemus who, according to Athenian myth, spread the good news about agriculture around the world.[54] Images of a dismembered young Pentheus distributed amongst the Bacchants allude to the origins of wine rather more brutally.[55]

There are many images of Heracles fighting centaurs on vases and in temple sculpture from the seventh century onwards; enough of them have sufficient indications that the fateful visit to the cave of Pholos is intended. The *Beazley Archive* pottery database comes up with 85 scenes with Herakles and Pholos, many referring to the story straightforwardly by showing a giant submerged *pithos* with its lid removed. One black-figure amphora in the Louvre (#7585) has the word *kentauros* curling from the rim like wine fumes; others show the battle itself; Dionysos is often to be found nearby.[56] There are rather fewer images on vases identifiable as the battle at the wedding of Pirithous and Hippodameia, but it is clear that the metopes on the south side of the Parthenon, for instance, refer to this event, not least because of the presence of women and of drinking vessels knocked over and even weaponised.

5 Milled Life

There is no birth of the pleasures of food to compare with births of love and of sex and inventions of wine and homosexuality. But there is one set of myths, rituals, and images often twinned with the invention of wine that plot the human consumption of food on a timeline. The most famous version of the myth is that told in the *Homeric Hymn to Demeter*, the story of the rape

301332, 301333 etc. are highly circumstantial. Near a shrine of Dionysus, appropriately at the entrance to the city near the Dipylon gate, Pausanias saw images of Amphictyon entertaining Dionysus and of Pegasus who brought the cult from Eleutherae (1.2,5).

53   *BA* 310403.

54   Robertson 1986, 83–8.

55   Especially popular in the early years of the fifth century e.g. *BA* 11686, 43279, 45070, 200077, 201114, 201963.

56   The most succinct discussion of the texts and images remains Gantz 1993, 390–2.

of Persephone, the grief of her mother Demeter, her residence in Eleusis, the temporary release of her daughter and the teaching of her Mysteries to the Eleusinians, including the prince Triptolemus.

Although in the *Hymn* the focus is on the revelation of the Eleusinian Mysteries and it seems clear, reading between the lines, that men had been sowing and ploughing—and indeed sacrificing—before agriculture was interrupted by Demeter's grief, in practice there was a fusion between the teaching of the Mysteries and the teaching of the secrets of the Neolithic revolution from an early date, not just ploughing and sowing, but also threshing and milling, so that Eleusis was celebrated as the origin of agriculture and Triptolemus as the man who spread the techniques of agriculture around the Greek world.[57]

Again one must try to assess the presence of such myths in the culture. The myths of the gift of grain would certainly have currency and vividness in Athens during the various long Eleusinian festivals. Images of Triptolemus' 'mission', sowing seeds of wheat from his flying chariot, became popular on Athenian vases from the mid-sixth century onwards, and that mission seems to have been described in some detail in Sophocles' lost early play *Triptolemus*, produced in c. 468 BCE, according to Pliny the Elder.[58] For the initiates at Eleusis it would have been difficult to avoid monuments to the primacy of Triptolemus. That primacy would have been reinforced even to those who had never made the trip to Eleusis or heard of Triptolemus when the Athenians produced their imperialistic demand that, as a due return for that great gift for mankind, other cities must or might like to pay a first fruits offering of grain to the two goddesses.[59]

There were other similar but more generalized allusions to belief in epochal advances in human alimentation. So we learn from several proverb-collections that there was a custom at Athenian weddings for a boy with both parents living—a *pais amphithales*—to put on a crown of thorns intertwined with acorns while carrying a winnowing fan full of loaves, repeating the formula 'I/They fled the bad; I/they discovered the better', ἔφυγον κακόν, εὗρον ἄμεινον— a formula also intoned in Bacchic initiations, according to Demosthenes, and therefore perhaps a well-known formula of ceremonies of transition in general.[60] Acorns had long been associated with a primitive diet and the paroemiographers and lexicographers explained the custom, not unreasonably, as

---

57 *Homeric Hymn* 2 *to Demeter* 305–313. Hayashi 1992.
58 Sophocles frr.596–617, Pliny *NH* 18.65.
59 *IG* I³.78, Xenophon, *Hell* 6.3,6, Isocrates, *Paneg.* 28–31, Plato, *Menex.* 237e–238a, Demosthenes 60.5, Smarczyk 1990, 224–252.
60 Demosthenes 18.259.

symbolizing that 'they have thrust away the savage (*agrios*) and ancient diet, and have discovered the civilised (*hēmeros* 'domesticated', 'cultivated', 'tame') form of nourishment'.[61] The *Suda* cites further proverbs and phrases that fill out for us this alimentary version of the Greek structural opposition of savagery to civilisation: 'For there are no thorns', used on two occasions by Aristophanes, comes 'from the transformation of life into something more civilised'.[62] 'The thorny way of living (*bios akanthōdēs*)': one which is difficult and harsh, the former way of living. And 'the milled way of living' (*alēlesmenos bios*). The easy and sweet.' 'It seems to recall the transformation in the way of life from the savage and thorny way of life that there was before, before there was cultivation of land and seeds'.[63]

The thinking behind such practices and proverbial phrases is also reflected in more intellectual treatments of human nutrition. When Plato discusses a simple way of life for his city in the *Republic*, he includes the toasting of primitive acorns as part of their 'feast', provoking Glaucon to comment that it is as if he is producing a city for pigs.[64] The author of the treatise *On ancient medicine*, writing around 400 BCE, offers a complete history of human nutrition:

> To trace the matter still further back, I think that not even the *diaita* and nourishment enjoyed at the present time (*hēi nun chreontai*) by men in health would have been discovered, had a man been satisfied with the same food and drink as satisfy an ox, a horse, and every animal except for mankind...., Yet I am of opinion that to begin with man also used this sort of nourishment. Our present ways of living have, I think, been discovered and developed (*tetechnēmena*) during a long period of time. For many and terrible were the sufferings of men from strong and bestial (*thēriōdēs*) diet when they consumed foods both raw and unmixed (*akrēta*) and potent ... For this reason the ancients too seem to me to have sought for nourishment that harmonised with their constitution, and to have discovered that which we use now. So from wheat, after steeping it, winnowing, grinding and sifting, kneading, baking, they produced bread,

---

61   Pseudo-Plutarch *Proverbia Alexandrina* 1.16 [*Paroemiographi*, I 323–4], cf. Diogenian 4.74, Zenobius 3.98, Suda epsilon 3971, with other references to the custom in Detienne 1977, 117, 188, nn. 82–4. Oakley and Sinos 1993, 29 and 136 nn. 39 and 40, noting that *likna* are shown in a wedding procession of 540–30 *BA* #310361 fig. 65, as noted already by Jane Harrison in her discussion of the custom, Harrison 1903, 313–7. On the significance of the acorn-eating Arcadians, see Burkert 1972, 84–5 with n. 1, Borgeaud 1988, 14–15.

62   Suda omicron 769, Aristophanes frr. 284, 499.

63   Suda beta 295, alpha 1183.

64   Plato, *Republic* 372d.

and from barley they produced *maza*. Experimenting with food they boiled or baked, after mixing, many other things, blending the strong and unmixed with the weaker components so as to adapt all to the constitution and power of man.[65]

6   Conclusion. The Pleasures of the Flesh and the Origins of Pleasures

It may seem a bit of an anti-climax to conclude a survey of the origins of pleasure with the pleasure of avoiding indigestion by no longer having to eat acorns, but there are interesting patterns in the way the Greeks plotted these pleasures of the flesh onto a secular timeline that also apply to those pleasures of the flesh that we might more easily associate with the word pleasure, i.e. drinking and sex.

In the first place it does seem peculiar that the origin of pleasures should be so much to the foreground and continually rehearsed in Greek culture. This is particularly true of wine, which was never drunk, it sometimes seems, without some small allusion to the fact of its discovering, in the endless epiphanies of Dionysus, reproducing some first epiphany, and the pervasive minatory images of the dangers involved in the first sip. But the birth of Aphrodite also seems to have been kept vividly in mind by pageants such as the courtesan Phryne's emergence from the sea at Aegina during the Aphrodisia and the artworks supposedly based on that re-enactment, Apelles' famous painting for the temple of Asclepius in Cos and Praxiteles's naked Aphrodite Euploia for the temple in Cnidus. One could argue that the familiar epithets Cypris, Cytherea and Paphia on their own conjure up an image of Hesiod's maiden-form figure materializing out of the foam on the shore, of the birth of sex, as much as the epithet Delian applied to Apollo calls to mind the endless birth pangs of Leto and the lighting up of the world at the moment they were relieved. And although Plato's allusions to the origins of Eros and of Himeros in *Symposium* and *Phaedrus* will hardly at first have had an impact beyond a small group of devotees, they nevertheless serve to confirm again the importance of origin-stories in Greek thinking about pleasure.

It is not just a tendency that can be discovered in the context of the origins of pleasure of course, as we have seen with the long lists of inventors produced by Pliny the Elder and Hyginus. In part this is the product of what we can call an etymological tendency in Greek thinking, the recourse to the rhetoric that it is at the origin of a thing that we can discover its true meaning, its essence

---

65   Hippocrates, *VM* 3.

or its most authentic form. But the obsession with firsts also draws attention to the way that the Greeks viewed the world-as-we-know-it as the result of a long accumulation of artefacts, institutions and forces. This worldview is in turn closely tied to the materiality of Greek polytheism, which envisions a composite creation with divided domains under the tutelage of different gods. Since religious festivals and cult demonstrate a powerful tendency to dwell on their own origins and foundations, if some pleasure or item of pleasure holds an important place within the domain of a particular divinity, then festivals and cult will tend to dwell on the origins of those pleasures and items of pleasure, thus confusing the discovery of wine and the arrival of the (mystic) cult of Dionysus, eliding the discovery of the secrets of the 'milled' way of life with the revelation of the Mysteries of Eleusis, the birth of *ta aphrodisia* with the cult of Aphrodite in Paphos. But if beginnings are a characteristic feature of Greek discourse and of Greek thinking in general, we need to ask how this feature manifests itself in the particular context of the pleasures of the flesh and whether this has consequences for the experience or the practices of pleasure.

The story of the birth of Eros as fourth thing in existence in Hesiod's *Theogony* serves at the very least to show Eros as a super-primordial force preceding the age of Ouranos, let alone of Cronus or Zeus, and therefore a central feature of the universe as we know it, to which all powers must bow—a kind of cosmic background noise carrying echoes, as it were, of the Big Bang. We can perhaps see a reflection of that priority in the image on an alabastron of winged Eros goading Zeus, who is chasing Ganymede, and it is at the very least highly suggestive that Aristophanes is able to allude to Hesiod's Eros in *Birds*, spelling out the logical necessity of his early birth as a prerequisite for theogony. In other words the centrality of Eros in Greek thinking and the overwhelming power of *erōs* in Greek experience is supported by his early placing on the timeline of Greek cosmogony.

The birth of Aphrodite might be directly connected to the experience of pleasure on at least one occasion: the festival of Aphrodite that seems to have concluded the festival of Poseidon on the island of Aegina. Here we learn there were courtesans present, as one would expect. The philosopher Aristippus is said to have spent two months a year at the festival with the courtesan Lais, and whoever was Phryne's admirer after she had risen from the sea during the festival could have had a somewhat direct experience of sleeping with post-natal Aphrodite.[66] This blending of the imaginary and the real is not merely facetious. In the representations of the birth of Aphrodite—supposedly inspired by Phryne's Aeginetan bath—and the commentary on them in ecphras-

---

66   Athenaeus 13.588e.

tic epigrams, the representations of the birth of the goddess of sexual love always inspire in the imagined viewer an appreciation of her charms, so that the realism of the image—'Where did he see me naked?', 'Olympus is bereft', 'Apelles watched Aphrodite', 'Apelles saw Aphrodite emerging from the waves', 'not painted but alive'—leads first to a sense of presence and then to a present desire in the onlooker—'let Ares' wrath be confounded'—one of whom, according to Pseudo-Lucian's famous account, actually left a sperm-stain on the Cnidian Aphrodite.[67] This confluence of presence and *jouissance* is very similar to the way that the mere passing of Aphrodite in the Homeric Hymn throws *himeros* into the wild beasts of Mt Ida—wolves, lions, bears and panthers: 'so that all at the same time mated two together in their shadowy lairs'.[68]

The original coming of Aphrodite out of the frothy sea therefore is aligned with the process of the coming of desire in the subject and ultimately—and this is more than a facetious pun—with the experience of coming. That the experiencing of the power of a god can be transposed onto the (mythical) history of (the cult of) a god was, of course, one of the important insights of Walter Friedrich Otto in his study of Dionysus, arguing that stories about the advent of Dionysus do not refer to the actual historical introduction of the cult in some folk memory, but reflect his essential character as a 'coming god'.[69] The emphasis on the first comings of the pleasures of the flesh in Greek culture reflects and provokes in the Greek subject an element of epiphany in the experience of pleasure, even of fresh discovery.

This sense of coming anew to pleasure, and the opportunity that goes with it to unthink the pleasures of the world and imagine a world not (yet) aware of them, is nicely elaborated in Herodotus's account of the expedition sent to the king of Ethiopia by Cambyses. The king is given wine for the first time and, alone of the products of the northern civilization, finds it exceedingly pleasant.[70] Even more striking perhaps is the episode of the Lotus-Eaters in the *Odyssey*, subjects of a pleasure—the honey-sweet fruit of the lotus—as far beyond the experience of the Greeks as wine from that of the Ethiopians.[71]

---

67   *Anthologia Palatina* 16.180.5–6, [Lucian] *Amores* 15, cf. Platt 2011, 170–211. An image of a wet undressed Aphrodite in a temple dedicated to Aphrodite of Fair Voyage, supposedly modelled on the courtesan Phryne coming out of the waves at Aegina, must automatically have recalled her successful original landing on Paphos. At any rate the conclusion of a ritual bath of the goddess/her statue in the sea, like the sea-bath of Athena Polias in Athens, would in Aphrodite's case inevitably have evoked her original emergence from the sea.

68   *Homeric Hymn to Aphrodite* 5.74.

69   Otto 1965, 97.

70   Herodotus 3.22.3.

71   Homer, *Od.* 9.83–105.

There is a powerful sense of contingency in Greek ontology and that sense of contingency applies also to its pleasures.

But as those of Odysseus's companions who are invited to eat of the fruit of the lotus soon discover, there are great dangers in these discoveries. Like the Cyclops or the centaurs or the Icarian shepherds *hoi prōtoi oinon piontes*, or like Laius 'the very first originator of love of males among the Greeks', the Ithacan lotus-eaters are overwhelmed by the new pleasure and forget themselves. So there is a second group of origin stories placed next in sequence to the birth/invention of pleasures that relate to their proper management. If images and discourse rehearsing the origins of wine and sex can be seen as by-products of the linkage of wine and sex to festivals and cults rehearsing the origins of Dionysus and Aphrodite, the discourse about the discovery of the proper *usage* of pleasure belongs to a narrative centred on politics and civilization. In Athens therefore it is an early king, Amphictyon, who lays down the rule that wine must always be mixed with water in order for alcohol to be safely consumed, although to be sure there are cults, e.g. Dionysus Orthos, and religious practices, e.g. a toast of neat wine for Agathos Daimon at the beginning of each Athenian symposium, that give the rules a ritual dimension.

An interesting case here is presented by the origin stories of homosexuality: Laius may have pioneered male homosexual *erōs*, according to Aelian/ Euripides or, according to Plato, pioneered the perversion (*diephtharkenai*) of natural lust, but the tragic hubristic catastrophic myth of Laius's rape of Chrysippus, at least in the version retold by (or invented by) Euripides, could never have been a foundation myth for socially acceptable Greek Love, i.e. the elaborate protocols and rituals, the *nomoi*, laid down for *dikaios erōs* in different cities, most notably in Athens.[72] Plutarch is surely more plausible when he says it was not Laius but the Theban Law-givers who invented Theban homosexuality, while, according to Aristotle, it was Minos who set up Cretan homosexuality and in the same way Xenophon makes Lycurgus the inventor of Spartan homosexuality, whatever that was.[73] This sense of political origins, *polis* origins, for the safe management of pleasures was reinforced by comparative Hellenic sociology inasmuch as citizens of one polity noticed and pointed out the differences in, say, proper drinking practices, between Sparta and Athens and Thessaly, or in proper pederastic practices between Crete, Sparta, Athens, Boeotia and Elis.[74]

---

72   Plato, *Laws* 636b, Davidson 2007, 469–70.

73   For some sordid speculations see Davidson 2007, 330–1.

74   There is a nice comparison of drinking-practices in Critias 88 B 33 D-K *ap.* Athenaeus 11.463ef, while the classic comparison of Greek pederastic practices is Plato, *Sym.* 182ac.

There is room to doubt that any lawgiver, Minos, Lycurgus or Amphictyon, ever laid down how citizens were to drink or practise Greek Love, but in the case of these stories, myths of origin serve to reinforce the sense of institutionalization of the management of pleasures, associating the proper way of drinking, the proper way of pederasty with an individual polis and that polis's institutions. The origin stories might also serve to account for another peculiar feature of Greek pleasure, the extraordinary elaboration of protocols, formulaic practices and pottery-assemblages with which in different cities basic instincts such as (homo)sexual lust and drinking alcohol are barnacled: the following of boys in a pack, the hanging outside doorways, the never-modifying formula of the *kalos* inscription or, on the other hand, the correct sequence of toasts, the mixing with water, the lying on couches, the equal pouring of wine, the singing of songs by turns, all always moving from left to right.

So perhaps the key to the experience of Greek pleasure which is revealed by thinking about the emplotment of pleasures and pleasure-ways onto a timeline is a double contingency, an awareness of the contingency of pleasures in the first place—that they have not always been around, that they remain un-enjoyed by others, that there may well be pleasures out there of which we know nothing—and then an awareness that in the protocols of pleasure, the management of appetites, other Greeks do it differently.

It is with this second group of origins that the *Homeric Hymn to Demeter* fits best in my view, a story about culture and institutions, *thesmoi*, rather than one about nature, a story about moving on from the Hippocratic author's unmixed, thorny, bestial way of life, to the tamed, milled and upright; but unlike same-sex *erōs* or drinking, the Mysteries of Eleusis/ bread were uniform, thanks to the successful mission of the Eleusinian Triptolemus.

CHAPTER 3

Must We Suffer in Order to Stay Healthy? Pleasure and Pain in Ancient Medical Literature

Véronique Boudon-Millot*

Plutôt souffrir que mourir, C'est la devise des hommes.

JEAN DE LA FONTAINE, *La mort et le bûcheron*

∴

Notions of pain or suffering may more readily come to mind in medical, and in particular therapeutic, contexts, but the idea of pleasure is hardly absent from ancient medical literature. In fact, the two notions are frequently evoked side-by-side and in the same contexts, notably in many lists of the 'passions' or *pathe* (according to the double sense of the Greek word *pathos*, meaning both ailment and emotion). Some medical authors even wrote about the therapeutic virtues of pleasure, not to mention the numerous recommendations regarding the pleasures of love (*aphrodisia*) given by physicians. More broadly, pleasure experienced by the patient in the course of a treatment or regimen—far from being censured or condemned—could even serve as an ally of the physician, and contribute to good health.

After surveying the different terms commonly used to express pleasure and pain in Greek, we shall focus on the roles played by each of these two concepts in ancient medical thought. We shall especially be looking for original medical perspectives on pleasure and pain, bearing in mind that Greek medicine lacked all powerful and truly effective means of anesthesia.

1   The Vocabulary of Pain and Pleasure

In the *Ars medica*, Galen cites six 'affections of the soul' (τῶν ψυχικῶν παθῶν), among which figure anger (ὀργῆς), distress (λύπης), joy (*gaudium*; the term

---

*   Translated by Caroline Wazer, with revisions by the volume editor and the author.

DOI:10.1163/9789004379503_004

omitted in the Greek manuscripts but used in the indirect Arabo-Latin tradition is most likely a translation of χαρά, pride (θυμοῦ), fear (φόβου) and envy (φθόνου).[1] In his *Les passions de l'âme*, Descartes also counts, to use his terminology, six 'primal' emotions. He notes that 'sadness is in some way primary and more necessary than joy, and hatred more necessary than love, because it matters more to reject harmful and potentially destructive things than to acquire things that could add some perfection that we can survive without'.[2] Ancient authors, however, were far from being in agreement regarding the nature and the role of pleasure (ἡδονή) and pain (λύπη). In particular, they diverged on the question of whether pleasure and pain were affections (πάθη), judgments (κρίσεις), or simply opinions (δόξαι).[3]

Galen himself echoed this debate in a passage from *On the Doctrines of Hippocrates and Plato*, in which he argues against the philosopher Chrysippus. Galen reproaches Chrysippus for having recognized, in the first book of his treatise *On the soul* (Περὶ ψυχῆς), the existence of both a desiderative power (ἐπιθυμητικήν) and a spirited one (θυμοειδῆ), and for having assigned a particular locality in the body to each affection. In his treatise *On the Affections* (Περὶ τῶν παθῶν), however, the philosopher seems to have changed his opinion. In fact, Chrysippus no longer seems to recognize this partition of the soul, to the extent that he now identifies some irrational power as the cause of affections (τινὰ δύναμιν ἄλογον ἐν τῇ ψυχῇ τῶν παθῶν αἰτίαν ὑπάρχειν), before further considering whether or not affections can be added to judgments in order to influence them. There is, however, a major contradiction in Chrysippus' reasoning according to Galen, for whom an affection must necessarily be a judgment

---

1 Galen, *Ars medica* 24.8 (p. 351 in the edition of V. Boudon-Millot [Paris, 2000]). It should be noted that, in the *Ars medica*, the ψυχικῶν παθῶν constitute the sixth term of a list of the necessary causes of change in the body, following: 1) ambient air; 2) movement and rest; 3) sleep and waking; 4) ingesting food and 5) material evacuated. Popularized by late Galenism under the name of six 'non-natural things', this list of 'non-natural' causes of physical illness would exert great influence over later medicine (see Rather 1968). For the present subject, it suffices to note that this list constitutes an explicit point of contact between the affections of the soul (i.e., those of a moral nature) and the maladies of the body (those of a physical nature).

2 R. Descartes, *Les Passions de l'âme*, art. 137 (trans. Jonathan Bennett) and also art. 69: 'But there aren't many simple and basic passions. Look over my list and you'll easily see that there are only six: wonder, love, hatred, desire, joy, sadness'. Descartes justifies reserving the primary place for sadness on account of its utility for the body, which it helps to guard against things that could hurt it by avoiding them in time. For Descartes, 'any of the bodily movements accompanying these passions can be harmful to health when they are very violent, though they may be good for it when they are only moderate' (art. 141). This idea of moderation is itself at the heart of ancient medical thought.

3 On emotions in Galen and in particular on the role of grief, see Boudon-Millot 2016.

(ἤτοι κρίσις), some irrational affection following on this judgment (ἢ κρίσεσιν ἐπιγιγνόμενον), or a runaway movement of the desiderative power (ἢ κίνησις ἔκφορος τῆς ἐπιθυμητικῆς δυνάμεως). And while Chrysippus deems it preferable to consider that affections are judgments, he seems to forget what he had written in the first book of his treatise *On the soul*, namely that love is an affection of the desiderative power, and bitter anger of the spirited.[4] Furthermore, casting aside the opinion of his predecessors, Chrysippus does not hesitate (according to Galen) to define distress as 'a fresh belief that evil is present' (τὴν λύπην ὁριζόμενος δόξαν πρόσφατον κακοῦ παρουσίας), fear as 'the expectation of evil' (τὸν δὲ φόβον προσδοκίαν κακοῦ), and pleasure as 'a fresh belief that good is present' (τὴν δ' ἡδονὴν δόξαν πρόσφατον ἀγαθοῦ παρουσίας). Chrysippus here has in mind only the rational part of the soul (τοῦ λογιστικοῦ τῆς ψυχῆς μόνου), in the sense that opinion and expectation (τὴν δόξαν καὶ τὴν προσδοκίαν) belong to this part, and forgets the desiderative and spirited parts.[5]

When he says that the affections are conations and opinions and judgments (ὁρμὰς καὶ δόξας καὶ κρίσεις), Chrysippus follows the doctrines of Epicurus and Zeno more closely than his own. In fact, when he defines distress as a 'shrinking' before what is thought to be a thing to avoid (μείωσιν εἶναί φησιν ἐπὶ φευκτῷ δοκοῦντι ὑπάρχειν) and pleasure as a 'rising' up at what is thought to be a thing to pursue (ἔπαρσιν ἐφ' αἱρετῷ δοκοῦντι ὑπάρχειν), both movements that he terms 'contractions and expansions' (καὶ αἱ συστολαὶ καὶ αἱ διαχύσεις), he speaks of affections of the irrational power which supervene on opinions (τῆς ἀλόγου δυνάμεώς ἐστι παθήματα ταῖς δόξαις ἐπιγιγνόμενα). This is the view of Epicurus and Zeno, but not that of Chrysippus, who professes in such matters a rather surprising position coming from a man who claims to offer a logical and precise doctrine.

Galen himself proposes several definitions of passions, which he ascribes generally to an irrational cause. His opinion seems in fact to have evolved on this issue, which interests him only insofar as the emotions have the capacity to cause a certain number of diseases in the soul and in the body or, conversely, the capacity to benefit health. But the conception of passion that prevails in the Galenic corpus is presented in *Diagnosis and treatment of the affections and errors of the soul*, where the passions (τὰ πάθη) are defined as having an origin

---

4   Galen, *De placitis Hippocratis et Platonis* IV 1. 14–17 (ed. De Lacy, CMG V 4, 1, 2, Berlin, 1981, p. 238). I have borrowed part of De Lacy's translation.
5   *Ibid.* IV 2. 1 (ed. De Lacy, p. 238).

that depends on the individual, and an irrational force as their cause.[6] In this sense, passion (πάθος) is the opposite of error (ἁμάρτημα).[7]

Within the category of affections, pleasure and pain—whether experienced by the patient or perceived by the physician, according to the relevant sensory organ—cover realities that may be expressed by means of a relatively varied vocabulary. When he reflects on the role of sensation at the beginning of *On the causes of symptoms*, Galen remarks that it makes little difference whether one describes a sensation as 'distressing, grievous, arduous, painful, or stressful', (ἀνιαρὰν ἢ λυπηρὰν ἢ ἀλγεινὴν ἢ ὀδυνηρὰν ἢ ἐπίπονον αἴσθησιν), just as it is irrelevant to refer to a disease by the terms 'affliction, grievance, pain, suffering, or distress' (ὥσπερ οὐδὲ αὐτὸ τὸ πάθος, ἀνίαν ἢ λύπην ἢ ὀδύνην ἢ πόνον ἢ ἀλγηδόνα).[8] But in *On the pulse for beginners*, among the causes of 'changes contrary to nature' (τῶν παρὰ φύσιν αἰτίων τροπαί), pleasure appears next to anger (θυμοῦ) and fear (φόβου), pleasure is cast as the opposite of grief (λύπης), which Galen, in the context of sphygmology and the symptoms attached to each of these manifestations, distinguishes from pain (ἄλγημα).[9] Similarly, in *On the doctrines of Hippocrates and Plato*, Galen concedes that to speak of pain (ὀδύνην) or of suffering (πόνον) is the same, but distinguishes between a dolorous disposition (πόνος) of the body and the sensation of pain (ὀδύνη) linked to this disposition.[10] Finally, although the lexical field of pleasure may appear less rich than that of pain, Galen employs the substantive χαρά (joy) alongside the noun ἡδονή (pleasure) and the adjective ἡδύς (pleasant), and distinguishes the pleasures of the body (ἡδοναῖς τε σωματικαῖς) from the joys of the soul (χαραῖς ψυχικαῖς).[11]

The vocabulary of suffering therefore refers to physical and emotional suffering (πόνος) and pain (ὀδύνη), both usually designated by the term distress (λύπη), and both likely to be at once symptom and cause of numerous physical and mental disorders. Similarly, pleasure (ἡδονή) of the body or pleasure (χαρά)

---

6   We should note that, in French as well, the term 'passion' can have multiple meanings, whether negative (and rather passive) when destructive passion is meant, or positive (and rather active) when it designates passion for something, for example sports or music. In Greek, it is the term *pathos* that best translates the first sense of the French word *passion*, while *himeros* better expresses desire for something.

7   Galen, *De animi cuiuslibet affectuum et peccatorum dignotione et curatione* (Kühn v, 1–103; I. Marquardt, *Scripta minora* I, Leipzig, 1884, pp. 1–81; W. de Boer, CMG v 4, 1, 1, Leipzig-Berlin, 1937, pp. 3–68; G. Magnaldi, Rome, 1999).

8   Galen, *De symptomatum causis* I, 6 (Kühn VII, 115).

9   Galen, *De pulsibus ad introducendos* (Kühn VIII, 473).

10   Galen, *De placitis Hippocratis et Platonis* VII 6. 34 (ed. De Lacy, p. 468, 25).

11   See Galen, *In Hippocratis Epidemiarum VI commentum* (Kühn XVIIB, 210, 11–12): καθάπερ γε κἀν τοῖς ψυχικοῖς πάθεσι, λύπαις καὶ φόβοις, ἡδοναῖς τε σωματικαῖς καὶ χαραῖς ψυχικαῖς.

of the soul, according to the intensity of its manifestations, can prove itself more or less beneficial or, to the contrary, harmful to the health of the patient.

2   Physiology of Pain and Pleasure

Pleasure and pain are of interest to the physician primarily as symptoms. It is no surprise therefore that a discussion of this subject is to be found at the beginning of *On the causes of symptoms*.[12] Pleasure and pain manifest themselves through sensation, although they manifest themselves differently according to the sense concerned: more weakly when vision is involved, but more strongly in the cases of touch, taste, and, following them, smell and hearing. The reason, as Plato noted in a passage of the *Timaeus* (64c8), cited by Galen, is that

> when an affection which is against nature and violent occurs within us with intensity it is painful, whereas the return back to the natural condition, when intense, is pleasant; and an affection which is mild and gradual is imperceptible.[13]

To Plato's opinion about pleasure and pain, Galen adds the even older perspective of Hippocrates in *Places in man*. Here, the coherence of all parts of the body, which explains how sensations can be transmitted from one part of it to another, is compared to a circle, according to an image that also appears in Plato's *Timaeus*.[14] Hippocrates says: 'For in each thing that is altered with respect to its nature, and destroyed, pains arise'.[15] Beyond *On the causes of*

---

12   Galen, *De symptomatum causis* I, 6 (Kühn VII, 115).

13   Using the *Timaeus* (64d1) and not Galen's text as in Kühn VII, 115 (τὸ μὲν παρὰ φύσιν καὶ βιαίως γιγνόμενον ἀθρόως ἐν ἡμῖν πάθος, ἀλγεινόν· τὸ δὲ εἰς φύσιν ἀπιὸν αὖ πάλιν ἀθρόον, ἡδύ· τὸ δὲ ἠρέμα καὶ κατὰ μικρὸν, ἀναίσθητον), but the direct tradition: τὸ μὲν παρὰ φύσιν καὶ βίαιον γιγνόμενον ἀθρόον παρ' ἡμῖν πάθος ἀλγεινόν, τὸ δ' εἰς φύσιν ἀπιὸν πάλιν ἀθρόον ἡδύ, τὸ δὲ ἠρέμα καὶ κατὰ σμικρὸν ἀναίσθητον. Trans W. R. M. Lamb.

14   Hippocrates declares at the beginning of *Places in man* (c. 1) that 'there is no beginning point of the body, but rather every part is at the same time both beginning and end, in the same way that in the figure of a circle, no beginning point is to be found', whereas Plato, in the *Timaeus* 64b, affirms: 'Whenever what is naturally mobile is impressed by even a small affection, it transmits it in a circle (κύκλῳ)'. On the image of a circle in ancient authors, see de Romilly 1975.

15   Hippocrates, *Places in man* c. 42. 1 (ed. R. Joly, pp. 71–72): τὴν γὰρ φύσιν διαλλασσομένοις ἑκάστοισι καὶ διαφθειρομένοις αἱ ὀδύναι γίνονται. Trans. Paul Potter.

symptoms, Galen cites this Hippocratic passage four further times in his writing, evidence that he accorded it particular importance.[16]

In essence, the feelings of pain and of pleasure are the results, respectively, of a change contrary to nature and a return to nature. Pleasure and pain are, therefore, the sign or symptom of a departure from and of a compliance with the natural (κατὰ φύσιν) state so desired by the patient and sought after by the physician. Galen also insists upon the importance of the rapidity and intensity of the change (τάχος τε ἅμα καὶ μέγεθος τῆς μεταβολῆς) that causes such pain. He then distinguishes among the different causes likely to bring about abrupt changes with respect to the different senses: for touch, intense cold or heat; for taste, an acid, sharp, or spicy flavor; for smell, pestilential odors; for hearing, rough, strong, and rapid sounds, such as a violent racket, which could bring about deafness; and for sight, intense lights of the sort that could cause a glare. While the cause differs, the process is always the same: pain is occasioned by anything that is capable of exposing, nicking, cutting, or injuring the substance of the body in some way, or, to put it simply, breaking its continuity (διαιρεῖ τὸ συνεχές) and unity, especially when such an event occurs suddenly (ἐπειδὰν ἀθρόως συμπίπτῃ).[17] Galen goes on to specify what he means by the expression 'suddenly' (ἀθρόως), which also appears in the passage from the *Timaeus* cited above. This adverb (or adjective) describes any change that is both intense and rapid, just as Plato indicates when he declares that the sensation of pain (τὴν ἀνιαρὰν αἴσθησιν) results from an affliction of the sensory organs that is both violent and immediate (ἐκ βιαίου τε ἅμα καὶ ἀθρόου παθήματος).[18]

Pleasure, according to Galen, results from the opposite cause: when a body risks rupture, an immediate return to the natural state produces pleasure.[19] Pleasure of the eyes thus results from the contemplation of a dark blue; that of the ears, from hearing a steady and slow voice rather than a raucous and

---

16   See Galen, *De placitis Hippocratis et Platonis* VII 6. 34 (ed. De Lacy, p. 468, 25); *De tremore et palpitatione* 6 (Kühn VII, 620, 6–8); *De inaequali intemperie* 3 (Kühn VII, 739, 9–10) and *In Hippocratis Epidemiarum VI comm.* (CMG V 10, 2, 2, p. 343, 3).

17   Galen, *De symptomatum causis* I, 6 (Kühn VII, 117): καὶ φαίνεται κοινὸν ἐν ἀπάσαις ταῖς αἰσθήσεσι τὸ ἀνιαρὸν πάθος, ἐκ διακρίσεώς τε καὶ διαιρέσεως τοῦ συνεχοῦς καὶ ἡνωμένου σώματος ἀποτελούμενον.

18   According to this point of view, the more an agent is formed from small particles (λεπτομερέστερος), the more easily it will cause damage in the body. Such an agent will penetrate more deeply, as it is true that what is fine is always more active than what is thick (*De symptomatum causis* I, 6 = Kühn VII, 119: ἀεὶ δ' ἐν τῇ φύσει δραστικώτερόν ἐστι τὸ λεπτομερὲς τοῦ παχυμεροῦς).

19   *De symptomatum causis* I, 6 (Kühn VII, 118): τὸ δ' ἐναντίον αὐτῷ τὸ ἡδὺ διὰ τὴν ἐναντίαν αἰτίαν. τοῦ γὰρ κινδυνεύοντος διασπασθῆναι ἢ εἰς τὸ κατὰ φύσιν ἐπάνοδος ἀθρόα τὴν ἡδονὴν ἀπεργάζεται.

fast one, which would be quite disagreeable. Here, Galen adds a clarification: the causes of pleasure can vary according to whether the sensory organ is in perfect health (ὑγιαινούσης ἀκριβῶς), fatigued (κεκμηκυίας), or, indeed, already sick (νοσούσης). Thus, a steady and slow voice is only agreeable if the ear is in good condition, while a tired ear will appreciate a voice that is also small (καὶ ἡ σμικρὰ προσφιλής) and a sick ear will prefer a very steady, very slow, and very small voice that is also rhythmical (ἡ εὔρυθμος). In the case of taste, pleasure results from anything sweet and fatty (πάντες οἱ γλυκεῖς καὶ λιπαροί). The reason, according to Galen, is that these juices (χυμοί) are specially adapted to the substances of the body that they help to unify (ἐκλεαίνουσι). More generally, pleasure is born from opposites: from heat when one is cold, cold when one is hot, moisture when one is dry, and dryness when one is wet. To give only one example, the tongue (in the sense of taste) will find one type of food or another pleasurable according to circumstance, meaning the disposition and the needs of the body.[20] The role of habit is equally important. Indeed, if people prefer certain foods according to their nature, and if food which is appropriate for the body is more agreeable to the palate (ἥδιον), that which at first seemed distasteful can become pleasurable through the force of habit.[21]

To summarize, the sensation of pain (i.e. suffering or unpleasantness) is the result of a break from nature, and the sensation of pleasure that of a return to the natural state.[22] The intensity of the pain or pleasure is proportional to the intensity and the speed of the change perceived by one or another sense. Still, it is necessary to avoid extremes, as excesses of pleasure can resemble forms of unpleasantness. As discussed below, this intensity must remain proportional (summetron). The pleasure derived from oil massages and baths, whether following physical exercise or in order to ease pain, can similarly be explained by their softening and relaxing effect on a body that has become tense and hardened by exertion or by suffering, for pain and pleasure are principally provoked by the sudden and massive (ἀθρόως) surge of opposite applied to opposite. To preemptively address a potential objection, Galen again quotes Hippocrates on tetanus:

---

20 *Ibid.* (Kühn VII, 123): ἥδεται μὲν οὖν ἡ γλῶττα κατὰ διαφέροντας καιρούς, ἄλλοις ἄλλοτε τῶν ἔξωθεν αὐτῇ προσπιπτόντων χυμῶν.

21 Galen, *De consuetudinibus* 2 (*SM* II, pp. 21–22).

22 Galen, *De symptomatum causis* I, 6 (Kühn VII, 125): ἡδόμεθα τοίνυν ἐν τούτῳ τῷ γένει τῆς αἰσθήσεως, ἁπλῶς μὲν εἰπεῖν, εἰς τὸ κατὰ φύσιν ἐπανερχόμενοι.

in the case of a muscular youth having tetanus without a wound, during the mid-summer, it sometimes happens that the sprinkling of a large quantity of cold water recalls the heat. Heat relieves these diseases.[23]

In such a case, some might think that the affliction (tetanus caused by the cold) had been relieved not by its opposite, heat, but by like, cold. This is not, however, the case, because in truth—and provided that the patient has no wound that would not tolerate the bitter cold—the sprinkling of cold water recommended by the physician is actually intended to produce heat meant to counteract and to relieve the coldness of the tetanus. Galen concludes this discussion with a somewhat paradoxical reflection on the role and the respective scales of pleasure and pain, feminine and masculine, in the sexual act:

> The sensation of the generative parts is affected in a specific and remarkable way in that it has a very strong power, in the male for expelling semen, while in the female there is such power in the ovaries and spermatic vessels, but also the attractive power in the whole uterus. For Nature has joined both powerful desire and pleasure to the emission and the taking-in of the sperm. But the distress when superfluous sperm remains within builds up gradually over a long time, and because of this, though it is very irksome ... it falls short in intensity of the pleasure which is present in sexual intercourse. When the separation of what is distressing occurs suddenly there is a correspondence between the speed of the return to what is natural and the magnitude of the pleasure.[24]

Galen, in essence, distinguishes the unique source of masculine pleasure (ejaculation) from the double source of feminine pleasure (emission and retention of semen). But, given that every sensation is much stronger if it arises 'all at

---

23   Hippocrates, *Aphorisms* v, 21 cited by Galen in *De symptomatum causis* I, 6 (Kühn VII, 125), but also in *In Hippocratis Epidemiae VI comm.* (Kühn XVIIA, 910, 6 = CMG V 10, 2, 2, p. 67, 8–10) and *In Hippocratis Aphor. comment.* (Kühn XVIIB, 806, 5). Trans. adapted from that of C. D. Adams.

24   Galen, *De causis symptomatum* I, 6 (Kühn VII, 126–127), trans. W. V. Harris: ἴδιον δέ τι πέπονθεν ἐξαίρετον ἡ τῶν γεννητικῶν μορίων αἴσθησις, ὅτι καὶ δύναμιν ἰσχυροτάτην ἔχει, κατὰ μὲν τὸ ἄρρεν γένος ἀποκριτικὴν τοῦ σπέρματος, κατὰ δὲ τὸ θῆλυ καὶ ταύτην μὲν ἔν τε τοῖς ὄρχεσι καὶ τοῖς σπερματικοῖς ἀγγείοις, ἀλλὰ καὶ τὴν ἑλκτικὴν ἐν ὅλῃ τῇ μήτρᾳ· συνῆψε γὰρ ἡ φύσις ὑπερέχουσαν ἐπιθυμίαν τε ἅμα καὶ ἡδονὴν τῇ τε προέσει καὶ τῇ συλλήψει τοῦ σπέρματος. ἀλλ' ἡ μὲν ἀνία, τοῦ περιττοῦ σπέρματος μένοντος ἔσω, ἀθροίζεται κατ' ὀλίγον ἐν χρόνῳ πλείονι, καὶ διὰ τοῦτο, καί τοι μεγάλα λυποῦσα (περὶ ὧν ἑτέρωθι λέξομεν) ἀπολείπεται τῷ μεγέθει τῆς ἡδονῆς, ἣν ἐν τοῖς ἀφροδισίοις ἴσχοι. ἡ δ' ἀπόκρισις ἡ τοῦ λυποῦντος ἀθρόως γιγνομένη τῷ τάχει τῆς εἰς τὸ κατὰ φύσιν ἐπανόδου καὶ τὸ τῆς ἡδονῆς μέγεθος ἀνάλογον ἔχει.

once' (ἀθρόως), the physician concludes that, for women, the resumption of
sexual relations after a period of abstinence and the considerable troubles that
result from that (Galen is clearly thinking here of the ravages of hysteria) does
not render pleasure less intense. On the contrary, because the accumulation of
sperm in the uterus has been progressive and therefore less painful, the pleasure of sexual relations, when they occur suddenly after a long period of abstinence, will be equally sudden and intense.

If the physiology of pleasure and pain can be explained by a brusque change
from a natural state to a non-natural state, the sensations thus caused, whether
they be agreeable or disagreeable, are all likely to have certain positive or negative effects on the body.

3   Etiology

Pleasure and pain, as we have already seen,[25] figure among the causes of certain
'changes contrary to nature' (τῶν παρὰ φύσιν αἰτίων τροπαί), alongside anger,
fear, sorrow, or any inflammation (φλεγμονῆς). In particular, these changes can
be diagnosed by the patient's pulse. They are recognized in the case of pleasure by a 'great and intermittent' (μέγας καὶ ἀραιός) pulse, and in that of pain
by a pulse that is 'small, slow, weak, and intermittent' (σμικρὸς καὶ βραδὺς καὶ
ἀμυδρὸς καὶ ἀραιός).[26] Hippocrates had already established a link between the
dispositions of the soul and the health of the body, and noticed their physiological effects, as in this passage of *Epidemics* VI. The details of its interpretation are certainly debatable, but the physician distinguishes between that
which pertains to the mind (ὁκόσα δὲ ἐκ θυμοῦ) (but 'temper' might be a better
translation than 'mind' here) and that which pertains to the body:

> Anger (ὀξυθυμίη) contracts the heart and the lungs and draws the hot
> and the moist substances into the head. Contentment (ἡ δ' εὐθυμίη)
> releases the heart and those substances. Labor (πόνος) is food for the
> joints and the flesh, sleep for the intestines. Intellection (φροντίς; 'reflec-
> tion' according to Littré) is a stroll for the soul in men.[27]

---

25   See *supra* n. 9.

26   See Galen, *De pulsibus ad introducendos* (Kühn VIII, 473) and also *De causis pulsuum* IV, 4
     (Kühn IX, 160, 5): Λύπης δὲ μικρὸς καὶ ἀμυδρὸς καὶ βραδὺς καὶ ἀραιός.

27   Hippocrates, *Epidemics* VI 5, 5, 1 (trans. W. D. Smith): ὀξυθυμίη ἀνασπᾷ καρδίην καὶ πλεύμονα
     ἐς ἑωυτά, καὶ ἐς κεφαλὴν τὰ θερμὰ καὶ τὸ ὑγρόν· ἡ δ' εὐθυμίη ἀφίει καρδίην. Πόνος, τοῖσιν ἄρθροι-
     σι καὶ σαρκὶ σῖτος, ὕπνος σπλάγχνοισιν. Ψυχῆς περίπατος, φροντὶς ἀνθρώποισιν. E. Littré (vol.
     5, of his edition, p. 317, notes the obscurity of the last part of this passage. Galen, in his

The Hippocratic treatise *Humours* likewise enumerates the disruptions of the spirit that can affect the body: sorrows, fits of rage, desires (οἷον λῦπαι, δυσοργη- σίαι, ἐπιθυμίαι), as well as anything that 'aggrieves the soul accidentally (τὰ ἀπὸ συγκυρίης λυπήματα γνώμης), whether by sight or by sound'. The author adds:

> Fears, shame, pain, pleasure, passion and so forth: to each of these the appropriate member of the body responds by its action. Instances are sweats, palpitation of the heart and so forth.[28]

Pleasure and pain, as Galen notes in the *Appendix* of *Regimen in Acute Diseases*,[29] belong to the series of those 'small causes' that Galen refers to most frequently under the name *prophaseis*, in order to distinguish them from the true and primary causes of disease, which depend upon the good or bad disposition (*diathesis*) of each individual. From this point of view, physical pain, like races, wrestling, and pancration, the pleasures of love, massages, warmth, cold, old age, outbursts of rage and fear with which it is often associated, is very often simply a precipitating cause, capable of tipping the balance of some *diathesis* toward disease or health, without, however, having a direct effect itself:

> But frequently, as I have said, due to the disposition of the body, this or that thing does not constitute a cause of the disease but rather its *prophasis*. Properly speaking, one might better term such causes *prophaseis*, not only because they are obvious, as they are often called when a visible lesion occurs in the body as a result of some obvious cause. Indeed, when no other unhealthy disposition is underlying, no significant disease ensues, and that which is the real cause is that which is responsible for the lesion that occurred in the body. Know, then, that the present discourse applies to causes such as those that harm the body, without being the cause themselves (i.e. not on their own initiative). And to put it in a word, these are in first place labours (οἱ πόνοι), of which there exist

---

commentary, understands that exercise is beneficial for the joints, while food and sleep benefit the viscera.

28 Hippocrates, *Humours* 9 (Littré 5, pp. 488–490; Overwien, CMG I 3, 1, p. 168, 11–13): Οἱ φόβοι, αἰσχύνη, ἡδονή, λύπη, ὀργή, τἆλλα τὰ τοιαῦτα. οὕτως ἐνακούει ἑκάστῳ τὸ προσῆκον τοῦ σώματος τῇ πρήξει, ἐν τούτοισιν ἱδρῶτες, καρδίης παλμός, τὰ τοιαῦτα. (trans. W. D. Smith).

29 On the part of *Regimen in acute diseases* designated by the editors as the *Appendix*, see R. Joly in his edition of 1972, p. 11, who notes that Galen believed it was inauthentic, but distinguished 'des passages dignes d'Hippocrate au point de vue à la fois du style et de la pensée, d'autres seulement pour la pensée ou pour le style, d'autres, enfin, indignes d'Hippocrate'.

many particular forms: races, wrestling and pancration, the pleasures of love (ἀφροδίσια), massages, warmth, cold, old age, outbursts of rage, grief (λῦπαι), fears.[30]

These 'small' causes, to use the Galenic terminology (which frequently pairs the adjective σμικρός with πρόφασις), are not to be underestimated, because the pain of the soul, or grief (λύπη)—just like physical pain—can be fatal. The effects of grief on health are described well by Galen in *On the avoidance of grief*, but also elsewhere. In *Diagnosis and treatment of the passions of the soul*, Galen reports the case of a young man who is distressed by every little thing (ἐπὶ σμικροῖς ἀνιώμενος) and for this reason suffers from insomnia.[31] The wife of Justus, on account of some grief or other (τι λυπουμένην) that she refuses to disclose, similarly lies awake all night, keeping her husband from sleep.[32] Galen later discovers, again while taking her pulse, that she is secretly in love with the dancer Pylades.

Yet more serious is the case of the grammarian called Kallistos (or Philistos or even Philistides) in the Arab sources. Galen, in the *Commentary on Epidemics VI*, tells us that he saw this man die of grief over having lost all his books in the fire of 192 at Rome.[33] The clinical presentation is the same as in the preceding cases: first insomnia, then fever, then death. Another grammarian, whose name is poorly established as Philides, and who may be the same man, is mentioned in *On the avoidance of grief* because he let himself die 'consumed by discouragement and grief' after the loss of his books in the same fire of 192. Others, Galen adds, 'went around for a long time dressed in black robes, thin and pale, like people in mourning'.[34]

The effects of pleasure are no less formidable. As is well illustrated in the example of the pleasures of love, all depends on the amount.[35] When

---

30   Galen, *In Hippocratis librum de acutorum victu* (Kühn XV, 903, 4 = Helmreich, CMG V 9, 1, p. 358).

31   Galen, *De animi cuiuslibet affectuum et peccatorum dignotione et curatione* I, 7 (ed. Magnaldi, pp. 43–44).

32   Galen, *De praecognitione* 6 (ed. V. Nutton, CMG V 8, 1, Berlin, 1979, p. 100).

33   Galen, *In Hippocratis Epidemiarum librum VI* (ed. E. Wenkebach-F. Pfaff, CMG V 10, 2, 2, Berlin, 1956, p. 486, 19–21, fragment preserved only in Arabic).

34   Galen, *De indolentia* 7 (ed. V. Boudon-Millot-J. Jouanna, p. 4, 6–8). On the possible identification of the two grammarians, see *ibid.*, pp. 41–42 (commentary).

35   See Hippocrates, *Epidemics VI* (Littré): πόνοι σιτία ποτὰ ὕπνοι ἀφροδίσια, πάντα μέτρια cited by Galen in his commentary on *Epidemics* (Kühn XVIIB, 84, 6); but also in his commentary on *Joints* (Kühn XVIIIA, 600, 5); in the *De consuetudinibus* (Dietz 127, 17); the *Protreptique* 14, 1 (ed. V. Boudon-Millot, p. 115); the *De sanitate tuenda* (Kühn VI, 84, 7); and the *De alimentorum facultatibus* (Kühn VI, 464, 12; ed. J. Wilkins, p. 11).

performed too frequently, sexual relations exhaust; when too rarely, they are injurious to health. In fact, and as Galen explains in the *Ars medica*, temperament is of the utmost importance. A hot temperament spurs the testicles to the pleasures of love (ἀφροδισιαστική τέ ἐστι), while a cold temperament does the opposite.[36] An individual with a hot and dry temperament will be fervently aroused to the pleasures of love, but also very quickly satisfied. Forced lovemaking will damage this individual. In contrast, someone with a hot and humid temperament will have the strength to support more frequent pleasures of love without any damage; only abstinence will damage such a man. Finally, a wet and cold temperament will arouse one to the pleasures of love only rarely, as will a dry and cold one. Contrary to the opinion of Epicurus, against which Galen argues, the practice of sexual relations is, therefore, not harmful provided that one indulges moderately and according to one's temperament, in such a way that one always feels relaxed when one gives oneself up to it and chooses a moment when one's stomach is neither too full nor too empty, and one's body neither excessively cold nor hot, nor immoderately dry nor wet.[37]

The idea of moderation and of balance being at the heart not only of medical thought but of ancient thought more generally was destined for a great posterity: the author of the article 'Passion' in the *Dictionnaire de médecine*, published in Paris in 1826, still considered that

> pleasure, therefore, cannot be continuous ... Moderate pleasure is the well-being of the brain [*enumeration of its positive effects on the body*]. If it is extreme, it produces on the brain a profound impression [*and negative effects*] ... Overly vigorous pleasure has been known to bring about death. History tells us that Sophocles died of pleasure while receiving a prize for his tragedy; that Dionysius the tyrant had the same fate, of which he assuredly was unworthy; that Diagoras died of pleasure while embracing his three sons who were victors at the Olympic games; that Polycrates, Chilo the Lacedaimonian, and Philipides died of joy ... All of these individuals were advanced in age, and the suspension of the action of their hearts and brains therefore more fatal. If moderate pleasure is frequently repeated, it will imprint happy modifications upon the body [*numerous examples of which, including plumpness, fully developed features, and a ruddy complexion, attest to a good state of health*] ... Pain, discomfort, distress, grief, sadness, dejection, and despondency produce changes of another type, when their amount exceeds our strength. Like pleasure,

---

36   Galen, *Ars medica* 13 (Kühn I, 339; ed. Boudon-Millot, 2000, p. 313).
37   *Ibid.* 24, 9 (Kühn I, 371–372 = ed. Boudon-Millot, p. 351).

pain produces immediate and secondary effects and can be sharp or light [*new list of symptoms*] ... If grief persists, a deathly pallor covers the face ... Violent grief frequently causes death.[38]

To achieve this balance of pleasure, a mark of good health, ancient Greek medicine already proposed a certain number of aphrodisiac recipes, such as the preparation based on hyacinth (περὶ βολβῶν), a bulbous plant described by Galen in *On the properties of foodstuffs* as being capable of producing, in those who have eaten to excess, 'a more abundant sperm that makes one desire sexual relations more strongly'.[39] But there also existed ingestibles that could curb sexual desires, such as *vitex agnus castus*, 'chasteberry', the properties of which Galen also reports.[40]

4   The Roles of Pleasure and Pain in Therapeutics

In light of the roles of pleasure and of pain in physiology and etiology described above, it should come as little surprise that, as a sign of the return to nature, pleasure—or at least the relief that comes from the suppression of pain—should be fully integrated into therapeutic aims. The ἤπια φάρμακα used by the centaur Chiron in the *Iliad*[41] and the gentle care provided by Democedes of Croton, according to Herodotus, are testimony to this orientation of Greek medicine against the idea that to be useful or efficacious a treatment must necessarily be painful. Furthermore, the doctor is ready to suffer to alleviate the pain of his patient. As the author of the Hippocratic treatise *On breaths* affirms, medicine belongs to the category of the painful arts that cause nothing but grief (λυπηραί) to their practitioners but are very useful (ὀνήιστοι) for their users:

> For the medical man sees terrible sights, touches unpleasant things, and the misfortunes of others bring a harvest of griefs that are peculiarly his; but the sick by means of the art rid themselves of the worst of evils,

---

38   Entry signed 'Rostan' (presumably L. L. Rostan, 1790–1866) in N. P. Adelon et alii, *Dictionnaire de médecine*, Paris, 1826, volume XVI, s.v. Passion, pp. 189–190.

39   Galen, *De alimentorum facultatibus* II, 64 (Kühn VI, 653 = ed. Wilkins, p. 172). On the 'pleasure prescription' and the different recipes for *aphrodisia*, see especially Ps.-Galen, *De remediis parabilibus* II, 27 (Kühn XIV, 486–489).

40   *De alimentorum facultatibus*. I, 35 (Kühn VI, 550, 11 = ed. Wilkins, p. 82).

41   *Iliad* IV, 194, 218–219.

disease, suffering, pain and death. For medicine proves for all these evils a manifest cure.[42]

In fact, kindnesses (αἱ χάριτες), which is to say, 'the list of particular attentions shown by the physician toward the patient in order to please him', are intended to alleviate the pain of the patient:[43] perfectly clean drink, food, and environment, softness of everything touched, a cool drink whenever possible, without however compromising the treatment of the patient. The author of the *Aphorisms* goes further still in his desire to please the patient:

> Food or drink which, though slightly inferior, is more palatable (ἥδιον), is preferable to that which is superior but less palatable (ἀηδεστέρων).[44]

Commenting on this passage, Galen offers the following justification:

> It is not only on account of the pleasure of the patient (οὐ διὰ τὸ κεχαρισμένον μόνον) that he should do this, but also in the belief that it will be more useful (ὠφελιμώτερον).[45]

In such cases, the physician does not aim simply to please the patient when he accords him a kindness that, while not directly useful to the treatment, at least does not negatively affect the good prognosis of his recovery.[46] Hippocrates affirms, to the contrary, that a better-tasting drink will be not only more agreeable to the patient, but also more useful for his treatment because, as Galen explains, a pleasant (ἡδέως) drink is easily (ῥᾳδίως) digested by the stomach and properly assimilated by the body.[47]

Physicians in ancient medical texts also regularly attempt to improve the taste of a great number of disagreeable, nauseating, or repugnant medications. The many recommendations given by the physician to improve (ἡδύνειν) the

---

42 Hippocrates, *Breaths* I. 2 (ed. Jouanna, pp. 102–103), trans. W. H. S. Jones.

43 On the 'kindnesses' of the physician toward the patient, see Hippocrates, *Epidemics* VI, 4, 7 and the analysis of Jouanna 1992, 190–192.

44 Hippocrates, *Aphorisms* II, 38 (Littré IV, 480, 17), trans. W. H. S. Jones.

45 Galen, *Commentary on Aphorisms* (Kühn XVIIB, 537, 7–8).

46 On the kindnesses that can be qualified as 'gratuitous', see Galen, *Commentary on Epidemics* VI (Kühn XVIIB, 136): ἐν δὲ τῷ νῦν προκειμένῳ λόγῳ γένους ἑτέρου καὶ πράγματος ἐμνημόνευσεν, ἐν ᾧ κεχαρισμένον τε καὶ ἡδὺ τοῖς νοσοῦσιν ὁ ἰατρὸς πράττει μηδὲν τῇ νόσῳ λυμαινόμενος, ὥσπερ ὅταν ἐπιτρέψῃ πρὸ τοῦ καιροῦ λούσασθαι καὶ πιεῖν καὶ φαγεῖν ὀπώρας τινὰς ἢ ψυχρὸν ὕδωρ πιεῖν.

47 Galen, *Commentary on Aphorisms* (Kühn XVIIB, 537, 9): ὅσα γὰρ ἂν ἡδέως προσενεγκώμεθα, περιστέλλεσθαι τούτοις ἡ γαστὴρ εἴωθε καὶ πέττειν μᾶλλον αὐτὰ ῥᾳδίως.

flavor of foods as well as drugs, in order to make them more agreeable to the
patient, are in fact far from rare in medical texts. Whenever possible without contravening the efficacy of the treatment, the physician seeks to act
in the interest of the pleasure (εἰς ἡδονήν) of the patient.[48] Seasoning with
different salts or herbs and the addition of wine or honey are also intended to
improve the taste of numerous medications, such as the famous theriac. This
is Dioscorides' advice:

> A living viper is put into a new pot, and with it salts (ἁλῶν) and some well-
> pounded dry figs, a pint of each, with six *kyathoi* of honey. The cover of
> the pot is tightly corked with clay and it is baked in an oven until the salts
> have carbonized. After this it is pounded into small pieces and stored.
> Sometimes it may agree better with the stomach (πρὸς εὐστομίαν) if some
> spikenard or malabathrum leaf is mixed in.[49]

We find the same recommendation to improve the recipe for theriac with the
addition of salts prepared, in part, for pleasure (τοῖς ἐσκευασμένοις εἰς ἡδονὴν
ἁλσὶν) in the writings of Galen.[50] As the pleasure of the invalid, whenever it
does not compromise the efficacy of the treatment, is mentioned with some
consistency, it is not surprising that, in parallel, the physician aims not only to
suppress the pain of his patient, but also to propose the least painful (ἀνωδύνως)
treatment possible.[51]

The *Commentary on Epidemics VI* provides Galen with the opportunity for
a detailed exposition of the role of pleasure and pain in therapeutics. In fact,
the debate on the role attributed to pain in treatment is embedded within
another debate on the necessity of 'treating opposites with opposites'. The
aforementioned passage of *Aphorisms* V, 21 concerning tetanus, a 'cold' ailment that Hippocrates recommends should be treated with the sprinkling of
cold water in certain cases, gives Galen the opportunity to focus on the role of
pain in treatment. Galen begins by restating the great Hippocratic principle

---

48   The expression εἰς ἡδονὴν appears twelve times in the Galenic corpus: four times in *De
     alimentorum facultatibus*, three times in the pharmacological treatises, and twice in the
     commentaries in the context of kindnesses granted to patients.

49   Dioscorides, *Materia medica* II, 18, 2, 1. Adapted from the translation of T. A. Osbaldeston.

50   Galen, *De simpl. med. facultatibus* XI, 1 (Kühn XII, 318, 16).

51   On the necessity of using the least painful treatment possible, an idea expressed with
     the help of the adjective ἀνώδυνος (used 278 times in the Galenic corpus), the substantive
     ἀνωδυνία (used 27 times), and the adverb ἀνωδύνως (used 18 times), see especially Galen,
     De methodo medendi IV, 7 (Kühn X, 296): 'Surely we must try to treat the sensory part
     in the most painless way possible' (τὸ μὲν οὖν αἰσθητικὸν μόριον ἀνωδύνως ὅτι μάλιστα χρὴ
     πειρᾶσθαι θεραπεύειν).

that 'opposites are cured by opposites', an inviolable principle that he repeats multiple times in his work.[52] In fact, in the case of tetanus, the sprinkling of cold water has no purpose other than to provoke, in reaction, a surge of heat in the body meant to counteract this 'cold' disease. Certain physicians, especially Empiricists and Methodists, did not accept this principle. In order to convince them, Galen even planned to write a treatise entitled *That Hippocrates was right to say that opposites are cured by opposites*, a project that he apparently never had the time to realize.[53] He does however proceed to deliver the principal arguments that he intended to employ against his adversaries. Some contend, for example, that in the case of patients suffering from 'sciatica' (ἐπὶ τῶν ἰσχιαδικῶν), for which one would perform a cauterization of the hip bone, pain would assuage pain (δι' ὀδύνης ὀδύνην ἰάσατο), something that Galen judges to be completely absurd (πρόδηλον ἔχει τὴν ἀτοπίαν):

> And those who see fit to treat a lesser pain with a greater pain err considerably. For it is not the pain that effects the treatment of pain, but the cure that works with pain that treats the condition causing the pain.[54]

Thus, in such cases, the treatment is not the pain itself, but rather the cauterization that accompanies the pain.[55] No physician has ever healed a patient simply by cutting, slicing, or burning him. In fact, if the pain were the cause of the cure, it would be possible to cure all patients, Galen quips. In reality, this is not the case, and if it were possible, for example, to extract a tooth without pain, a toothache would be cured without suffering (ἀνώδυνος). Treatment consists of one single thing: to eradicate the source of the disease, whether without pain or, if that is impossible, with pain.[56] The first solution is, however, always

---

52   On this famous formulation as one of the fundamental principles of Hippocratic therapeutics, see Galen, *De methodo medendi* VIII, 9 (Kühn X, 588–590); XI, 2 (Kühn X, 739–740) and especially 12 (X, 767–773), where Galen cites the Hippocratic precept 'opposites heal opposites' four times in the same chapter, after having already cited it once in chapter 9 (Kühn X, 761). In Hippocrates, see *Breaths* c. I, 5 (ed. Jouanna, p. 104, 11): τὰ ἐναντία τῶν ἐναντίων ἐστὶν ἰήματα and the note of Jouanna in his CUF edition (p. 131).

53   *Ibid.* (Kühn XVIIA, 914): τὸ δὲ γενησόμενον βιβλίον ἐπιγραφήσεται Περὶ τοῦ καλῶς ὑπὸ <τοῦ> Ἱπποκράτους εἰρῆσθαι τὰ ἐναντία τῶν ἐναντίων ὑπάρχειν ἰάματα.

54   Galen, *In Hippocratis Epidemiarum VI comm.* II, 9 (Kühn XVIIA, 910–911): οὐ γὰρ ἡ ὀδύνη τὴν θεραπείαν ἐργάζεται τῆς ὀδύνης, ἀλλὰ τὸ σὺν τῇ ὀδύνῃ βοήθημα τοῦ ποιοῦντος αὐτὴν πάθους.

55   *Ibid.* (Kühn XVIIA, 911, 10–12): οὐ γὰρ διὰ τὴν ὀδύνην ἐθεραπεύθη τὸ πάθος, ἀλλὰ διὰ τὴν καῦσιν, ᾗ συμβέβηκε κατὰ τύχην ὀδύνη.

56   *Ibid.* (Kühn XVIIA, 912, 11–13): ἓν γὰρ μόνον ἐστὶ τὸ ἰώμενον, ὅπερ ἂν ἐκκόπτῃ τὴν διάθεσιν ὁπωσοῦν, ἐάν τε χωρὶς ὀδύνης, ἐάν τε σὺν ταύτῃ.

preferable, since pain can exacerbate (παροξύνειν) the condition.[57] Therefore it is absurd to contend that like cures like, just as much as if a bald physician were, by chance, to succeed at treating an equally bald patient, a physician with a pointed head to cure a similar patient, or a crippled physician to heal a cripple.

This polemic seems, however, to indicate that not all physicians shared Galen's opinion, according to which pain not only has no role in treatment, but, further, threatens to exacerbate disease. The anthology assembled by Stobaeus, in the section titled *On health, and the foresight to preserve it*, mentions the opinions of different authors on this question.[58] Thus, according to Xenophon, Socrates, who did not neglect his body and who condemned those who neglected their own,

> disapproved of over-eating followed by over-exertion, but approved of taking as much hard exercise as the soul can take with pleasure. He said that this habit not only insured good health, but also did not hamper the care of the soul.[59]

To derive pleasure from what one eats is, therefore, not only not reprehensible, but even beneficial for health, so long as one avoids excess. Socrates, according to Stobaeus, also limited himself to recommending that those who feared appearing intemperate 'avoid all that drives them to eat when they are not hungry, and to drink when they are not thirsty'.[60] To support this principle of temperance, Stobaeus then cites the famous Hippocratic adage frequently repeated by Galen: 'food, drink, sleep, the pleasures of love, all in moderation'.[61] Among these philosophers and physicians, however, the orator Gorgias raises a dissenting voice:

---

57 *Ibid.* (Kühn XVIIA, 913–914): ἐπεὶ δὲ <πολλοὶ> πολλάκις ὑπό τε τῶν ἐμπειρικῶν καὶ τῶν μεθοδικῶν λόγων παραγόμενοι διαβάλλειν ἐπιχειροῦσιν αὐτό, παραπλησίους λέγοντες λόγους οἷς ἄρτι διῆλθον, ἴσως ἄμεινόν ἐστι μετὰ τὸ συμπληρῶσαι τὴν ἐξήγησιν τοῦ προκειμένου ποιῆσαί τι βιβλίον, ἐν ᾧ δειχθήσεται 'τὰ ἐναντία τῶν ἐναντίων ἰάματα' ὑπάρχοντα μόνα πρώτως τε καὶ καθ' ἑαυτά.

58 Stobaeus, *Anthology*, IV, 37, 19.

59 Xenophon, *Memorabilia* I, 2, 4, cited by Stobaeus.

60 *Ibid.* I, 3, 6. This opinion of Socrates is also reported by Plutarch (*Precepts of health* 124D8; *On gossip* 513D1; and *On curiosity* 521F3).

61 See Hippocrates, *Epidemics* VI, 6, 2 (Littré V, 324) where the quotation begins with πόνοι (toils), omitted by Stobaeus: πόνοι σιτία ποτὰ ὕπνοι ἀφροδίσια, πάντα μέτρια. The complete passage is cited by Galen in the *Protrepticus* 11 (Kühn I, 28; ed. Boudon-Millot, p. 107, 6–7, and in *De alimentorum facultatibus* (Kühn VI, 464, 11; ed. Wilkins, p. 11, 17–18), and in *De consuetudinibus* (Dietz 127, 16).

Asked what diet he had adopted in order to reach extreme old age: 'I never did or ate anything', he responded, 'for pleasure (πρὸς ἡδονήν)'.[62]

This declaration of the sophist—who was, surely, eager to challenge the prevailing opinion—remains, however, isolated in ancient Greek medical thought. Far from sharing the idea that later would be promoted by a subset of Judaeo-Christian thought, i.e. that a remedy necessarily had to be disagreeable in order to be efficacious, Greek physicians did not shy away from affirming the benefits of pleasure for health.

5   Conclusion

The physiology of pleasure and of pain, as it explained by Plato, particularly in the *Timaeus*, and then taken up by Galen, has as a necessary corollary the idea that what is agreeable to the senses (touch, taste, smell) is equally good for the health and the conservation of the body. Conversely, that which is bad or disagreeable to the senses is equally offensive or harmful for health. Further, that which is produced by nature or is the manifestation of a return to nature, in the case of recovery after illness, for example, is sensed as agreeable and a source of pleasure. Better still, pleasure granted to the patient can be a part of treatment and can even facilitate recovery. By contrast, and in opposition to a poorly understood Stoicism, pain is never the ally of the physician, who must seek to fight it by all means despite a modest therapeutic arsenal. In stark difference to the famous commandment in Genesis condemning women to 'give birth in pain',[63] ancient medical thought expressed gentleness as its deepest originality, especially when compared with Egyptian medicine.

We must concede, however, that Greek physicians had very little by way of an answer when they were confronted by the dissenting voices that recognized a role for pain that was, if not beneficial, then at least sometimes positive. In particular, a convincing physiological explanation for the pain of childbirth is to be found nowhere in Galen. And it is clear that he was little concerned with this domain of medicine. Traditionally abandoned to midwives, it is made relevant by the problem of justifying how such a natural act could bring about such suffering. But above all, and beyond this one case, a recent study undertaken

---

62   Stobaeus, *Anthology* IV, 37, 21, adapted from translation by Josiah Renick Smith: Γοργίας ἐρωτηθεὶς ποίᾳ διαίτῃ χρώμενος εἰς μακρὸν γῆρας ἦλθεν 'οὐδὲν οὐδέποτε' ἔφη 'πρὸς ἡδονὴν οὔτε φαγὼν οὔτε δράσας'.

63   *Genesis* 3, 16.

by researchers from the University of Bristol, University College London, and the Universities of Udine and of Ferrara could well support Gorgias against the physicians. This team has explored the effects of 'Substance P', a chemical substance released by the nerves in response to a wound or to pain, on the process of tissue healing following thrombosis or even cardiac arrest.[64] The researchers concluded that, in mice and also in humans, pain response is important in the process of recovery, and that to block it—or to block it too much—may be harmful. No doubt, however, ancient physicians would readily have agreed with the conclusion of the contemporary researchers that, ideally, medications should be effective in managing pain without impeding the process of recovery.

---

64   Amadesi et al. 2012.

CHAPTER 4

Pain and Medicine in the Classical World*

W. V. Harris

1 Introduction

'I would rather stand three times in the line of battle', says Medea famously, 'than bear a child a single time'.[1] Whatever else we may think about this passage, it will serve to remind us that ancient life was physically very painful by modern standards. Most women experienced unmitigated labor pains, on average at least five or six times, not counting miscarriages, if they survived till menopause. Men who 'stood in the line of battle'—and that was a very large segment of the male population until the Roman peace arrived—could expect painful wounds. Most people who did physical work could expect aches and pains if not traumas in consequence. Slaves could expect frequent pain, since severe corporal punishment and other forms of ill treatment were their common lot, not to mention crucifixion. Everyone could expect toothaches, digestive pains, and, if they lived long enough, arthritis and the assorted discomforts of old age. And in most cases there was little or nothing that anyone, doctors included, could offer in the way of analgesics.

The 1840s were a revolutionary decade in human history—the time when ether and chloroform were first used to anesthetize patients before surgery.[2] In earlier times, having your leg amputated or your 'stone' removed was mainly a matter of endurance and, if you were fortunate, alcohol. Another important date in this history was 1899, the year in which the first effective analgesic based on salicylic acid (which is found in willow bark) became commercially available in the form of aspirin. I simply mention these dates to underline the possibility of very large experiential and attitudinal differences with respect to physical pain between us—citizens of mostly prosperous modern countries—and the ancients.[3]

---

* I should like to thank Véronique Boudon-Millot, Kathleen Coleman and Vivian Nutton for their comments on an earlier version of this paper.

1 Euripides, *Medea* 250–1. See the exegesis of Mossman 2011, 238–9.
2 This was the result of experimentation in Britain, France and the USA. The story tends to be told from a national point of view. A good account, from a French perspective, can be found in Rey 1995 [1993], chapter 5.
3 For a lucid account of modern knowledge of the way that the human nervous system works with respect to pain see Heinricher and Fields 2013.

My intention in this brief essay is to contribute to a discussion of the ways in which Greeks and Romans, and in particular Greek and Roman physicians, reacted to and dealt with physical pain. An immediate difficulty confronts us: how much *generalization* is in fact possible? Pains themselves differ, and not only in intensity.[4] And we scarcely need ancient authors to tell us that different kinds of humans react differently to pain; but they do tell us so—the Hippocratic writers knew it,[5] and Aristotle observes, when he discusses pain and pleasure in the *Nicomachean Ethics*, that individual human reactions to them differ.[6] So let us proceed with proper caution when we say that 'the Greeks and Romans' thought or did any particular thing about the experience of pain.

There is anguish entirely unconnected with ill health, but my subject here is flesh-and-blood physicality. What, practically speaking, did Greeks and Romans do about physical pain, and did they ever succeed in alleviating it or overcoming it? Or was the sufferer always or usually left to his or her own psychological powers of resistance? And we may wonder whether, during the many centuries of learned or rationalistic Greek medicine, much—or any—new knowledge accrued in this area. Then there is the matter of anesthesia during surgical procedures, with the same ensuing question as to whether there was any progress. Finally, we come to the question of resistance, what it amounted to, how robust it was, a question which leads in turn to impossible questions about the subjectivity of pain—can we say whether Greeks and Romans felt more or less pain than we do when certain things happened to them?

All these problems put together are much too large for a single paper, and all I can hope to do here is to sketch the landscape. The subject is all the more challenging because it ideally requires an author with a deep knowledge of both pharmacology and pain-theory; I have read as much as possible in these fields in the time available, but I fully expect to be corrected.

In a recent paper I have argued at length that we cannot understand Graeco-Roman healthcare unless we make ample space for popular medicine (which

---

4   On Greek awareness of this fact, and Galen's efforts to describe the differences see King 1999, Roby 2016.

5   E.g. *De morbis* 1.22: 'When younger men suffer from one of the ailments that were said to arise from exertions they suffer in more ways and more severely, and feel more pain (*algeousi*) than do others ... older men ... suffer more mildly', etc. I return to this matter in the last section of this paper.

6   A different point, obviously. *Nic.Eth.* 7.7.1150a: 'With regard to the pleasures and pains and appetites and aversions that arise through touch and taste ... it is possible to be in such a state as to be defeated by those of them which most people master, or to master even those by which most people are defeated', etc.

I was at some pains to define) as well as rationalistic medicine.[7] In this paper on the other hand, while I shall pay some attention to the popular origins of physicians' pharmacological knowledge, I shall concentrate on the most effective measures and treatments that were available, without any implication that physicians were always more helpful than drug-sellers (*pharmakopô-lai*) when it came to providing analgesics. And we shall not forget that in all periods people will have looked to divine help and to amulets for pain relief. In Campbell Bonner's great work on amulets, he analyses in detail their use for medical purposes (ailments of the digestive tract were apparently the main evil to be guarded against),[8] and popular remedies for pains represent a substantial subject for research; but that must wait for another occasion.[9]

From the beginning of classical Greek textuality[10] it is commonly assumed in certain contexts that *pharmaka*—substances—exist that can alleviate pain.[11] When Menelaus is wounded by an arrow in *Iliad* 4, Agamemnon assures him that a doctor will apply effective *pharmaka* to the wound that will relieve the 'black pains' (4.190–1); the doctor is Machaon, and the *pharmaka*, we are told, came to Machaon's father from Cheiron (4.218–19). Doctors are *poluphar-makoi*, ready with many medicines (*Iliad* 16.28). At the end of *Iliad* 11, when Eurypylus is dealing bravely with an arrow wound in his thigh, he encounters Patroclus:

> 'Take me back to my black ship.
> Cut this shaft from my thigh. And the dark blood—
> wash it out of the wound with clear warm water.
> And spread the soothing healing salves (*êpia pharmaka*)
> across it, the fine drugs they say you learned from your
> friend Achilles, who in turn learned them from Cheiron,
> the most humane of the Centaurs ...'[12]

---

7   Harris 2016.

8   Bonner 1950, chapters 3 and 4.

9   For some useful remarks see McNamara 2003–4, 17.

10   It seems sensible not to assume that substances whose medical usefulness was more or less known in ancient near-eastern cultures (*Papaver somniferum*, for instance, was used in second-millennium Egypt: Nunn 1989, 23) were also known to pre-Hellenistic Greeks unless there is specific evidence to that effect. Yet there was probably some trade in medical drugs between Babylonia and Egypt on the one hand and Greeks on the other.

11   For the wide meaning of *pharmakon* see among others Lloyd 1979, 44, Salazar 2000, 54, Fausti and Hautala 2009, 2–5. The latter, unfortunately rather inaccessible, article provides a valuable bibliography on Greek and Roman pharmacology. For a brief survey of the surviving pharmacological texts see Totelin 2011, 219–20.

12   This translation is much indebted to R. Fagles.

Patroclus complies, and he 'crushed a bitter root and covered over the gash to kill his comrade's pain, a cure that fought off every kind of pain (*odunêphaton, hê hoi hapasas esch'odunas*)'.[13] This is the wonderful mythical world, where heroes can get effective though unspecified pain relief. Similarly, once again, in tragedy: Philoctetes, in Sophocles' version of his story, is imagined as having found on Lemnos an effective pain-killing *phullon*—a leaf, or is it a plant? its name is not given—and he made use of it (*Philoctetes* 649–50).

It can be argued that Homer and Sophocles would not have written in these ways unless some of their contemporaries had at least some minimal knowledge of effective pain-relieving *pharmaka*, even though it is fairly well recognized that humans have a vast capacity for believing in materially useless remedies.[14] And it appears from the story that Herodotus told (perhaps in the 420s) about the famous physician Democedes of Croton that the ideal Greek physician claimed, in some circumstances at least, to use relatively 'gentle' methods (3.130).[15]

2   Hippocratic Medicine

Our instinct may be to look at once for *pharmaka*, but that would be to ignore the view of at least some Hippocratic doctors that 'all the causes of pain (*ponos*) can be reduced to the same one, namely that it is the strongest foods that hurt a person most, whether he is healthy or ill' (*Vet. Med.* 6).[16] Hence the obvious treatment was to correct the sufferer's diet, and dietetics were always a major part of ancient medical therapy.[17] But most serious pains needed some other treatment beyond a light diet, and so we turn now to the drugs known in Hippocratic times.

---

13   11.828–32, 846–8.
14   As to why this is so see especially Stannard 1982.
15   Democedes was the most skillful doctor of his time (*fl.* 520), Herodotus says (3.125). When Darius sprained his ankle, his Egyptian doctors failed to relieve the pain, but Democedes, using 'Greek cures' that were 'gentle' (*êpia*), enabled the king to get some sleep.
16   According to another Hippocratic view, not incompatible with this one, pain is a consequence of an imbalance of the 'humours': 'pain is felt (*algei*) when one of these elements is in defect or excess, or is isolated in the body and is not compounded with all the others. For when an element is isolated and stands by itself, it is inevitable that the place which it left becomes diseased, and that the place where it stands in a flood must, because of the excess, cause pain (*odunên*) and suffering (*ponon*)....' (*De natura hominis* 4). The author of this treatise, almost certainly Hippocrates' son-in-law Polybus, later discusses the role of regimen in the aetiology of illness (ch. 9).
17   Nutton 2004, 96.

Plato's Socrates supposed that midwives possessed *pharmakia* (little drugs) and spells that could ease the pangs of childbirth (*Theaetetus* 149cd). We may guess that the drug that midwives mainly used, when they could obtain it, was made from dittany or 'false dittany'. About the former plant (*origanum dictamnus* L.) Theophrastus says (*History of Plants* 9.16.1) that it

> has marvelous powers ... and is especially useful for women in child-birth ... they use the leaves ... they use it against difficult labour, for they say that it either makes childbirth easy or at least by general agreement it makes the pain cease. It is given as a drink in water. But it is scarce ...

and it was peculiar to Crete. The plant called 'false dittany' (*ballota pseudo-dictamnus* Bentham), so Theophrastus says (9.16.2), was useful for the same purposes (and not confined to Crete) but was much weaker. If either plant had any such effects they were probably all in the mind.[18]

What about other kinds of pain? Hippocratic physicians could extract an arrow and bind up a wound (though even in these cases they could do fatal harm), but they claimed to be able to do a great deal more. They claimed among other things to know of effective pain-remedies, though it is seldom clear exactly how much they are claiming for the remedies in question. It is even less clear how much they were believed.

Aphorismi 5.25 says that 'swellings and pains in the joints, when not caused by a wound, are relieved in most cases by the pouring on of cold water ... for numbness in moderation removes pain', a sensible basic remedy.[19] But the Hippocratic work *De affectionibus*, above all, is packed with pain remedies, per-haps because it is addressed in part to laypeople (*idiôtai*).[20] The author offers

---

18   The Hippocratics claimed that dittany speeded childbirth but not that it made it oth-erwise less painful: see the references given by Amigues 2006, 196. Contemporary Greek scientists who have enthused about dittany (Liolias et al. 2010) have not pro-vided any clinical evidence that substances from either plant would have such effects. Nor have I found such evidence elsewhere. Cf., concerning dittany, http://www.ema .europa.eu/docs/en_GB/document_library/Herbal_-_HMPC_assessment_report/ 2013/08/WC500147179.pdf, pp. 12–13.

19   According to *De locis in homine* 42, pain arises from heat and from cold and is cured by its opposite; the author also seems to say that there is remedy for the pain associated with each disease, but he gives no details.

20   But Potter 1988, 4, has shown that they were not the only audience. —In my view Horden 1999, 297–302, demonstrated that the Hippocratic writers do not distinguish system-atically between their principal words for pain—*odunê, algos, algêma* and *ponos*—and I cannot see any systematic distinctions between them in later medical writers either.

pain remedies from head to foot (I omit therapies that are aimed at illnesses and not specifically at pains):

> Headaches (ch. 2): washing, sneezing, cleaning out *phlegma*,[21] regimen of gruel and water, if necessary bleeding, cutting the head, cauterizing the veins.
>
> Earaches (4): washing with hot water, steam-bath, if necessary drink an unspecified *pharmakon* to draw the *phlegma* upwards.
>
> Toothaches (4): if decayed, extraction; otherwise, dry by cautery; things to chew (*diamasêmata*) also help.
>
> Side pains caused by pleurisy (7): give the patient 'something' that will remove *phlegma* and bile, clean the 'cavity' (*koiliê*) and cool it with an enema; drinks and gruel; later, warming.[22]
>
> Back or side pains because of pneumonia (9): the remedy for pleurisy listed in the [lost] book *Pharmakitis* (*Medication Book*).[23]
>
> Midriff pains (10):[24] as with pleurisy; warm the patient and give a medication for the 'cavity'; give any drink except wine.
>
> Whole-body pain in fever (14):[25] evacuate downwards with an unspecified *pharmakon*, an unspecified potion, or gruel.
>
> Hypochondrium and heart pains in the summer (15): a drink of melicrat [a mixture of honey and water], warming, induce vomiting; if necessary an enema, fomentations (*chliasmata*); medications from the *Pharmakitis*.
>
> Wandering pains in the 'cavity' (15): something to drink from the *Pharmakitis* 'or whatever else you think suitable'; if necessary, evacuation downwards and withhold food.
>
> Sudden pains without fever (16): wash and warm.
>
> 'Cavity' pains caused by dysentery and colic (23): clean out the patient's head, evacuate the 'cavity' with boiled milk, wash the area below the navel, administer nourishment from the *Pharmakitis*.

---

21   *Phlegma* is not phlegm or any other specific substance recognized in modern medicine.
22   *Koiliê* does not correspond to any modern anatomical concept: sometimes it is the thorax, sometimes the gastro-intestinal tract.
23   Which will of course have been accessible to very few.
24   The term is *phrenitis*, which in this context we must treat as a physical rather than a mental disorder.
25   *Ponoi*, not as is usual with this author *odunai* or *algêmata*.

'Cholera' pains (27) (the reference is to a digestive complaint that was not cholera): give what is written in the *Pharmakitis* again, moisten the 'cavity', soften the body with hot baths.[26]

Strangury pains (28): the *Pharmakitis* once more, the section concerning diuretic *pharmaka*.

Sciatica (29): soften the affected part with baths, fomentations and a vapour-bath *(puria)*, evacuate the cavity downwards, refer to the *Pharmakitis*.

Arthritis (30): apply cooling agents, evacuate downwards, give the patient whatever gruel and drink you think suitable.

Gout (31): the same treatment as for arthritis. If pain persists in the toes, cauterize the veins a little above the knuckles.

We may conclude that Hippocratic doctors were seriously concerned about pain and were expected by their patients to have at least some capacity to help, but that their ideas ranged from what was both painful and dangerous (cauterizing veins) to what was futile (evacuation, one of the ancient physician's stand-bys) to what may have been mildly helpful (warming) to, very occasionally, what would really have helped (extracting decayed teeth, with obvious risks). Futility dominated. Other less systematic texts in the Hippocratic corpus seem to point in the same direction.[27] Without the text of the *Pharmakitis* a full evaluation is impossible, but *De affectionibus* seems evasive. That would not be surprising since well-regarded recipes were financially valuable,[28] in consequence of which we shall sometimes encounter a certain secretiveness in other authors too.

Meanwhile some Hippocratics implicitly or explicitly acknowledge that in particular circumstances there was nothing effective that they could do to alleviate pain. The harrowing case-reports in *Epidemics* book 7, for example, while

---

26   In this case and in chapter 29 the *Pharmakitis* book is referred to as *Pharmaka*. Schöne 1920 showed that a surviving 'Hippocrates' fragment—not in Littré's edition—, which he reprinted, is likely to be part of the introduction to this work, though he also suggested (435 n.2) that the *Pharmakitis* was not written by the author of *De affectionibus*. The text is also in Monfort 2002. Why did the work not survive in full? It was presumably considered obsolete in later centuries.

27   *Epidemics* Book 6 (6.6.3) recommends as treatments for unspecified pains cautery and excision (both of them very painful in themselves), also 'heating, cooling, sneezing, the juices of plants appropriate for the pain in question, and *kukeôn*'. *Kukeôn* was a mixed drink of sometimes fabulous properties (*Odyssey* 10.316, etc.); the word simply means 'mixed drink' but it generally seems to have consisted of wine, cheese and honey— medicinal value, nil. For the ineffectiveness of Hippocratic analgesics cf. Byl 1992, 214.

28   Cf. Mattern 2013, 260—referring to a much later ancient period.

they occasionally mention treatments that more or less alleviated pain, more frequently avoid any such claims.[29] There is no mention of opiates.

But very large claims have sometimes been made about classical Greek knowledge of opium. The

> harvesting, preparation, distribution, and application [of the opium poppy] in general pharmacy and medical therapeutics all were sophisticated and as precise as was then possible. Our ancient sources attest repeatedly to this deep sophistication in the grasp and understanding of the opium poppy, and Hellenistic and Roman medicine had refined a lengthy and venerated tradition of multiple uses.[30]

Yet this author shades the evidence: he immediately tells us that the passage in the *Odyssey* (4.220–30) in which Helen makes everyone extra happy at a Spartan banquet by lacing their wine with some unspecified *pharmakon* is a reference to the opium poppy—but the poet does not mention poppies and is clearly imagining a drug of quite unheard-of properties.[31] Nor does anything else that this scholar has to say about Hippocratic pharmacology justify his strong language (as to Hellenistic and Roman times, I will discuss them separately). John Riddle—well-known for his claim, which initially convinced me but then encountered serious objections, that the herbal contraceptives and abortifacients recommended by ancient medical writers were to a great extent effective—,[32] is the other leading scholar who entertains a high opinion of Hippocratic pharmacology.[33] He reports that ninety per cent of the 257 drugs recommended for assorted purposes in the corpus of Hippocratic

---

29   A degree of success: 7.1.5, 7.2.7, 7.3.1, 7.4, 7.8.

30   Scarborough 1995, 4. The author is a classicist who has made a life-long study of the history of pharmacology.

31   See Heubeck, West and Hainsworth 1988, 206–7, though even they do not perhaps make enough room for the poet's imagination. To be clear: no Greek author prior to the Hippocratics mentions the analgesic effects of any poppy-derived substance. The notion that Helen was administering opium has a long history, appearing for example in Guido Majno's splendid *The Healing Hand* (Majno 1975, 144). But opium is a soporific; mandragora, on the other hand, might have made the party livelier.

32   See, from a biochemical point of view, King 1998, 147–51. Frier has shown, by reference to the ages of mothers at childbirth in Roman Egypt, that artificial means of contraception were little used, if at all, by ordinary married couples there (Frier 2001, 153).

33   His most important papers are to be found in Riddle 2002.

writers are also mentioned in standard modern pharmacological texts, which leads him to the conclusion that the Hippocratics 'knew' a great deal.[34]

That is theoretically possible. Human beings in the Middle East, and presumably in Bronze Age Greece too, had been using plants for their healing qualities for thousands of years before Hippocrates, and, while we should not suppose that they 'tested' them in any modern sense, they may indeed have learned at least something about the pain-killing properties of those (few) plants that possess them. There is also the matter of placebo effects, to which I shall return later (there were probably some such effects, but not on a large scale).

But the obstacles in the way of the ancient development and use of effective drugs were formidable and should by now be familiar.[35] Not only were the preconditions of modern science largely lacking, the materials themselves— their preparation and conservation—were exceedingly hard to control. Rightly if rhetorically, Vivian Nutton has asserted that the world of medical drugs in antiquity was one of 'travelling salesmen, unscrupulous traders, adulteration, confusion and neglect'.[36]

And our investigation is difficult too. In the first place, it is often (not just occasionally) hard to know exactly which species of plant an ancient writer had in mind, if indeed he had one in mind. (For the confusion about poppies and about hellebore see below). The identification of plants in classical texts is often a very intricate matter, and the identifications in Liddell and Scott, still the supreme work of philological authority, now seem to be quite often misleading.[37] Secondly, it is quite often difficult to know what the illness was that the drug was intended to counteract: it is enough to look back at the conditions listed in the summary of Hippocrates' *De affectionibus* given above.

Hence we need a more focused statistical enquiry. It is not a question whether the plants recommended by the Hippocratics had some medicinal value, but whether they had the effects actually attributed to them. It will not do to pick out an isolated passage or two in which a Hippocratic writer recommends poppies for pain relief and conclude that the classical Greeks 'knew about the

---

34   Riddle 1987, 37. Yet this author also says (1992, XV, 18) that 'we should never evaluate the
      [medical] past on the basis of what modern science and cultural values regard as truth',
      somewhat contradicting his own practice.

35   See Nutton 1990, 7–8, for a clear statement.

36   Nutton 1990, 8.

37   Lloyd 2002, 110–11, following Raven 2000, 5–10.

pain-killing properties of poppy-juice'.[38] A team of medical scientists led by
Plinio Prioreschi has in fact tried a statistical analysis, reviewing all the passages they could find in the Hippocratic corpus that describe forms of pain
relief and concentrating on the poppy, since it is the one substance that these
authors often mention that undoubtedly had analgesic properties.

Prioreschi and company consciously weighted their research in favour of
the Hippocratic writers by supposing that when they recommend the use of
poppies they and their readers are thinking of *Papaver somniferum* and/or
Papaver setigerum (whereas most species of the genus *Papaver* contain no opi-
ate at all). They concluded nonetheless that 'the Hippocratic physician did not
recognize the analgesic property of poppy'.[39] They counted 97 passages in the
Hippocratic corpus in which the writer offers a prescription for the relief of
pain, and in 16 of these prescriptions poppies are an ingredient.[40] There has
to be some suspicion admittedly that these Hippocratics were somewhat confused about which part of the poppy was useful.[41] (I optimistically assume for
the sake of argument that the author intended to recommend the use of one of
the poppy species that actually includes opium).

In my view the correct conclusion is that (some of) the Hippocratic physicians did in fact recognize the analgesic properties of opium, but only very
dimly and distantly (the author of *Affections*, who saw himself as an expert on
pain-management, clearly set no particular store by it). It might be guessed

---

38   This kind of procedure is regrettably common, e.g. in Zanchin 2014. Opium was quite
      widely used in ancient Egypt, but for a variety of medical purposes: Crawford 1973, 231–2.
      There is room for further work here. Merlin 2003, 302–12, gathered uncritically a good deal
      of Neolithic and Bronze Age evidence for the use of poppies, but much of it may have
      been culinary (cf. Zohary 2012, 109) or psychotropic. The texts are in this sort of case the
      best guide to what the ancients knew.

39   Prioreschi et al. 1998, 328. In Prioreschi's view, 'in antiquity, progress in pharmacological
      knowledge was practically impossible', because of the number of variables (1998, 310). My
      conclusion in this paper is different.

40   There are some minor inaccuracies in their list, and I count 101 passages in which works
      in the Hippocratic corpus tell the reader how to relieve one pain or another. The sixteen
      passages in which the use of poppy is recommended are in fact fifteen: *De morbis* 3.16,
      De muliebribus 1.64, 1.105, 2.117, 119, 129, 149, 201, 206 (twice), *De natura muliebri* 15, 38, 44,
      De diaeta acutorum, Appendix 30 Littré = 63 Potter, and *De internis affectionibus* 40. It is
      possible of course that the book *Pharmakitis* strongly recommended opiates. —In all the
      cases listed here the recipes include other ingredients. The significance of the fact that
      poppy is mostly recommended for women is unclear.

41   It is usually not specified. *De muliebribus* 1.105 and 2.206 speak of juice (*opos*) of the
      poppy. *De natura muliebri* 38 refers to the seeds, which is on target, but chapter 15 of the
      same work refers to the rind or peel (*lepuron*) and *De muliebribus* 2.119 refers to the pod
      (*keluphos*). That is not encouraging.

that patients received some relief from pain in roughly one case out of six, but that is merely a guess, and the patients of many Hippocratic physicians will have received no pharmaceutical relief at all. It is clear that most such physicians, seeking to ease pain, were more likely to prescribe *ptisanê*, a drink made out of barley that came in various forms[42]—which contains various nutrients but is not an analgesic.[43]

What happened to the other patients, it is important to notice in any case, was not often merely neutral: some remedies put into effect by doctors were obviously harmful, like the treatment inflicted on an unfortunate man in the Hippocratic *Epidemics* 5.7 who, suffering from major pains in his right hip and groin, was subjected to severe bleeding and died a few days later. The author of the Hippocratic *De diaeta acutorum*, having recommended bleeding for the relief of pain (21), further recommends a scary mixture of herbs, including black hellebore, to induce evacuation; he claimed that hellebore and a plant that is called *peplos* were effective pain-killers. On the most likely identifications of these plants they are both as it happens seriously toxic.[44]

The history of hellebore supports a pessimistic view of Hippocratic analgesics. Hellebore is the medicine that the Hippocratic authors recommended more than any other (118 hits in the TLG), for all sorts of conditions.[45] In reality black hellebore (*Helleborus niger* L.) is poisonous, while so-called white hellebore (*Veratrum album* L.) is effective mainly as an evacuant.[46] Patients whom the Hippocratic doctors treated with hellebore must either have died in consequence (and sometimes we know that that was the result), or at best suffered effects that helped them not at all. The fact that the doctors of the late fifth century believed that they had learned a lot about the correct use of hellebore makes this case an especially intriguing one.[47]

---

42   Cf. Jones 1923, 60.
43   Theophrastus, *HP* 9.16.8, reports that one Thrasyas of Mantinea—apparently a contemporary—had invented a lethal drug that was painless; its ingredients included hemlock and poppy-juice, so it seems that Thrasyas had some understanding of the analgesic or soporific potential of the latter.
44   The second seems to be *Euphorbia peplus* L.
45   Cf. Aliotta et al. 2003, 126–8.
46   See Girard 1990. Lloyd 1983, 127, wonders whether the physician readers always knew whether black or white hellebore was meant.—Herophilus, who was an enthusiast for drugs (Pliny, *NH* 25.15, with Von Staden 1989, 400), seems to have had a real passion for hellebore, if Pliny (*NH* 25.58) understood him correctly (Herophilus compared hellebore to a vigorous general, a *fortissimus dux*).
47   Oribasius, *Coll.med.* 8.8 quotes Ctesias, himself a doctor, to this effect (*FGrHist* 688 F68); cf. Grmek and Gourevitch 1985, 5.

Before leaving the Hippocratics one must say something about mandragora (mandrake)—which will require a more detailed discussion later.[48]
Mandragora's roots contain alkaloids that have hallucinogenic and narcotic
effects.[49] The Hippocratic doctors from time to time recommend its use,
in eight passages altogether, but never as an analgesic—though *De locis in
homine* recommends it for sick persons as an antidote to suicidal thoughts.[50]
Theophrastus seems to be somewhat better informed. He reports that it was
used both as an aphrodisiac and as a cure for insomnia;[51] more importantly, he
tells us that it is 'useful' against gout (*ta podagrika*) as well as against erysipelas
(*History of Plants* 9.9.1).[52] It is a reasonable assumption both that this 'usefulness' consisted of pain relief and that physicians of Theophrastus' time, some
of them at least, shared his beliefs about mandragora's properties. It was also
well known in the fourth century that mandragora could induce sleep.[53] But
medical men may have held back from trying to anaesthetize patients with
mandragora before performing painful procedures because they knew, like
Theophrastus (*Causes of Plants* 6.4.5), that an excessive intake would be lethal.

3   Roman-Era Physicians

Did later Greek doctors know more? There were certainly plenty of obstacles
in the way of pharmacological progress, in the shape of the factors that are
generally recognized as having slowed down scientific research in antiquity, in
particular the lack of statistical reasoning and the lack of a scientific community. Here in any case we encounter the most frustrating aspect of the history of
Greek medicine, the relative poverty of the Hellenistic sources. It seems impossible to gain any reliable idea as to whether Diocles of Carystus or Herophilus,
to mention two of the relatively well-known figures, really knew any more than

---

48   The best account of ancient uses of plants of the genus mandragora may still be that of
      Steier 1928. See also van den Berg and Dircksen 2008.
49   For the effects of ingesting mandragora see further Ramoutsaki et al. 2002, 45 (but it
      should be noted that none of the historical remarks in that paper are trustworthy).
50   *De locis in homine* 39. For the other references see Moisan 1990, 382–3.
51   Mandragora's aphrodisiac effects had a long history, including Genesis chapter 30 and
      Machiavelli's sex-farce *La Mandragola*.
52   'For they say [note the distancing; cf. Lloyd 1983, 122–5] that its leaves, used with meal,
      are useful for treating wounds, and that its root, when scraped and steeped in vinegar, is
      useful for erysipelas, gout and insomnia and as an aphrodisiac. It is administered in wine
      or vinegar …'.
53   Demosthenes, *Philippic* 4.6, Aristotle, *On Sleep* 3.456b30 (like poppy, wine and darnel);
      cf. Plato, *Republic* 6.488c.

the Hippocratics in this department.[54] Herophilus is generally credited with a major advance in the understanding of the nervous system,[55] but neither he nor any other ancient scientist could make any therapeutic use of this new knowledge. Yet there is good reason, as we shall see, to think that there was in fact some real pharmacological progress between the time of Theophrastus and that of Celsus.

If we knew more about the teaching and practice of Asclepiades of Bithynia (whom, following Pliny, I prefer to date to the time of Pompey, not to the rather earlier date preferred by some scholars), he might be a significant witness here. On the one hand he seems to have been reluctant to inflict painful treatments on his patients, famously saying that it was the duty of the physician to treat the patient 'safely, swiftly and pleasantly (*iucunde*)' (Celsus, *On Medicine* 3.4.1), and on the other hand he was evidently for the most part against administering drugs.[56] One may suspect therefore that in his time it was still reasonable to doubt the analgesic properties of the main substances that the doctors believed in, which does not, however, signify that there had been no progress at all (but Asclepiades certainly had his eccentricities and was not always reasonable).

With the first century AD, if not earlier, there begins a new age of relative confidence among doctors, with respect to pain-management at least. It may be a sign of this new attitude that the epitaph from the city of Rome of a doctor named Nicomedes claimed, some time in the second century, that he had 'saved many people with pain-relieving *pharmaka*'.[57] The medical profession continued to have a thoroughly mixed reputation,[58] but a claim such as that of Nicomedes cannot have seemed altogether ridiculous. It was also probably less ambitious than it seems, because lesser pains hardly counted as pains— so it appears. Scribonius Largus (writing under Claudius) gives us a hint here:

---

54 Galen mentions Diocles among thirteen major pharmacological authorities (XI.795K), and the existing fragments refer to opium (frr. 147 and 148a van der Eijk), but the passages in question were selected by Galen and we cannot know how well Diocles understood opium's properties. However it is to be noted that the only medical writer to whom Caelius Aurelianus attributes a treatment of liver disease that includes poppy juice is also Diocles (*Chronic Diseases* 3.62 = fr. 120) (but his overall treatment would probably have been lethal).

55 See Von Staden 1989, 159–60.

56 When, according to Celsus (3.4.2), he 'did away with medications' ('medicamenta sustulit'), the specific context is the treatment of fevers. His hostility to analgesic drugs is also visible elsewhere, however (Celsus 3.18.14, concerning the treatment of *phrenitis*). From Scribonius Largus, *Comp. praef.* 7–8, it appears that Asclepiades did not altogether disapprove of drugs, but Largus had a vested interest in asserting that.

57 *IG* XIV.1879 = *IGUR* 1283, Samama 2003, no. 476.

58 Cf. Harris 2016, 10 n.39.

describing a dental procedure that would have been acutely painful to a modern sensibility, he assures the reader that it can be carried out 'painlessly' ('sine ullo ... dolore') (*Compositiones* 53).[59]

It is plausible to suppose, however, that there were some advances in pharmacological knowledge by the first century AD, for when the learned Galen looked backwards—and he notoriously revered the far-distant Hippocratics— he privileged the pharmacologists of roughly the last century before his own time, in particular Andromachos the younger (who flourished under Nero),[60] and Asclepiades Pharmakion (the Pharmacist, datable to the last quarter of the first century AD). He takes recipes from still earlier writers, all the way back to Diocles, but it is the moderns (relatively speaking) who win his confidence.[61]

And in fact non-medical writers very strongly suggest that by Vergil's time at the latest some of the medicinal powers of opium were widely recognized. The earliest such references presuppose that poppies were regarded as capable of producing either a soporific effect (*Aeneid* 4.486, Ovid, *Amores* 2.6.31, *Tristia* 5.2.24, *Met.* 11.605) or were a cause of forgetfulness (*Lethaea papavera, Georgics* 4.545), or both at once (*Georgics* 1.78).[62] None of this means that the analgesic property of opium was fully recognized, but it hints at a degree of recognition.[63]

Two papyrus documents of the early first century AD allude to the use of opium without indicating its precise properties. A document of the year 37 from Euhemereia (*P. Rylands* II.141, lines 21–22) refers to the sale of opium,

---

59   'So even when the tooth is partly decayed, I do not recommend that it should be pulled at once, but that the area where it is hollow should be cut out with a surgical chisel (*scalpro medicinali*), which is done painlessly'.

60   See Fabricius 1972, 66 and 185 (on Andromachos' date). The earliest pharmacological writers whom Galen cites frequently are Heras (20 BC–20 AD?) and the mysterious Apollonius the follower of Herophilus (whose chronology is afloat; some locate him as early as the first half of the first century BC); see Fabricius 66, 181–5, etc. Galen's other favourites, Archigenes, Damokrates and Kriton, are Neronian or later. The recipes themselves may of course be much older.

61   Jouanna and Boudon 1997 showed with what finesse Galen expressed his profound respect for Hippocrates in his pharmacological works without actually adopting his medications.—See further below.

62   The two effects are amalgamated in Ovid, *Ars Am.* 3.647–8, where, however, the nature of the *medicamina* is not specified.

63   What a curious but uncritical layman thought he knew about poppies and opium three generations later can be seen in Pliny, *NH* 20.198–209: at first sight, all his knowledge of opium as an analgesic is inaccurate, but he includes a tantalizing reference to the 'famous drug' *dia kôduôn* (200).

while a recipe from Oxyrhynchus (*P.Oxy.* VIII.1088, lines 66–67) describes a soporific made of henbane, anise and opium.[64]

Returning to medical writers, let us consider first of all Celsus—leaving aside the question whether he actually practised medicine. The usual concerns arise—does he refer to the right species of the plant in question, does he know which part of the plant is useful, does he know appropriate dosages? These questions are usually unanswerable. And very often Celsus is plainly groping in the dark, like his Hippocratic predecessors: when, for example, he sets out remedies for pain in the *nervi*—by which he seems to mean sinews or tendons—he offers the reader a series of actually useless suggestions (3.27.2).[65] Pain in the kidneys elicits the recommendation that you should rub together specific quantities of cucumber seeds, pine kernels, almonds and a little crocus, and administer them in milk (4.17). Pains in the liver, spleen and 'sides' elicit still more complex but equally useless recipes (5.18.3–5), and then there is the recipe of Apollophanes, which 'relieves all pains' (5.18.6).[66]

But Celsus' most interesting chapter about pain relief concerns pills (*catapotia*):

> Those which relieve pain by means of sleep they call 'anodynes'.[67] Unless there is extreme necessity, it is inadvisable (*alienum*) to use them. For they are made of powerful medicaments that are alien to the stomach (5.25.1).[68]

He then describes a single exception to this advice, with five ingredients including what he calls 'poppy tears' (*papaveris lacrimae*). But what is most significant is that of the nine complex pain-alleviating recipes that are described in

---

64 Trismegistos 12927 and 63118.

65 '... the part should be wetted with water containing soda, but not oil, then wrapped up, and under it should be placed a brazier containing some glowing charcoal with sulphur.... Cups may also be applied ...'. Etc.

66 'Turpentine-resin and frankincense soot, each 4 *denarii* (about 16 grams), *bdellium*, *ammoniacum*, iris, calf's or goat's kidney-suet, mistletoe juice, each 4 *denarii*'. Quite costly, no doubt.

67 There is a strong hint here of one of the limitations of ancient analgesic drugs: even at their best they could not reliably alleviate pain without inducing unconsciousness.

68 It could be argued that Celsus' reluctance to recommend drugs reflects his predilection for the Methodist sect, for which see Scarborough 1991, 204. The legal liability that, in Roman law, stemmed from a lethal overdose (Grmek and Gourevitch 1985, 12–13) may also have made practitioners more cautious.

this chapter (5.25.1–9) no fewer than six include 'poppy tears' or mandragora.[69] The implication seems to be that there had indeed been some serious progress in pain-control since Hippocratic times. If you went to a doctor of Celsus' time complaining of pain, he might tell you that your pain was not severe enough to run the risk of medication, but if the pain were intense you had a notably better chance of receiving effective medication than you would have had 400 years earlier—always supposing that you could afford it. But it was still a great lottery: when Celsus tells his readers how to alleviate toothache, 'which can be counted among the greatest of torments', he recommends opium and mandragora, but they are merely minor elements in a long list of largely useless advice (6.9).

The list of remedies completed by Scribonius Largus between 43 and 48 has not always been well served by recent scholarship, as far as analgesics are concerned.[70] He was apparently somewhat conservative in this department—so at least his silence about mandragora suggests. He is the earliest extant writer to have used the term opium (*Compositiones* 22 and 93), and he knows which part of the poppy produces it (*Comp.* 22); his warning against bogus opium (*ibid.*) also implies some expertise. But the value of his remedies for pain has in any case been absurdly exaggerated by some recent scholarship: it is drastically false to say that Scribonius' remedies 'can be held to be mostly in line, or at least not contradictory, with respect to those which modern medicine makes use of'.[71] Scribonius, who gives ample space to magical remedies,[72] offers approximately 110 recipes that are specifically supposed to relieve pains.[73] Some 21 (19 per cent) of these recipes included some substance with genuinely analgesic potential such as opium or henbane. But that may give an excessively optimistic view of Scribonius' knowledge, for quite apart from his 89 or so useless recipes, some of those that do include opium or henbane include such overwhelming proportions of other ingredients that their analgesic effect is

---

69   One of the six also includes *hyoscyamus* (henbane); hyoscyamine is recognized as anti-cholinergic/antispasmodic drug.

70   For the text of Scribonius Largus see now Jouanna-Bouchet 2016.

71   Mantovanelli 2012, vi. The vagueness of this claim is evident. Buonopane 2014 is confused. Fabbri 2017, 23–4, also gives an unduly optimistic account of Scribonius' knowledge in this area.

72   Capitani 1972, 128–32. See for example chs. 12, 13, 16, 17, etc., etc. At the same time he was well aware that testing remedies was important (e.g. *Epist.* 1, *Compos.* 98), and he distances himself a little from some particularly absurd remedies (e.g. ch. 14).

73   I have restricted myself to cases where pain is explicitly the target, since it is at least possible that in the case of other remedies for painful conditions it is the condition itself not the associated pain that is the target. In some cases it is unclear how many separate remedies are being proposed.

likely to have been negligible.[74] In short, Scribonius seems to be scarcely better informed than the Hippocratic writers of four centuries earlier.

Roughly half a century elapsed between Celsus' *De medicina* and the completion of Dioscorides' catalogue of *materia medica*. This work lists nearly 200 species of plant that are said to alleviate pains of one kind or another, plus 27 animal-derived substances.[75] One might therefore suppose that his book was merely a repository of superstitions, but matters are not so simple: *Papaver somniferum* (4.64) and mandragora (4.75) receive more attention from the author than any other supposedly analgesic substances, and *hyoscyamus* (henbane, 4.68) receives a relatively detailed treatment too. Willow bark also makes a minor appearance (1.104).[76] The implication of Dioscorides' work has to be that the patient who found an effective analgesic in this period was still a very fortunate one, but that the patient had significantly better prospects than before.[77] One notes with great interest that the *materia medica* detected in the excavation of the Roman camp at Neuss in the Rhineland included *hyoscyamus*; the most likely closing date of the destruction level in question is 69/70 AD.[78]

A good deal also depended on which sect your doctor preferred. If you encountered a 'Methodist', you would probably find him, like Asclepiades of Bithynia,[79] very reluctant to prescribe pain-alleviating drugs. Thus Caelius Aurelianus, basing himself on the second-century Soranus, who was a Methodist, takes a negative view of the use of pain-killing medicaments to counteract toothache (*Chronic Diseases* 2.79–83): 'many' of the 'old physicians', he says, recommended treating toothache with 'drugs that the Greeks call *anôduna* [pain-killers] and which we [Latin-speakers, that is] will call *indoloria*', but he is sceptical and he explains why.[80] His lengthy discussion of chronic

74 Opium makes up less than 5 per cent in the recipes given in chs. 23, 26, 30, 31, 121, 126, 147, and 173. Some of Scribonius' recipes have absurd numbers of ingredients (42 in ch. 177 seems to be the extreme case). One should not think of Scribonius' book as simply a textbook or handbook, but also as an advertisement and perhaps as a fantasy.

75 The passages in question are conveniently listed in Beck 2005, 500. The plant species are listed in Books I to IV, the animal substances in Book II.

76 *Salix* sp. L. (Greek *itea*).

77 What role Dioscorides himself played in this development cannot be known. His statement that he had 'led a soldier's life' (1 pr.4) has led to much speculation.

78 Knörzer 1965.

79 For the relationship between Asclepiades and the Methodists see Vallance 1990, 131–43. As to the extent of the influence of the various medical sects see Leith 2016.

80 The passage is too long to be quoted in full here. 'The fact is that such drugs remove the sensation of pain, but not the affection itself. These writers also prescribe fumes for the teeth … but it would be better to avoid these substances because they congest the head,

headaches, which canvases every kind of remedy known in antiquity, including bleeding, cupping and specific diets, also tends to exclude drugs (*Chronic
Diseases* 1.4–50). If the condition persists, one may in the end use hellebore
(white hellebore, presumably) (1.43), but those exponents of other sects who
recommend *fomenta* (fomentations, 1.45) and *malagmata* (emollient plasters)
are mistaken.[81] In his discussion of diseases of the liver he mentions three
anodynes that other people prescribe, the 'two peppers' (*dia diôn pipereôn*),
the 'fever-allaying' (*lêxipureton*) and the 'ground pine' (*chamaepityn*) (*Chronic
Diseases* 3.58–9), but he dismisses these recommendations as erroneous (3.62).
Drugs play a minor role at most (see for instance 2.155 on limiting dosages).

The position of Aretaeus of Cappadocia in this history is mysterious, and
not only because his career may belong to virtually any period in the first two
centuries (he was perhaps a somewhat older contemporary of Galen's, born
therefore in the early years of the second century).[82] His medical procedures
sometimes seem especially hair-raising—see, for instance, his proposed ways
of treating chronic headaches (*Treatment of Chronic Diseases* 1.2)—, and he
treats pain relief as such in an offhand manner; the only drug he mentions
in this connection is the juice of the plant thapsia (*thapsia* sp.).[83] But what is
strangest is that when he refers to pain-killers in *Treatment of Acute Diseases*
2.5, à propos of ileus—which is, he says, so painful that its victims desire to
die—his treatments are the usual mixture of bleeding, evacuation and so on.
But also: 'give a drink of cumin or rue or of sison, or, with these, some of the
pain-killing drugs—there are many thousands (*muria*) of them that have come
to be trusted, some by some, some by others, as a result of experience (*peira*)'.[84]
He shrugs the matter off, leaving a curious impression of evasiveness. Perhaps,

---

and to substitute warm mead (*mulsum*) (80) or some other soothing fluid. (80) ... And
these writers prescribe that the teeth be covered over with the juice of poppy (*opium*),
galbanum, pepper, laserwort, sulphurwort or ... spurge.... Because of all their acrid properties, all these preparations would be more appropriate for the intervals of remission,
though even then a great abundance of drugs should be avoided. (81) ... according to the
Methodist sect, the period of exacerbation is not the time for irritant drugs ...'.

81   It is interesting that Caelius believes that there has been medical progress in this area
      since the days of Themison (first century BC): 1.50.

82   For an exhaustive discussion of Aretaeus' date see Oberhelman 1994, 941–59.

83   Also mentioned by Dioscorides 4.153 as having analgesic properties among others.

84   Much has been written about whether *peira* came to mean something like 'experiment' or
      'experimentation', and not just 'experience'. See van der Eijk 1997, 56, and the bibliography
      referred to there. On the limits of experimentation in ancient pharmacology Grmek and
      Gourevitch 1985 remains essential reading.

like the Methodists, he had in fact little real confidence in analgesic drugs; perhaps he wished to keep information to himself.[85]

Another medical writer who floats chronologically over a long period is usually known as the Anonymus Parisinus.[86] He refers generically to analgesic 'powers' (*dunameis*) that can counteract colic (XV.4), and he recommends among other things a draught of poppy juice and mandragora as one treatment among several for the victims of *phrenitis* (I.7), but in general his pain remedies would have been ineffectual, and they seem to take us back to the haphazard days prior to Celsus.

So we come finally to Galen and in particular to the approximately 2,700 pages of his four major works on pharmacology.[87] An important passage in *De methodo medendi* 12.1 (X.816–19K) discusses pain-killers (*anoduna*), warning against overdoses and recommending generous doses for the terminally ill. But what is crucial is that Galen knows and states quite straightforwardly which drugs can alleviate pain: they are 'those that are made out of poppy juice, *hyoscyamus* seeds, mandragora root, storax [Gk. *styrax*], and such materials' (X.816K).[88] A thorough statistical analysis must await another occasion, but if we take the passage in Galen's works that gathers together the greatest concentration of analgesic recipes, *De compositione medicamentorum secundum locos* 7.5 (XIII.85–97), all but two of the 27 recipes include at least one substance that is now recognized as having genuinely analgesic properties—if it is prepared and administered properly—, namely poppy/opium, henbane and mandragora. Poppy/opium is present in 93 per cent of the recipes, henbane in 56 per cent, mandragora in 14 per cent (and storax in 19 per cent).[89]

---

85   Yet, as Amber Porter has pointed out (Porter 2016, 301 n.52), Aretaeus 'exhibits a very pronounced emotional reaction to the pain and suffering of patients'; she instances *Causes of Acute Diseases* 1.6.

86   Re-edited by Garofalo 1997.

87   *De simplicium medicamentorum temperamentis et facultatibus* (XI.379–892K and XII.1–377K), *De compositione medicamentorum secundum locos* (XII.378–1007K and XIII.1–361K), *De compositione medicamentorum per genera* (XIII.362–1038K), *De antidotis* (XIV.1–209K). None of the contributors to the volume entitled *Galen on Pharmacology* (Debru 1997) took any interest in the efficacy of Galen's remedies.

88   Of storax Dioscorides 1.66 says that it 'has heating, emollient and digestive properties [Galen says the same in *De simp. med.* 8.17.42 = XII.131K] ... it is combined profitably with emollients and analgesics'. I have not found any evidence that anything derived from any of the species that might have been known to Dioscorides or Galen under that name had any real analgesic properties.

89   For Galen's knowledge of the plants in question see respectively *De simp.med.* 7.12.13–15 (XII.72–6K), 8.20.4 (XII.147–8K), 7.12.4 (XII.67K) and 8.18.42 (XII.131–2K).

The obvious conclusion is that Galen, and presumably the more informed among the other physicians of his time, had a much better knowledge of effective analgesics than the Hippocratics and a distinctly better knowledge than that of the physicians of the first century AD (though all this needs to be tempered by the fact that Galen avowedly took some of these recipes from predecessors of earlier generations). A rare—to this date, practically unique— scientific evaluation of an analgesic described by Galen, an ointment for athletes that he calls the 'grey (ointment) of the Olympic victor', seemed to add some confirmation: it would have worked (though it may well have been addictive too), because of its opium ingredient.[90] But I am authoritatively told that 'the conclusions [of the paper in question] are pharmacologically unwarranted, because one cannot create an equivalence between transcutaneous delivery of a water-soluble opioid drug' and 'what would be an appropriate intravenous or intramuscular dose',[91] which seems obviously correct.

The analgesic that most arouses Galen's enthusiasm, however, was known as *philôneion* after its inventor Philo of Tarsus, who boasted of its fabulous effects and described its composition, somewhat cryptically, in thirteen elegiac couplets, which Galen transcribes and explicates (*De compositione medicamentorum secundum locos* 9.4 = XIII.267–276K). The clearest reference to it in another source one finds in Galen's older contemporary Aelius Aristides (*Orations* 49.29),[92] who attributes positive effects to it. According to Galen, in any case, it was known to every doctor (*Ad Glauconem de medendi methodo* 2.8 = XI.114K).[93] The ingredients include henbane and opium; he also warns that it will have (*not* may have) harmful side-effects (ibid.). Galen regarded opium as the main anesthetizing ingredient (XIII.273K) and explained the role of other ingredients too. It would be interesting to know when Philo concocted this remedy; he is usually dated to the first century AD, but Galen's statement

---

90   Bartels et al. 2006. I owe this reference to Vivian Nutton. The authors conclude on the other hand that the other analgesically interesting ingredients, frankincense and *crocus sativus* L., would have had no detectable effects. The text in question is *De comp.med.sec.loc.* 4.8 = XII.753K.

91   Professor R. Holzman, pers. comm.

92   The *philôneion* may well correspond to the recipe of 'Philo' given differently by Celsus 6.6.3 (and Galen says that it came in various forms, XIII.273K), and it may also be the recipe of Philo mentioned by Aretaeus of Cappadocia, *Treatment of Chronic Diseases* 2.5.

93   It produced an astonishingly effective cure of a case of liver disease (testimony of Philo himself, accepted by Galen XIII.201K). In *De locis affectis* 2.5 (VIII.84K) it is the first effective analgesic that comes to mind, and the reader is assumed to be familiar with it (so too in *Comment. VI in Hipp. Epidemiorum lib. VI* 5 = XVIIB.331–2K).

that he worked 'in olden times' (XIII.267K) should probably take him back a little further.[94]

What all this meant for practical healthcare is of course a very large question. Did 'all doctors' really know of, and know how to prepare, the *philôneion*? Could their patients afford it? How many people will have taken their aches and pains to doctors in the first place? Certainly there were plenty of sceptics. Let's take Lucian's playlet about podagra (gout) as a parting example. Podagra, personified, boasts that all medicines, including henbane and poppy, are powerless against her (lines 145–71). Syrian doctors appear who have an ointment that they claim will conquer the pains of gout, but they are ignominiously defeated. In short, nothing works.

And people knew that the preferred analgesic substances could be dangerous. The elder Pliny believed that if you smell too much mandragora you will lose the power of speech and if you drink too much of it you will die (*NH* 25.150; but see below for its use in surgical practice). He also believed that drinking henbane could lead to insanity (*NH* 28.74).

But wait—what of placebo effects? Did ancient patients sometimes experience relief from pain because they believed that the mainly useless medicines they had taken were actually effective? The research of recent decades has shown that placebo effects in general are in some circumstances real (the bibliography is very long). Not surprisingly such effects vary from condition to condition, but there can be no doubt that some pains are genuinely affected.[95]

We have to ask, though, whether placebos only work in a world in which both doctors and generally available medicines have a fairly high success rate, and hence generate confidence. Greek doctors sometimes claimed that confidence in the skill of the physician could on occasion lead to a real improvement in the patient's condition,[96] and we should I think believe that, even though the confidence was largely misplaced.[97] From Hippocratic times onwards, the reputation of doctors was more equivocal than is often recognized,[98] but whether they were behaving like traditional shamans or more or less like modern physicians they undoubtedly laid claim to a great deal of prestige—most

94 I realize that it is unsatisfactory to stop this diachronic survey with Galen, and that it would be very much worth considering Oribasius, Aetius, Paul of Aegina and others from this point of view, but Galen must be the terminus for the time being.

95 For a summary see Wager and Fields 2013. The role of the patient's expectations is brought out by Benedetti et al. 2005.

96 [Hippocrates], *Praecepta* 6, where there are problems with the text. This work might be Hellenistic.

97 [Hippocrates], *Epid.* 6.5.7 advises a conscious deception to dispel earache.

98 Harris 2016, 9 n.39.

rulers listened to them, most Greek cities showed them a certain amount of respect.

And we make a crucial mistake if we conclude from their rate of failure that they could not claim to be competent. In early nineteenth-century America, when medicine was still heavily Galenic, physicians could not cure many illnesses, by the standards of 2018, but they could very often do what they, and their patients, believed was necessary. They 'believed that nearly all of the prevailing diseases were overstimulating, tipping the patient's vital balance to a dangerously overexcited condition'. So they bled, cupped and used mercury-containing drugs, and 'no one could doubt that the violent purging and debility that followed a large dose of calomel were the sequelae of giving the drug',[99] and so the physician's prestige survived, whatever happened in the end to the patient. An important factor in the effectiveness of placebo treatments is conditioning: has the patient's previous experience led him/her to expect improvement? Ancient patients will not have been like modern ones in this respect, but they may, like modern ones, have been influenced by suggestibility and the sheer desire for relief.[100]

The question then spills over into another: if people believed that Asklepios, or some other god, could bring them pain relief, did this belief sometimes trigger a measure of real relief? Hence an old and complex debate about the famous healing inscriptions from the temple of Asklepios at Epidaurus. It is hardly to be doubted that there were at least a few psychosomatic effects.

4   Anesthesia

So far, I have been discussing the pains that come with sickness or trauma. While the writers of the *Corpus Hippocraticum* write incessantly about pain, it is almost invariably the pain felt by the patient because of his/her illness or trauma, *not* the pain caused by amputation, cauterization or other medical procedures.[101] In the whole Hippocratic treatise *In the Surgery*, there is only one reference to the pain the patient may experience: the physician is recommended to operate quickly, 'easily' and 'painlessly' (*aponôs*) (*In the Surgery* 7)—though nothing at all is said about how to produce this result.[102]

---

99   Warner 1990, 194 and 195.

100   On the importance of these factors see Wager and Fields 2013, 369–70.

101   An exception: [Hippocrates], *Medicus* 5.

102   During the cauterization of hemorrhoids, [Hippocrates], *Haem.* 2, not surprisingly advises using assistants to hold the patient down. If he cries out, so much the better: it makes the target area more accessible.

Was it simply taken for granted that surgery was very very painful and that there was really nothing that could be done to alleviate the pain except getting it over with quickly? Actually there may have been a sort of conspiracy of silence.

In Hippocratic surgery there simply was no anesthesia, as far as we know[103]— you hold the patient down, or tie him/her up, and begin to cut. The earliest mention of anesthesia is an unspecific one in a fragment of the Academic philosopher Crantor, writing about 300 BC, but then we hear nothing until the first century AD. Crantor's view, preserved in slightly different versions by Cicero and by Plutarch,[104] was that if he were to undergo surgery, he would not want to be anesthetized because that would make him in some way less than human. This has been taken to mean that effective anesthesia was actually available,[105] but it should rather be taken as a theoretical view suggested by the famous passage in *Iliad* XI, discussed earlier, in which the Homeric heroes make use of fabulous pain-killing drugs.

What we encounter some 350 years after Crantor is an apparent contradiction. On the one hand Dioscorides tells us quite clearly that you can anesthetize a patient with white mandragora (4.75):[106]

Some boil down the roots with wine until reduced to one third, strain, and store, administering one *cyathos* [45.6 ml.] to insomniacs, to those in much pain, and to those undergoing surgery or cauterization whom they wish to anesthetize.... From the skin of the root they also make, without boiling, a wine: one must cast three *mnai* [1.3098 kg.] of root skin into one *metrêtês* [39.36 l.—this looks like industrial production!] and give three *cyathoi* of it to those about to undergo surgery or cautery ... for they become unaware of the pain because they sink into deep sleep.

There is another recipe too (4.75.7):

They say that it stupefies when as much as one *drachma* [3.411 gr.] is drunk [with wine] or when eaten in a lump of barley or in prepared food.... Physicians about to perform surgery or cautery use this one too.[107]

---

103 Cavenaile 2001, 29.
104 Cicero, *Tusc.Disp.* 3.6.12, Plutarch, *Consolatio ad Apollonium* 3 (*Moralia* 102D) (= Crantor fr. 3 Mette = Mette 1984, 17), pointed out by Cavenaile 2001, 30–1.
105 Cavenaile 2001, 31.
106 Translation and measures from Beck 2005.
107 But in 5.71 one *cyathos* drunk in wine is lethal. For an optimistic view of the usefulness of mandragora in surgery see Willer 2015, 283.

Pliny, just a little later, confirms that mandragora was used in his time as an anesthetic in surgery (*NH* 25.150),[108] and also tells us that it was not obtainable everywhere (sect.149).

Celsus, on the other hand, omits all mention of the matter from his book on surgery (*De Medicina* VII). As we saw earlier, he seems to reflect a degree of progress in the use of analgesics, but he clearly does not believe that any drug can diminish surgical pain. He recommends that the surgeon should 'be pitiful (*misericors*), so that he wishes to cure his patient,[109] but not so that he is moved by the patient's screams (*clamor*) to go too fast or to cut less than is needed. So he should do everything just as if he were completely unaffected by the other's cries of distress' (pr. 4).[110]

How to explain this apparent divergence in the evidence?[111] I doubt that it is the result of mere divergence in the practice of individual surgeons. A more likely explanation is that at the time Celsus wrote (*De Medicina* VII can best be dated under Tiberius) the use of anesthetic drugs in surgery was wholly marginal.[112] The fact that, half a century later, mandragora was available in some places but not others (Pliny) reflects changing practices. Dioscorides, probably writing in the time of Vespasian,[113] and Pliny (who dedicated his *Natural History* in 77) are credible witnesses to a new world of surgical practice. Dioscorides was the first extant writer to use the word *anaisthesia* to refer to insensibility during surgery (5.140).[114] Aelius Promotus of Alexandria, who probably wrote in the second century, has two recipes for surgical anesthetics that include in one case henbane and mandragora, in the other henbane, mandragora and poppy seeds (*Dynameron*, ch.61).[115]

---

108   It is a mistake to dismiss this statement of Pliny's as a 'tale' (Prioreschi 1998, III, 240); Pliny is ignorant about chemistry but not about social practices.

109   On pity in medical writers of the imperial age see Porter 2016, though she does not discuss this passage.

110   Elsewhere he describes how exactly to hold down a surgical patient for a certain operation (7.26).

111   Salazar 2000, 63, sees the problem but not the solution.

112   Celsus' date: Nutton 2004, 373 n.63.

113   Dioscorides' date: in 1 pr.4 he refers to Laecanius Bassus, probably but not certainly the consul of 64, as a living person of great distinction; the latter died not very long before 77 (Pliny, *NH* 26.5, 36.203).

114   He does so à propos of 'Memphitic stone', which 'ground up and smeared on areas about to be operated or cauterized ... is reported [note the distancing again] to produce harmless *anaisthesia*'. Similarly Pliny, *NH* 36.56. I have not encountered a convincing identification of this mineral.

115   This text was published by Daria Crismani in 2002. The rest of Promotus' advice about analgesics is mostly terrible, which tends to undermine the progressive narrative being suggested here, all the more since Alexandria should have been advanced if any city was.

But it was a dangerous world, and that is what we see in Galen. When the patient is suffering extreme pain, you can render him or her insensible with medicines based on opium, mandragora or henbane, but if you use too much (he does not say how much) the patient will die (*Comment. II in Hippocratis lib. VI Epidemiorum* 5, XVIIA.903–4K).[116] Galen's extant writings about surgery never explicitly allude to the use of anesthetizing drugs; that may be insignificant, or it may indicate that Galen himself thought them too dangerous, or it may indicate that most physicians of his time were of that opinion. I incline to the first of these three views. It is evident in any case that, in cities at least, quite numerous operations were performed—which leads to further questions.

5   Resistance and the Experience of Pain

Did ancient people have stronger powers of resistance to pain than people like us who live in an era of relatively powerful and reliable analgesics and anesthesia? What does a power of 'resistance' actually mean in this context? In the chapter of the *Nicomachean Ethics* mentioned earlier (7.7) Aristotle says that Philoctetes, in the play about him by Theodectes, could be forgiven for being 'defeated' by the pain resulting from his grievous wound, because he at least 'resisted' (the verb is *antiteinein*). Does that simply mean that, in that play, Philoctetes did not *complain*, or was some other form of self-mastery involved? Elsewhere—for example, in the Hippocratic *Affections* 13—being 'defeated' by illness probably means dying of it. But I suppose that what we normally mean by the ability to resist pain, as distinct from illness, is the ability to go on functioning in the face of it. Is that what the ancients, philosophers and others, meant when they encouraged each other to fight against pain? It seems in any case a reasonable guess, though nothing more, that classical Greeks and Romans generally surpassed us in this respect.

Some of them famously theorized resistance, the Stoics taking the boldest line: 'dolorem malum esse negant' (Cic. *Tusc.Disp.* 2.17)—'they deny that pain is a bad thing'.[117] It would take us too far afield to consider in detail the likely effects of such doctrines, best considered perhaps as rationalizations of a survival technique. Certainly the effects spread out far beyond those who professed loyalty to Stoic philosophers. Galen claims, believably, that he despises

---

116   Pp. 63–4 in the *CMG* edition by E. Wenkebach. See further the warnings in *Comp.Med.Loc.* 8.3 (XIII.157K) and *Comment. II in Hipp. Aph.* 17 (XVIIB.478K). None of these three passages refers explicitly to surgery.
117   But the Stoics never denied that pain was painful.

(*kataphronei*) bodily pain but draws the line at the notorious torture, the bull of Phalaris (*De indolentia* 71). He prays not to have to demonstrate his powers of physical endurance (*karteria*) (ibid. 74).

There is a separate question. Did the Greeks and Romans, because they were accustomed to pain from childhood onwards, suffer less in some sense than we soft-living moderns do? How could we possibly tell, given that no one can feel anyone else's pain? This question is not about whether people *behaved* stoically, but about what they actually felt. What makes this problem especially delicate is that there has traditionally been a tendency to claim that out-groups that are looked down upon 'suffer less'. Joanna Bourke showed in detail in her recent book *The Story of Pain*, how at various times, until quite recently, this tendency has led to callous treatment of black people and children, among other categories.[118]

A standard medical text of the recent past tells us that physical pain 'is not simply a function of the amount of bodily damage done. Rather, the amount and quality of pain we feel are also determined by our previous experiences and how well we remember them, by our ability to understand the cause of the pain and to grasp its consequences'.[119] It is a topos of contemporary thinking about pain that cognitive and affective processes influence the individual's perception of pain.[120] Many such claims are unproven, to say the least: Hippocrates and his patients did not 'understand the causes' of most of their illness pains, but that is hardly in itself a reason to think that their pains were either more intense or less intense than those of a modern person. It is generally and reasonably supposed that when the adrenalin of combat or of athletic competition is flowing, some of the combatants and competitors feel less pain than their injuries or exertions would lead one to expect. Galen, as we now know, was well aware of this puzzle: 'why inflammations are less painful to those who are occupied with something else, while those who are not find that their pain not only does not subside but actually increases' (*De motibus dubiis* 8.21).[121] He goes on to offer two possible explanations, and to describe the case of an acquaintance who noticed that he felt more pain from his injured leg while he was in bed at night than while he was distracted during daytime.

None of this tells us anything definite about whole populations. Yet it *may* be true that populations that are accustomed from childhood to pains that

---

118   Bourke 2014, 194–7, 275–6.
119   Melzack and Wall 1996, 15 (a self-quotation). These authors' classic *Textbook of Pain* has now been superseded by McMahon 2013.
120   Bourke 2014, 20, 229.
121   Ed. Nutton (2011). Nutton firmly established the authenticity of this work.

cannot be alleviated by any means not only behave more stoically, but actually suffer less.[122] The idea that populations that are used to pain suffer less in consequence was already known to Greek physicians.[123] Some ethnographic literature, on the surface at least, appears to support such a view. One may think, for example, of the inhabitants of Tierra del Fuego as they are described by Darwin in *The Voyage of the Beagle* (chapter 10), who lived in the most wretched conditions when he was there in the 1830s. But do we really have any basis for thinking that the Fuegians, freezing, undernourished, brutalized by each other and without medicines, felt their pains any less than any other humans?[124]

To return, however, to the classical Mediterranean, here is a suggestive story about surgical pain. C. Marius suffered from varicose veins, so Plutarch tells us (*Marius* 6), and he disliked this unsightliness (*amorphia*). He therefore subjected himself to surgery, without an anesthetic presumably, to have them removed, but after the doctor had done one leg Marius said that the cure was worse than the defect, and refused to have the other leg done. Plutarch cites his behaviour as an example of toughness, not because Marius chose to undergo the operation but because he refused to be tied down for it, and did not grimace or groan. Pliny (*NH* 11.252) cites Oppius (that is C. Oppius, the supporter and biographer of Marius' nephew Caesar) as his source for the claim that Marius was the only Roman ever to have undergone this operation while standing, which implies that others submitted to it but allowed themselves to be tied down (also that there was no effective anesthetic available, at least in Marius' time). Such a story naturally attached itself to a famous military man. What to conclude from this? Some Romans voluntarily and routinely underwent acutely painful surgery for merely cosmetic reasons.

As far as I know, Galen only once gives any indication of the volume of surgery that took place in his time. In *De simpl. med.* 10.2.3 (XII.256K), discussing the use of dove's blood, he says that he had seen it used in 'vast numbers' (*murious*) of cases of trepanation at Rome, which remains a most remarkable report even when we make allowance for exaggeration and for the ideas that led people to undergo this procedure.[125]

---

122   For people who have propounded views like this see Bourke 2014, 199–206. Cf. Green et al. 2003, 284: 'ethnic differences in laboratory pain response have been reported in multiple studies using different pain stimuli'.

123   See, for example, [Hippocrates], *Vet.Med.* 3.4, speaking of an earlier age of human history ('probably'). For a Hippocratic view of the difference between young men and old see [Hippocrates], *De morbis* 1.22 (quoted above, n.5).

124   It is beyond my competence to discuss the possible evolution of endogenous opioids.

125   On this phenomenon cf. Harris 2016, 8 n.32.

6　　Conclusions

From the earliest times Greeks imagined that pain-alleviating drugs existed, and by Hippocratic times some of them had an inkling of an idea, but no more than an inkling, that opium was useful for this purpose. By the time of Theophrastus some knew something about the analgesic properties of mandragora. By the first century AD, much more was known about the analgesic effects of opium, mandragora and henbane; this was probably the result of widespread trial and error, though it is also possible that individuals such as Apollonius the follower of Herophilus made large contributions. By the time of Galen the best physicians, though they still often responded to pain with useless or harmful treatment, knew well that opium was effective and were aware of the analgesic properties of mandragora and henbane. As far as anesthesia is concerned, it was unknown until roughly the period 40 to 60 AD; but even after that its use was limited, even among those who could afford the substances in question, by a well-justified fear of a lethal overdose. The doctor's dose might kill not only the pain but also the patient.

CHAPTER 5

Pleasure and the *Medicus* in Roman Literature

Caroline Wazer

In a short biography of the physician Asclepiades of Bithynia, the purported founder of the Methodist medical sect or *hairesis*, Pliny the Elder reports the following:

> He used to attract men's minds by the empty artifice of promising the sick, now wine, which he administered as opportunity occurred, while now he would prescribe cold water ... He devised also other pleasures [*blandimenta*], such as suspended beds, so that by rocking them he could either relieve diseases or induce sleep; again, he organized a system of hydropathy, which appeals to man's greedy love of baths, and many other things pleasant and delightful to speak of [*alia multa dictu grata atque iucunda*] ...[1]

Celsus, writing several decades before Pliny, also connects the physician with pleasure. According to him, Asclepiades used to say that the duty of a physician was 'ut tuto, ut celeriter, ut iucunde curet': to treat the patient as safely, swiftly, and pleasantly as possible.[2]

Asclepiades seems to have made his name in the early first century BCE.[3] Originally a struggling sophist, he decided to begin a career in medicine despite having no training in the field. According to Pliny, Asclepiades's methods of treatment became extremely popular due to the pleasant cures described above—rocking beds, baths, and wine, which contrasted sharply with traditional Hippocratic medicine:

> The success of Asclepiades owed much to the many distressing and crude [*anxia et rudia*] features of ancient medical treatment ... then for the first time were used hot-air baths, heated from below, treatment of infinite pleasure. Besides this he did away with the agonizing treatment employed in certain diseases; for example in quinsy, which physicians

---

1   Pliny, *Historia Naturalis* XXVI.8.14–15. Trans. W. H. Jones.
2   Celsus, *De medicina* III.4.1 Trans. W. G. Spencer.
3   On the dating of Asclepiades' arrival at Rome and death, see Nutton 2013, 167.

DOI:10.1163/9789004379503_006

used to treat by thrusting an instrument down the throat. He rightly condemned emetics also, which were at that time employed unduly often.
He disapproved also of administering draughts that are injurious to the
stomach, a criticism which is to a great extent true.[4]

As is the case for medical practitioners of all types, Pliny seems to have held
a complex and sometimes self-contradictory opinion of Asclepiades and his
followers, including the celebrated Antonius Musa, who cured Augustus in
23 BCE by adjusting his bath regimen and diet.[5] Their Greek origins and claims
to authority on the subject of health were repugnant to the Roman encyclo-
pedist, but he approved of their rejection of the brutal aspects of traditional
Hippocratic medicine. Pliny also relied heavily on the (now lost) Methodist
writers Dionysius and Themison in his medical books, citing their remedies,
mostly drug recipes, without qualification.

Pliny's conception of the Methodists as pleasure-givers was not universal.
While Celsus, writing earlier in the first century CE, acknowledges the existence of their reputation for pleasurable cures, he notes that this reputation
did not reflect the truth of Methodist practice:

> Asclepiades ... did not clyster the bowel with such frequency but still he
> generally did this in every disease; but the actual fever he professed to use
> as a remedy against itself: for he deemed that the patient's forces ought
> to be reduced by daylight, by keeping awake, by extreme thirst, so that
> during the first days he would not allow even the mouth to be swilled
> out. Therefore those are quite wrong who believe that his regimen was a
> pleasant one in all respects [*Quo magis falluntur, qui per omnia iucundam
> eius disciplinam esse concipiunt*]; for in the later days he allowed even
> luxuries to his patient, but in the first days of the fever he played the part
> of torturer.[6]

Rather than by a difference in treatment, Celsus explains, the Methodists were
distinguished by their different understanding of the causes of health and disease. Methodists believed in atomism, as Caelius Aurelianus' fifth-century CE
adaptations of the writings of Soranus make clear. Health and disease were
therefore determined by the ability of atoms to move about properly within

---

4 Pliny, *HN* XXVI.16–17 (translation adapted from that of W. H. Jones).
5 On Antonius Musa: Pliny, *HN* XIX.38, XXV.38; Suetonius, *Divine Augustus* 58, 79; Cassius Dio,
   Roman History LIII.30.3–6.
6 Celsus, *De medicina* III.4.2–3. Trans. W. H. Jones.

the human body. Whereas physicians of the Hippocratic schools had to produce a diagnosis based on painstaking study of the composition of each individual patient's humors before treatment could start, Methodists believed that excessive tightness or looseness produced reliable and recognizable symptoms in all patients, and that any patients presenting the same symptoms could be treated in the same way.

As Celsus points out, the medical theory of the Methodists did not preclude them from using what Pliny calls 'distressing and crude' treatments when they thought it appropriate. What little we have of the Methodists' writings indeed suggests that treatments used by Methodist doctors were not always or even often pleasurable for the patient. In the only surviving complete book written by a known Methodist, Soranus' *Gynecology*, treatments such as bleeding and purgatives were occasionally recommended.[7] It is curious, then, that Pliny emphasizes the pleasurable aspects of Methodist medicine despite Celsus' refutation of that belief decades earlier, and the fact that practicing Methodist physicians like Soranus continued to use 'distressing and crude' treatments during and after Pliny's own lifetime.

Was Pliny's adherence to the seemingly spurious association of Methodism with pleasure unusual, or might it have accurately reflected the popular perception of these physicians? In a recent paper, David Leith has argued that the medical 'sects' were not limited to theoretical and elite medicine, but instead that many physicians treating the general public in the Roman world proudly advertised their affiliation with a *hairesis*, including the Methodist one.[8] Would a Methodist physician have been associated with pleasure to a greater degree than his non-Methodist competitors? This paper aims to assess the extent to which Pliny's accusations against the Methodist sect—that its members were quacks who attracted patients with false promises of pleasurable healing—are represented in non-medical literature of roughly the same time period covered by Pliny's treatment of the Methodist school, the last century BCE and the first century CE.

1   Medical Pleasure in Roman Literature

The *medicus* was a fairly common character in Roman literature. In novels of the second through fifth centuries, as Amundsen has noted, physicians

---

7   E.g., Soranus, *Gynecology* III.11, III.38, and III.43.
8   Leith 2016. See also Nutton 2013, 190–1, who offers a theory as to the popularity Methodism may have had among urban non-elites.

performed three notable roles: first, they diagnosed lovesickness; second, they provided (or refused to provide) poison to a would-be murderer; and third, they resuscitated seemingly dead people.[9] Stock characterizations of physicians appeared in other genres of Roman writing as well. In political histories, physicians could be a force for good or for ill: they could save an important man's life, as Suetonius and Cassius Dio describe Antonius Musa curing Augustus in 23 BCE,[10] or they could become involved in court intrigues up to and including murder by poison, as in Tacitus' implication of the imperial physician Xenophon in the death of Claudius.[11]

A common trope that crossed genres was that of the physician as money-grubbing quack, a characterization that appears in texts as diverse as Pliny's *Natural History*, Phaedrus's *Fables*, and Plautus's *Menaechmi*.[12] Nearly as common and even more damning of the profession was the characterization of the *medicus* as a thoughtless killer: an executioner (*carnifex*), undertaker (*vispillo*), or gladiator (*oplomachus*).[13]

By modern standards, these stereotypes were largely justified. We can infer from the corpus of ancient medical literature that many common treatments, including but not limited to cauterization and bleeding, would have caused significant pain in the patient beyond any discomfort resulting from their disease. For an example, in the following passage the career invalid Aelius Aristides describes the pain caused by his physicians in one of the many treatments he underwent in order to cure his mysterious and lengthy ailment:

> And for that the physicians began cutting me, starting from the chest and going in order all the way down to the bladder. And when the cupping instruments were applied, my breathing was completely stopped, and a pain, numbing and impossible to bear, passed through me and everything was smeared with blood, and I was excessively purged.[14]

---

9   Amundsen 1974.
10   Suetonius, *Augustus* 59, Cassius Dio, *History* 53.30.
11   Tacitus, *Annales* 12.67.
12   Pliny, *HN* XXIX.22; Phaedrus, *Fables* I.14; Plautus, *Menaechmi*, V.3–5. See also Baumbach 1983.
13   Pliny, *HN* XXIX.12: the physician Archagathus earns the epithet 'carnifex'. Martial in *Epigrams* I.30: 'Chirurgus fuerat, nunc est vispillo Diaulus'; I.47: 'Nuper erat medicus, nunc est vispillo Diaulus', and VIII.74: 'Oplomachus nunc es, fueras opthalmicus ante'.
14   Aelius Aristides, *Or.* 48.63 K. (trans. Israelowich 2012, 109).

Other texts play the stereotype of physicians' lack of concern for their patients' comfort for laughs, such as one of several jokes about doctors attributed to Hierocles and Philagrius:

> A certain person coming to a peevish physician said, 'Master, I am not able to recline, nor to stand, nor to sit down.' And the physician replied, 'There is nothing left for you but to be hung up'.[15]

In a small number of texts from the high Roman Empire, however, certain physicians are associated not with pain, but with pleasure.

The poet Martial mocks physicians in about a dozen of his epigrams. In the majority of cases, the poet employs the common tropes of physician as quack, charlatan, or executioner.[16] In two epigrams, however, Martial engages with the idea of medical pleasure in distinct and noteworthy ways. In the first, Martial plays with ideas of the role of sexual pleasure in women's health.

> Leda told her aged husband that she was hysterical,
> and regrets that she needs to be fucked;
> yet with tears and groans she says her health is not worth the sacrifice,
> and declares she would rather choose to die.
> Her husband bids her live, and not desert the bloom of her years,
> and he permits to be done what he cannot do himself.
> Immediately male doctors come in, and female doctors depart,
> and her feet are hoisted. Oh, what burdensome treatment![17]

In this case, the cure for Leda's hysteria is literal sexual pleasure, something that a husband would normally be expected to provide. The joke, presumably, is that Leda's infidelity is excusable on account of it being a cure for a medical issue and performed by professional physicians. Because Leda's desire is framed as a disease, her husband actually encourages her to stray.

The involvement of *medici* gives Leda's infidelity a veneer of respectability that relies on ideas about the role of sexual pleasure in women's health

---

15   *Philogelos* 183: Δυσκόλῳ ἰατρῷ προσελθών τις εἶπε· Σοφιστά, ἀνακεῖσθαι οὐ δύναμαι οὔτε ἑστάναι, ἀλλ' οὐδὲ καθῆσθαι. καὶ ὁ ἰατρὸς εἶπεν· Οὐδέν σοι λείπει ἢ κρεμασθῆναι (trans. Bubb). Other jokes in the collection with punchlines hinging on physician stereotypes include numbers 139 (moneygrubbing), 142 (thievery), 175a (moneygrubbing), and 176 (incompetence).

16   Incompetence: I.30, I.47, V.9, VI.53, VIII.74, X.77, XI.28. Greed and immorality: VI.31, VIII.9, IX.96, XI.60, XI.74. On doctors in Martial more generally, see Henriksén 2012, 364.

17   Martial, *Ep.* XI.71 (translation adapted from that of W. C. Ker).

that are genuinely represented in medical theory. One of the longest more-or-less contemporary expositions of this concept comes from Soranus, who explains arguments for and against female celibacy. While he notes that some physicians believe that abstinence is harmful for women's health because it interferes with menstruation and causes a buildup of undesirable material in the woman's body, Soranus himself is convinced that 'permanent virginity is healthful' not just for women but 'in males and females alike'.[18] Soranus, it is worth repeating, was a Methodist, a follower of the doctrine that Pliny so strongly believed relied on the promise of pleasure to attract patients.

In the second epigram of Martial that we will consider, a *medicus* is presented as the giver of pleasure that is gustatory, not sexual.

> To relieve your throat, Parthenopaeus,
> which is incessantly inflamed by a severe cough,
> your doctor prescribes honey, and nuts, and sweet cakes,
> and everything that is given to children to prevent them from being unruly.
> But you do not give over coughing all day long.
> A cough is not your malady, Parthenopaeus; it is gluttony.[19]

It seems reasonable to assume that physicians were sometimes willing to indulge their wealthy patients in such a fashion, but physicians did not have a universal reputation for prescribing sweets. In the *Satyricon*, while arguing that physicians have one of the most unenviable professions, Petronius' Trimalchio notes his distaste for the foods recommended by his own doctor.

> The doctor's [profession is the hardest] because he knows what poor men have in their insides, and when a fever will come—though I especially detest them because they so often order me to live on duck.[20]

As is made clear by the difference between the diets prescribed by the physicians of Parthenopaeus and Trimalchio, the effect of pleasurable food on health was a contentious matter in ancient medicine. A dialogue in one of Plutarch's *Quaestiones Convivales* centers on this debate: at a dinner party thrown by the

---

18   Soranus, *Gynecology* 1.7.32.
19   Martial, *Ep.* XI.86, trans. Bohn.
20   Petronius, *Satyricon* 56: 'medicus, qui scit quid homunciones intra praecordia sua habeant et quando febris veniat, etiam si illos odi pessime, quod mihi iubent saepe anatinam parari' (translation adapted from that of M. Heseltine).

physician Philo, a group of guests refuses to partake of the luxurious meal on the grounds that plain, tasteless foods are easier to digest and therefore healthier according to mainstream medical wisdom. Their leader Philinus stops short of calling Philo the physician a hypocrite for feeding his guests food that will make them unhealthy, but only just. In response to Philinus' claim that Socrates condemned eating for pleasure, another guest defends Philo's luxurious spread:

> What kind of pain, what deprivation, what sort of poisonous [sc. drug] can solve a disease as easily and simply as a bath taken on the nick of time, or wine administered when the patients needed it? Food too, if taken with pleasure, can solve all the complaints and restore nature to its proper course, as when good weather and calm waters return. But the remedies which work through pain accomplish little with great labours, they enforce themselves viciously and do violence to nature. Hence, Philinus should not condemn us if we don't run away from pleasure both sails on: we will try instead to unite the pleasant and [the] healthy more harmoniously than some philosophers [unite] the pleasant and the noble.[21]

In other words, pleasures reinforce health by maintaining balance in the body. Not partaking in these restorative pleasures, on the other hand, makes the body more vulnerable to disease and, importantly, to the pain and discomfort caused by physicians.

What of the Methodists? Tecusan tentatively identifies the host of the dinner party as a Methodist of the same name mentioned in a fragment of Galen, and notes that the themes and assertions of the dinner-party passage are 'consistently Methodist'.[22] There is no hard evidence of this connection, however, and the term 'Methodist' does not appear anywhere in Plutarch's writing, or in any of the non-medical texts discussed here.

Despite the above-mentioned evidence for broad popular awareness of medical sects, physicians appear largely undifferentiated by doctrine in non-medical Roman literature. The most obvious reference to the impact of the Methodist sect in Latin poetry must be Horace's *Epistle* 1.15. Published around 20 BCE, just a few years after Antonius Musa's cure of Augustus brought fame to the Methodist school, the poem includes a parenthetical aside that calls out Augustus' Methodist physician by name.

---

21   Plutarch, *Quaestiones Convivales* 4.1, 662A–D (Tecusan 2004 fr. 268, trans. Tecusan).
22   Tecusan 2004, 52.

> ... Since I'm
> Prescribed cold baths in winter, Antonius Musa
> makes visiting Baiae pointless, yet ensures I'm
> frowned on there. Of course the town sighs. Its myrtles
> are being abandoned, its sulphur baths scorned that
> rid the sinews of lingering disorders, indignant
> at patients who dare to subject head and stomach
> to Clusium's springs, or make for Gabii's cold fields.[23]

Horace humorously laments that the warm waters of Baiae had been replaced among the fashionably health-conscious with cold springs, in imitation of the cold baths to which Augustus credited his dramatic cure. Musa's cold-water treatment seems to have sparked a true medical fad in Italy; Wallace-Hadrill goes so far as to credit it as the impetus for momentous (and permanent) changes in bath architecture.[24] From Horace's perspective, Musa's success seems to have made popular health treatments *less* pleasurable, and not only because of the switch from hot to cold water. In addition to its famous hot springs, Baiae also had a reputation for being a place of relaxed morals and sexual promiscuity.[25] Around 29 BCE, six years before Musa's cure of Augustus, the elegiac poet Propertius had begged his beloved Cynthia to return home from the notorious resort town:

> Just leave corrupt Baiae as soon as possible.
> Those shores will bring divorce to many,
> shores unfriendly to chaste girls.
> Go to hell, waters of Baiae, you crime against love![26]

By endorsing cold baths over hot, Musa made obsolete the socially acceptable excuse for visiting Baiae: that physicians believed it beneficial for physical health.[27] To make things worse, the two towns with cold springs mentioned

---

23 Horace, *Ep.* 1.15.2–10 (trans. A. S. Kline).

24 Wallace-Hadrill 2008, 183: 'The precipitous collapse in fashion of the *laconicum* (and the conversion of the Stabian Baths) were surely the direct result of Musa's success'.

25 On the medicinal benefits of the Baiae springs, see Celsus, *De medicina* II.17.1 and Pliny the Elder, *HN* XXXI.4–5. The massive popularity of Baiae among health-seekers earlier in the first century BCE may itself have been the result of Methodist influence, namely Asclepiades' advocacy of hot baths as described by Pliny at *HN* XXVI.15.

26 Propertius, *Elegies* I.11 27–30, trans. V. Katz.

27 Horace may have been gratified to know that the seedier aspects of Baiae survived the vagaries of popular health wisdom: around 65 CE, Seneca complained about the immorality of the seaside town in *Epistulae morales ad Lucilium* LI.

by Horace, Clusium and Gabii, were far less glamorous than Baiae. Gabii in particular was considered a depressing backwater in the Augustan era—in another Epistle, Horace himself uses it as an example of an extremely desolate spot.[28] As with the marital infidelity of Martial's Leda, medical theory had provided cover for sexual licentiousness at Baiae, until popular ideas about the health benefits of springs were changed, ironically enough, by one of the most famous members of the very sect accused by Pliny the Elder of peddling phony but pleasurable cures.

2   Conclusion

At least insofar as we can glean from the small number of sources discussed here, Roman popular ideas about the relationship between physicians and pleasure were not as simple as what Pliny describes. Pleasure certainly could play a role in Methodist cures, such as the hot baths prescribed by Asclepiades, but Musa's celebrated adoption of the opposite extreme suggests that pleasure was not the defining feature of any Methodist treatment. Soranus' belief that sexual intercourse is unhealthy for both sexes sits at odds with the medical theory underpinning Martial's raunchy joke about Leda. That epigram, in turn, is evidence of significant currency of the theory that sexual pleasure *is* necessary for health among laypeople and, presumably, some substantial subset of physicians.

Medical pleasure in Roman literature, then, seems to have had little if any relationship to the reputations of different medical sects. Far more visible are ideas both positive and negative about the authority of physicians and the intimacy of their privileged positions with regard to the patient's body. In the majority of the above cases, an active role is taken by a canny patient, who exploits the authority of the doctor to provide cover for behavior that might otherwise seem self-indulgent or even immoral. Martial's Leda and Parthenopaeus fall into this category, while Horace is annoyed by the fact that he could no longer take advantage of his doctor's advice in order to enjoy an annual seaside vacation guilt-free.

Pliny's criticism of Asclepiades' reputation for pleasure therefore finds little outside corroboration. His decision to emphasize pleasure in his discussion of the Methodists is better understood not in the context of genuine popular ideas about physicians and pleasure, but rather as an essential part of the argument against professional medicine to which he returns several times over the

---

28   Horace, *Ep.* 1.11.7–8: 'Gabiis desertior atque Fidenis vicus …'.

course of the *Natural History*. Infused with rhetoric about the degeneracy of the Greek race, Pliny's invective focuses on the danger to the collective health of Rome posed by the rise of foreign doctors in Italy and a perceived decline of traditional Latin folk medicine. His explanation for the initial popularity of Methodist medicine foregrounds its contrast with the crude and painful methods of other, equally Greek, physicians. In other words, Pliny is warning his compatriots that Greek physicians are not to be trusted regardless of whether they inflict pain or give pleasure. The texts discussed above are evidence of the futility of Pliny's efforts: Romans of the early Empire were eager to know what professional physicians thought of many aspects of everyday life, and especially potentially pleasurable activities.

CHAPTER 6

What is Hedonism?[1]

Katja Maria Vogt

1 Introduction

When philosophers use the term hedonism, they usually imply the pursuit of
something lowly, as if the best a human being can aim for was like the life
of grazing cattle.[2] And yet there are philosophers who endorse hedonism.
To them, it seems that hedonists must not be destined for a lowly life at all.
Instead, they argue for a life of reasoning and friendship.[3] Given these discrep-
ancies, what then is hedonism?[4] This question bears, I propose, not only on the
reconstruction of ancient views that self-identify as hedonist. More generally,
it bears on how we understand ancient ethics. Compared to modern moral
philosophy, the ancients are greatly—some may say, excessively—interested
in pleasure and pain. As will emerge, I think that ancient ethics benefitted
from the presence of hedonism as a contender. In response to hedonism, Plato
and Aristotle seem to get something right: ethics needs to get clear about the
role of pleasure and pain in human psychology, the nature of pleasure and
pain, and its value.

The first premise of hedonism, I propose, is that pleasure is the only good
that does not derive its value from another good (section 2). This premise is
justified, in ways that explicitly reject the charge of a naturalistic fallacy, by an
appeal to nature: because pleasure is by nature pursued, it should be pursued

1　I am grateful to William Harris for inviting me to present at the conference that lead up
to this publication, and to all participants for interesting comments and discussions. Giulia
Bonasio, Sam McVane, and Isabel Kaeslin provided helpful feedback on a draft. Jens Haas
offered invaluable feedback, both for the version that I presented at the conference and for
the paper.
2　That hedonism is often understood as advocating a life like that of grazing cattle is Plato's
concluding remark in the *Philebus*. 'And did not pleasure turn out to receive fifth position,
according to the verdict we reached in our discussion?—Apparently.—But not first place,
even if all the cattle and horses and the rest of the animals gave testimony by following pleasure.' (Plato, *Philebus* 67a11–b2) Cf. *NE* 1095b16–23.
3　Epicurus says one should care more who one is eating and drinking with than what one eats
and drinks. To 'feed' without a friend is the life of a lion and a wolf. (Seneca, *Letters* 19.10).
4　On the pleasures of reasoning as well as the role of reasoning in the pursuit of pleasure
cf. Warren 2014.

(section 3). Sophisticated hedonism, as I call the kind of theory formulated by Epicurus, develops ideas that Plato employs (section 4). Critics of hedonism differ in how they respond to hedonism's first premise. Anti-hedonists, as I use this notion, endorse its opposite, namely that pleasure is bad. Non-hedonists, as I call them, reject hedonism while admitting that there are good pleasures (section 5). The well-known objection against hedonism, that there are *good and bad* pleasures, thus cannot count as anti-hedonist; neither hedonism nor anti-hedonism can account for both good and bad pleasures (section 6). The hardest problem for hedonism, on my account, lies elsewhere: in the variety of pleasure. Pleasures may differ so deeply that there is no unified notion of pleasure. Without such a notion, hedonism does not get off the ground (section 7).[5]

My distinction between hedonism, non-hedonism, and anti-hedonism addresses an inauspicious tendency in the literature. Often, the views of Plato and Aristotle are labeled as anti-hedonist, while on my account they are non-hedonist.[6] Terminology aside, this matters because there is room for markedly more negative views of pleasure than Plato and Aristotle hold, views that diverge sufficiently from their proposals to merit a different designation. It is an ordinary intuition, today and in antiquity, that wanting one's life to be pleasurable is not the same as pursuing pleasure for its own sake.[7] Ethics should accommodate this distinction, and refrain from classifying too many views as anti-hedonist. More than that, non-hedonism may well provide a model for ethical theorizing. Informed by psychology, it proposes norms that are distinctively norms for beings with our kind of mental life.

2   Only Pleasure is Non-derivatively Good

Ancient discussions of hedonism tend to start with one of the following exchanges, or a mix thereof:[8]

---

5   An influential account of hedonism today is offered in Feldman 1997 and Feldman 2004.

6   Recent contributions that ascribe anti-hedonism to Plato are Figal 2008; Evans 2008; Harte 2008; Shaw 2015. Moss emphasizes the ways in which Aristotle characterizes pleasure as deceptive and misleading (2012). Rapp describes Aristotle's positive assessment of pleasure in *NE* VII.13, 1153b8–15 as 'shocking' (2009); on my reading, it is not.

7   Thucydides employs his distinction, seemingly picking up on fifth century discussions. In his terms, it is one thing to want to live in a way that is accompanied by pleasure, καθ'ἡδονήν (History of Peloponnesian War, II.37.2) and another thing to live for the sake of pleasure, διὰ ἡδονήν (I.120.4). Cf. de Romilly 1966. I owe this reference to Giulia Bonasio.

8   *Philebus* 11a–12a as well as *Nicomachean Ethics* (*NE*), Book I treat these questions as near-equivalent.

'What is the best life?'—'The life of pleasure.'
'What is the good?'—'Pleasure.'

Ancient hedonists claim that 'the life of pleasure is good' and/or 'pleasure is the good.' For present purposes, the differences between these claims can be set aside. The upshot, in both cases, is that pleasure is the only non-derivative good. Whatever else may be good is made good via its relation to pleasure, deriving its goodness from the goodness of pleasure. For example, hedonism may admit that friendship is good, or that knowledge is good.[9] But it accounts for this goodness via the more fundamental goodness of pleasure: friendship, knowledge, etc., are good insofar as they are conducive to pleasure or insofar as they are pleasurable. Let's put the first premise of hedonism as follows:

NON-DERIVATIVE GOOD: Pleasure is the only non-derivative good.[10]

This claim identifies pleasure and goodness: pleasure and the non-derivatively good are one and the same.[11] This identification bears on one of the deepest questions in ancient ethics, namely whether there are several kinds of positive valence. Here is what the Socrates of Plato's *Philebus* grants in conversation with Protarchus, his interlocutor who defends hedonism: 'what takes pleasure, whether it is rightly pleased or not, can obviously never be deprived of really taking pleasure.' (37b2–3)[12] Socrates seems to ascribe positive valence to pleasure; he seems to admit that whoever is pleased is experiencing this positively. On this view, what is positive about all pleasures is that they are pleasant. But being pleasant and thereby of positive value does *not* make them good. This argument presupposes that there are genuinely different kinds of value.[13] The

---

9   Cf. Evans 2004.

10   According to Feldman, hedonism is the claim that pleasure is intrinsically good (1997). I refrain from this formulation because (i) it is controversial whether there is a shared sense of intrinsicality between contemporary and ancient discussions and (ii) Feldman's formulation is compatible with there being several intrinsic goods.

11   Cf. Plato's *Protagoras*, where Protagoras formulates the hedonist claim that pleasure and the good are the same (τὸ αὐτὸ ἡδύ τε καὶ ἀγαθόν, 351e5–6). Cf. Moss 2014.

12   My translations from the *Philebus* are adaptations, with changes, of Frede 1993, included in Cooper 1997. Cf. also Hackforth 1945 and Frede 1997.

13   Plato's *Gorgias* contains two arguments to the effect that pleasure and pain cannot be good and bad because good and bad are opposites; qua opposites they cannot be compresent in the same thing; but in thirst and the relief of thirst there is both pleasure and pain; hence pleasure and pain on the one hand and the good and the bad on the other hand differ (495e–497d).

three candidates that ancient thinkers consider are goodness, beauty (*kalon*), and pleasure.[14] These may be distinct values, each with its own account, such that beauty and pleasure are not kinds of goodness, but values other than goodness. Hedonism does not admit any such distinction. Pleasure and the good are identified, rather than being two kinds of value.

3   Psychological Hedonism and Normative Hedonism

What lines of justification does hedonism offer for NON-DERIVATIVE GOOD? Consider the premises NATURE and NORM:

> NATURE: Pleasure is pursued as the good in an uncorrupted, natural condition.
>
> NORM: Pleasure should be pursued.

It is a fact about human psychology, or so it is argued, that we pursue pleasure. This can be observed when we look at human beings who are as of yet uncorrupted by acculturation, and it can also be observed in the behavior of animals.[15] Here is how Epicurus, in Cicero's report, puts this:

> We are investigating what is the final and ultimate good [...] Epicurus situates this in pleasure, which he wants to be the greatest good with pain as the greatest bad. His doctrine begins in this way: as soon as every animal is born, it seeks pleasure and rejoices in it as the greatest good, while it rejects pain as the greatest bad and, as far as possible, avoids it; and it does this when it is not yet corrupted, on the innocent and sound judgment of nature itself.
>
> CICERO, *De finibus* 1.29–30[16]

---

14   Cf. the opening lines of the *Eudemian Ethics*, where Aristotle says that the very same thing, namely *eudaimonia*, has all three properties in the superlative: it is best, most beautiful, and most pleasant (1214a1–8). *Kalon* has ethical and aesthetic dimensions; the term can also be translated as admirable, noble, or fine. For present purposes, I adhere to the traditional translation, 'beautiful,' in a quasi-technical sense: as the designated translation of *kalon*. Cf. Konstan 2014a for a different perspective.

15   Cf. *Philebus* 67a11–b2, where Socrates presupposes that hedonists refer to cattle, horses, and so on, as providing *testimony* on what is good.

16   Long and Sedley 1987 [= LS], fragment LS 21A, translation LS with minor changes.

NORM is inferred from NATURE. Because pleasure is pursued as good in uncorrupted natural states, pleasure actually is good. In other words, 'should' is inferred from 'is': one *should* pursue that which is pursued, and no justification is needed other than that it *is* pursued. This inference seems suspicious, to the extent that it is often considered a naturalistic fallacy. Hedonism is a kind of naturalism: it aims to infer from natural features of human motivation and behavior how we should act, and what really is good. Here is Epicurus's defense of the inference:

> Hence he says there is no need to prove or discuss why pleasure should be pursued (*expetenda*) and pain avoided (*fugiendus*). He thinks these matters are sensed (*sentiri*) just like the heat of fire, the whiteness of snow and the sweetness of honey, none of which needs confirmation by elaborate arguments; it is enough to remind us of them. For there is a difference between an argument and conclusion reached by reasoning and a simple observation and reminder. The former discloses certain hidden and as it were obscure matters, the latter judges what is directly accessible and evident. Since man has nothing left if sensations are removed from him, it must be the case that nature itself judges what is in accordance with or contrary to nature. What does it perceive or what does it judge except pleasure and pain as a basis for its pursuit or avoidance of everything?
>
> CICERO, *De finibus* 1.30[17]

For Epicurus, the goodness of pleasure is perceived and thereby evident. Sense-perceptions as well as pleasure/pain are, according to his larger philosophical framework, criteria of truth.[18] Whatever theory one is putting forward about the good (or about anything), it must agree with these criteria. If pleasure is perceived to be the good, then a theory which disputes this fails to meet basic methodological standards.

Though ancient hedonists embrace both NATURE and NORM, these premises can be taken to express two kinds of hedonism, sometimes called psychological (NATURE) and normative (NORM).

---

17 The text continues in ways that attest to discussions about precisely this line of argument. Epicurus mentions that others in his school hold slightly different views, only to reiterate afterwards that it is unnecessary and misguided to do so.

18 Epicurus, *Letter to Menoeceus* 129.3–4 speaks of the pathos of pleasure as the yardstick by which we judge every good thing (ὡς κανόνι τῷ πάθει πᾶν ἀγαθὸν κρίνοντες) (LS 21B); cf. DL 10.31 = LS 17A.

Psychological hedonism [PH]: All human motivation is for pleasure.
Normative hedonism [NH]: Pleasure should be pursued.

To see how PH amounts to a kind of hedonism, compare it with a weaker claim, one that can be ascribed to Plato and Aristotle: all motivations involve pleasure/pain. Aristotle thinks that pleasure and pain accompany all distinctively human activity. Say, you get up in the morning tired, which you find unpleasant. You have a cup of coffee and like that it wakes you up. You start reading the news and find much of it dreadful. But there's a message from a friend, with a photo that makes you smile. And so on. In these ways, pleasure and pain accompany all activity and thereby affect motivation: one aims to hold on to pleasure, prolonging activities that provide it (say, having another cup of coffee, but not a third one, for then it would no longer come with the pleasurable sense of waking up), and avoiding activities that are painful (say, calling back your bank whose customer service is hit and miss).

On this (broadly speaking) Aristotelian view, things other than pleasure can motivate the actions that are accompanied by pleasure and pain. Say, an agent may be motivated to read the news because she aims to know what is going on. This desire for knowledge and its role in a good life are the primary motivations to refer to in an analysis of her action. That the action is accompanied by pleasure/pain and that this accompaniment has a motivational role does not exhaust the analysis and is not the most basic component of it. PH makes a more radical proposal. Whatever is pursued as good is pursued on account of its relation to pleasure. When it seems that people pursue knowledge or honor or beauty or some other value, what they really pursue is pleasure. This is not by itself a normative position—it does not put forward any claims on what one should pursue or on what is good. It can nevertheless count as a kind of hedonism. If it is true that nothing other than pleasure motivates human beings, then no normative theory that recommends otherwise is plausible. There is no evidence that any ancient hedonist held PH without also holding NH. But it is worthwhile to consider PH by itself, because Plato and Aristotle take PH a lot more seriously than NH: it is conceivable that human psychology simply is such that we are motivated, pervasively, by pleasure. If this is conceivable, and if one aims to defend a non-hedonist normative ethics, a close look at the workings of pleasure in human motivation is needed.

NH on its own (that is, without PH), is also a conceivable position. One might think that people are confused and misguided when they care about honor or beauty or other values as non-derivatively good. Really, they should aim at pleasure as the only non-derivative good. Though this position is conceivable, and has been held later in the history of thought, it does not seem that ancient thinkers entertain it.[19] To Plato and Aristotle, NH would likely seem ill-conceived, and not only because by their lights hedonism is false. They would argue that people do not need to be told to pursue pleasure. As Aristotle puts it, pleasure is 'dyed into' our psychology.[20]

4   Sophisticated Hedonism

Sophisticated hedonism is the type of position Plato envisages in the *Protagoras* (351b–358e). Hedonism, according to the *Protagoras*, is strictly a single-value theory. Unlike other approaches in ethics, which admit a plurality of values, it posits only one non-derivative good: pleasure. Hence reasoning about one's choices and pursuits is aggregative. In other words, a hedonistic deliberator aims for as much pleasure and as little pain as possible. This is why scholars speak of a pleasure-pain 'calculus'. Decision-making, on this picture, is quasi-mathematical. In Plato's terms, it is an art of measurement (356d). This art, however, is not concerned with momentary pleasure, but with the agent's life as a whole. It secures the most pleasure and the least pain in the long run. This makes correct calculation difficult: it must overcome perspectival mistakes that we are prone to (356a–357b). Typically, that which is temporally near looms disproportionally large in our minds, and that which is temporally distant appears disproportionally small. For example, when the visit to the dentist comes temporally closer, it may look more and more scary to the extent that the tooth does not seem to hurt all that much anymore.

Epicurus's instructions about choosing some pleasures over others echo the *Protagoras*. The sophisticated hedonist examines pleasures with a view to their long-term effects. But in Epicurean ethics, this line of study pushes beyond the aggregative model. Epicurus introduces distinctions between kinds of pleasures. Some pleasures are natural (φυσικαί) and others are empty (κεναί); and among those that are natural, some are merely natural and others necessary. Among the necessary, some are necessary for happiness, others for the body's

---

19   Sidgwick 1907 holds NH without holding PH.

20   '[...] for pleasure both is something shared with the animals, and accompanies all the things falling under the heading of choice. For in fact what is fine and advantageous seems pleasant. Again, pleasure is something we have all grown up with since infancy; the result is that it is hard to rub us clean of this impulse, dyed as it is into our lives (ἐγκεχρωσμένον τῷ βίῳ). (Aristotle, *Nicomachean Ethics* II.3, 1104b34–a3; all passages from the *NE* are cited in Rowe's 2002 translation, with changes).

freedom from stress, and others for life itself.[21] The task is to observe these (and further) distinctions, and that is, to do more than aggregative reasoning:

> Since pleasure is the good which is primary and congenital, for this reason we do not choose every pleasure either, but we sometimes pass over many pleasures in cases when their outcome for us is a greater quantity of discomfort; and we regard many pains as better than pleasures in cases when our endurance of pains is followed by a greater and long-lasting pleasure. Every pleasure, then, because of its natural affinity, is something good, yet not every pleasure is choiceworthy. Correspondingly, every pain is something bad, but not every pain is by nature to be avoided. However, we have to make our judgment on all these points by a calculation and survey of advantages and disadvantages. For at times we treat the good as bad and conversely the bad as good.
>
> EPICURUS, 129–130, *Letter to Menoeceus*, LS 21B, tr. LS

Two formulations in this text are especially noteworthy, because they put pressure on the premise that all pleasure is good. Epicurus says that though all pleasures are good, they are not all choiceworthy. And he says that at times one should treat the good as bad and the bad as good. That is, though all pleasure is good, there are reasons not to choose certain pleasures and not to avoid certain pains. The guide in choosing and avoiding is reason. This, too, pushes against the limits of hedonism. Epicurus goes so far as to call prudence the greatest good, though its value is derivative: prudence and sober reasoning *produce* the pleasant life, and their value derives from the value of pleasure.[22] In effect, Epicurus's proposals are surprisingly close to Plato's arguments in *Republic* VIII–IX, recommending simple pleasures and warning against luxurious habits.[23] He even endorses a version of Plato's proposal that reason can judge the relative merits of different pleasures (*Rp.* IX, 582a–583a).

---

21   Throughout this section, I am referencing Epicurus, *Letter to Menoeceus* 127–132. Epicurus employs a further distinction, between so-called static and so-called kinetic pleasures, which arguably supports the claim that, as long as pain is absent, one is in pleasure (namely, static pleasure). On this contested distinction, cf. Mitsis 1988.

22   Cf. *Protagoras* 356e, on the art of measurement as our 'savior'.

23   *Letter to Menoeceus* 130–132. Cf. Warren 2014. In Plato's third argument for ranking the pleasures of reason highest, Socrates proposes that what is—in the ambitious metaphysical sense of his notion of Being—satiates in a deeper and more lasting way than anything in the realm of becoming (585a–587b). Epicurus does not engage with the relevant metaphysics. But his distinction between empty pleasures and natural/necessary pleasures arrives at similar conclusions about the pleasures of reasoning.

Nevertheless, Epicurus' distinctions are ways of making hedonism more sophisticated, rather than ways of departing from or rejecting hedonism. Prudent reasoning is not by itself valuable; it is valuable because it helps one secure the most pleasure. No pleasures, on his account, are mere illusions. All pleasure is real and all pleasure is good. Plato's discussion of the pleasures of reason in the *Republic* introduces three models of how pleasure and pain relate (583b–585a), and his *Philebus* mentions a fourth model, ascribed to grumpy people with an inordinate hatred of pleasure (44c6–7). These models are worth laying out here because they help characterize Epicurus's position further:

Two Stage Model
(1) Pleasure
(2) Pain

Three Stage Model
(1) Pleasure
(2) Neutral, in-between state: neither pleasure nor pain
(3) Pain[24]

Qualified Three Stage Model
(1) Pure Pleasure (not the cessation of pain; example: the scent of a flower; the agent was not in pain before she walked by the flower)
(2) Neutral, in-between state that misleadingly seems to be pleasurable (cessation of pain) and painful (cessation of pleasure)
(3) Pain

Anti-Hedonistic Two Stage Model
(1) Pain
(2) Pleasure is the absence of pain in a way that makes pain primary. In a sense, there *is no* pleasure; what people call pleasure just is absence of pain.

Epicurus endorses the Two Stage Model. In his words, 'The removal of all pain is the limit of the magnitude of pleasures.'[25] Pleasure and pain, on his account, are equally real. They are each other's removal, without one of them being primary. The Plato of the *Republic* endorses the Qualified Three Stage Model,

---

24 On the question of whether there is a neutral state in between pleasure and pain, cf. *Philebus* 44a–b.
25 Epicurus, *Key doctrines* 3 = LS 21C. Cf. Cicero, *De finibus* 37–9.

which singles out a class of pure pleasures—those taken in reasoning—
that do not involve prior pain and do not mistake the cessation of pain for
pleasure.[26] Plato here captures an idea that both he and Aristotle explore in
various fashions: some pleasures merely seem to be pleasures without really
being pleasures.[27] In the *Republic*, the illusion comes about via a transition:
we take ourselves to be in pleasure when really we are merely relieved from
pain. This idea is pushed to its extreme in the Anti-Hedonist Two Stage Model,
which takes pain to be primary and pleasure to be nothing but the absence
of pain.[28]

5   Non-hedonism and Anti-hedonism

Critics of hedonism reject hedonism's first premise, that pleasure is the only
non-derivative good. On my proposal, this rejection comes in two guises. Anti-
hedonists endorse the opposite of hedonism, arguing that all pleasure is bad.
Non-hedonists hold that there are good and bad pleasures. The following non-
hedonist views correspond roughly to the hedonist's premises.

> POSITIVE VALENCE VS. GOODNESS: Pleasure is pleasant, and 'pleasant'
> is an experience with positive valence. But that does not make plea-
> sure good. There are good and bad pleasures.
> MOTIVATION: Pleasure and pain figure pervasively in our mental lives
> and in motivation.
> GOOD LIFE: Pleasure is an ingredient of a good life that no one would
> choose to do without (Plato). Pleasure is also part of the very best,
> divine life (Aristotle).

---

26   The question of whether ignorance is painful, and the seeking of knowledge a way of aim-
      ing to get rid of the pain of not-knowing, is difficult. Arguably, Plato goes back and forth
      on it, admitting this kind of pain in the *Symposium* and not admitting it in the *Republic*.
27   Pleasures other than the pleasures of reasoning are, for both Plato and Aristotle, prone
      to mislead. They are 'mindless advisors,' as a passage in the *Laws* has it (644c4–d3); in
      Aristotle's words, they are appearances of the good (*NE* 1113a33–b2). Cf. Moss 2012 and
      Sauvé-Meyer 2012 on these ideas.
28   Moss 2002 argues that Plato engages with pleasure as much as he does because he is in-
      terested in its deceptiveness: 'I will argue that Plato's suspicion of pleasure is systematic
      and philosophical, and tied to his most central views. Pleasure is dangerous because it is a
      deceiver. It leads us astray with false appearances, bewitching and beguiling us, cheating
      and tricking us.'

On this reconstruction, Plato and Aristotle count not as anti-hedonists but as non-hedonists. They never seem to call into question that pleasure is a positive experience. Habituation as the *NE* has it and education in Plato's *Republic* 'works with' the way our psychologies are. Both texts discuss how pleasure/ pain attitudes can be shaped and directed. The virtuous agent, who enjoys being moderate or just, is supported in her virtue by enjoying it (*NE* II.1–6).

Plato's *Philebus* ends with an analysis of the ingredients of a good life.[29] This life, according to the *Philebus*, contains pleasure. No human being would choose a life without it. A better life is conceivable, a divine life, and it would not contain pleasure. But ethics is about the good for human beings. A good human life does not contain all pleasures, because some pleasures are inherently bad. It contains certain pleasures, such as the pleasures of thinking, and these are among the causes of the goodness of a good human life (*Philebus* 66c). Aristotle's *Eudemian Ethics* starts with the claim that happiness (*eudaimonia*) is at once the best, the most beautiful (or most fine, *kalon*), and the most pleasant (1214a1–8). Along the same lines, according to the *NE*, the virtuous person enjoys her virtuous actions and the agent who engages in contemplation enjoys thinking (VII.11.1152b1–6). The life of contemplation is, in its purest form, a divine life. This life, and here Aristotle disagrees with Plato, is pleasant. A god continually enjoys a 'single and simple pleasure' (1154b26), namely the pleasure of contemplation.

Scholars often discuss Aristotle's two 'treatises' on pleasure, *NE* VII.11–14 and *NE* X.1–5, with a view to the differences between his positive proposals. What is perhaps more striking, however, is that *NE* VII.11–14 and to a lesser degree *NE* X.1–5 critically engage with arguments against hedonism. Aristotle reconstructs a set of arguments, presumably by Plato or others in the Academy, that are meant to defeat hedonism; and he pulls them apart, aiming to demonstrate their weaknesses.[30] Are these arguments flawed, such that Aristotle replaces them with more forceful and compelling ways to refute hedonism? It does not seem so. Rather, Aristotle seems more invested in refuting arguments against hedonism than in refuting hedonism.[31] He adduces considerations that

---

29 Cf. Vogt 2010.

30 On Aristotle's rejection of Academic anti-hedonist arguments, cf. Rapp 2009. Scholars traditionally pay much attention to Aristotle's rejection of an account he ascribes to Plato, according to which pleasure is a restoration and thus a change. The *Philebus* starts out with the restoration-account Aristotle objects to; but it ends with ideas about pleasure in a good life that Aristotle does not mention. On the difference between the restoration account and Plato's considered position, cf. Aufderheide 2011. Cf. D. Frede 1992 and Warren 2009.

31 Cf. Frede 2009.

distance him from the more negative assessment of pleasure he ascribes to Plato.[32] For example, he argues that the badness of pain suggests that pleasure must in some way be good (*NE* VII.13), and (along the lines of my introductory reference to Plato and the life of cattle) that disproportionate attention to bodily pleasures has given pleasure an inappropriately bad name (*NE* VII.14). Aristotle recognizes pleasure as an ingredient of virtue and an ineradicable feature of human motivation. He carves out space for a non-hedonist position that ascribes value to pleasure and takes seriously that pretty much everyone 'weaves' pleasure into happiness (1153b15; cf. 1152b6–7).

What, then, about passages where Plato and Aristotle talk about hedonism dismissively? One thing to say is that this is compatible with the picture I defend: non-hedonism, of course, disagrees with hedonism. Another thing to say is that, at different moments in their discussions, Plato and Aristotle target different opponents. At times, say, when Plato talks about the life of cattle at the end of the *Philebus*, he has in mind a brutish and unreflective kind of hedonism. But in the same dialogue, Socrates talks in civil ways and seemingly with genuine philosophical interest with Protarchus, whose task it is to defend hedonism.[33] At the beginning of Book x of the *Nicomachean Ethics*, Aristotle engages with Eudoxus, a philosopher in the Academy who holds a version of hedonism. Commentators discuss why Aristotle is so respectful, engaging with Eudoxus' views in earnest. One speculation, widely accepted, is that Eudoxus seems to have lived in ways Aristotle finds noble.[34] Like Epicurus, he seems to have been a sophisticated hedonist, someone who takes pleasure in activities that Plato and Aristotle approve of—virtuous action and thinking. His presence in Aristotle's arguments is, on the picture I defend, just one example of the way in which hedonists push ancient non-hedonists to refine their views.

Consider then the premises of anti-hedonism, corresponding (roughly) to the three premises of hedonism, NON-DERIVATE GOOD, NATURE, and NORM:[35]

---

32   Cf. Frede 2009 and Rapp 2009.

33   Along similar lines, both Plato and Aristotle ascribe the view that pleasure is the good to 'the many', which may suggest that they hold this view in disdain. And yet, according to the *Philebus* and according to the *NE*, both views—that pleasure is the good and that wisdom is the good—are flawed in the same fundamental way: they identify one value as 'the' good, rather than understanding that a good human life (*eudaimonia*) is the good. Cf. Vogt 2011.

34   Broadie 1991, 347.

35   Aufderheide 2011 defines anti-hedonism as the claim that no pleasure is good by itself, and argues that this is Plato's 'official view' in the *Philebus*.

BAD: Pleasure is bad.

IRRATIONAL: Pleasure is pursued in a state of illusion or in a corrupted condition.

ERADICATE: Pleasure should be recognized as illusory and/or eradicated from one's psychological life.[36]

Who counts, on this way of looking at things, as anti-hedonist? In the *Philebus*, Socrates refers to a group of harsh people. As they see it, there is pain and the removal of pain, which on their account is misclassified as pleasure. This is the Anti-Hedonistic Two Stage Model: pleasure is the absence of pain in a way that makes pain primary; pleasure is by itself nothing, and it is pervasively mistaken for something good. Hence with respect to these 'harsh people' it is not exactly right to say, as my premise BAD has it, that pleasure is bad. More precisely, pleasure is mistakenly viewed as good, while really it is not good, and it is not good on account of not even genuinely being in existence (44b10–11). Still, Plato describes the proponents of this view as anti-hedonists, or in his words, as haters of the power of pleasure who on account of this hatred refuse to acknowledge anything healthy in it (44c–d). Scholars have not been able to identify these thinkers; apart from their grumpiness and hatred, Plato ascribes to them a tremendous reputation in natural science (44b9). Either way, he introduces them in order to signal who the true enemies of hedonism are (44b6–7). It is in this spirit that I classify them as anti-hedonists.

A more straightforward candidate for counting as anti-hedonist is Stoic philosophy. The Stoics ascribe positive affective states to the wise person. But they see no place for pleasure in a good life as they conceive of it. For the Stoics, pleasure is one of the four generic emotions (*pathê*). These emotions are defined as excessive movements of the mind, as impulses for ill-conceived actions, as irrational and 'mad'.[37] This assessment is part of a larger framework, often called psychological monism. According to the Stoics, the soul is one, not in any way divided into reason and desire. Any tumultuous state, on this picture, disrupts our abilities to think. And pleasure is paradigmatically an irrational state of mind. On the Stoic picture, the person who is in an emotional state of mind is not enjoying it, even though she may claim she does. The turmoil in her mind is experienced negatively, or so the Stoics argue. This does

---

36   The Stoics, who on my classification count as anti-hedonists, ascribe motivations other than pleasure to newborns. First impulse, they argue, is for self-preservation and for the preservation of those closest to us. Thus the Stoics start with a different set of presumed observations. But like hedonists, they infer norms from what they take to be natural. Cf. LS (1987) fragments in chapters 57 and 59.

37   Stobaeus 2.88,8–90,6 (= LS 65A); cf. all fragments in LS chapter 65.

not make the ideal Stoic agent affectless. The wise person has 'good feelings' of joy, well-wishing, and caution (DL 7.116). That is, she experiences positive affective states. But she does not take pleasure, not even in virtue.[38]

As I see it, those who characterize Plato and Aristotle as anti-hedonists lack a principled way of distinguishing the positions Plato and Aristotle formulate on the one hand and the Stoic (as well as 'haters of pleasure') position on the other. A mere dichotomy between hedonism and anti-hedonism makes everyone who is not a hedonist an anti-hedonist. To signal how misleading this is, consider a lively debate among later Stoics, Galen, and others. They discuss psychological monism and pluralism precisely with respect to the question of whether pleasure can be 'tamed'. According to Plato and Aristotle, a molding of pleasure/pain attitudes that makes them fit into a good life can be attained. According to the Stoics, pleasure/pain attitudes are inherently irrational, no matter what. On my proposal, anti-hedonists hold that pleasure/pain cannot be made into something good, whatever efforts one undertakes via education, habituation, and so on. To them pleasure is not only such that it can mislead or typically misleads. It is thoroughly bad, in every instance and in an unsalvageable fashion. Anti-hedonism construed this way genuinely holds the opposite of hedonism.

6   The Bad Pleasure Problem

The best known line of attack against hedonism's first premise, that pleasure is the only non-derivative good, asks 'what then about bad pleasures?'[39] Here is an outline of the argument:

> Hedonism: Pleasure is good.
> Objection: There are good and bad pleasures.
> Objection Granted: Hedonism does not dispute the distinction between good and bad pleasures.
> Opposites (suppressed premise): Nothing has, in the same respect, at the same time, etc., opposite properties.
> Defeat: Hedonism must, *per impossibile*, assume that some pleasures are good *and* bad.

---

38   Cf. Sam McVane's contribution to this volume on the affective states of the wise person.
39   This objection is mentioned in the *Republic* as so well-worn that it is hardly worth repeating. 'What about those who define the good as pleasure? Are they any less full of confusion than the others? Or aren't even they compelled to admit that there are bad pleasures?' Plato, *Republic* VI, 505c6–8 (tr. Reeve 2004).

In reply, hedonists insist that all pleasures are inherently good, even if they are taken in bad activities.[40] This is, then, how hedonism rejects Defeat:

> Distinction: All pleasures are good qua being pleasures, and some pleasures are bad qua their object/cause.

This distinction preserves the unity of pleasure: all pleasure is alike insofar as it is good; it differs merely in its object. Protarchus, Socrates's interlocutor in the *Philebus*, famously puts this as follows: 'pleasures come from opposite things. But they are not at all opposed to one another. For how could pleasure not be, of all things, most like pleasure?' (12d7–e2). To see how the debate continues, consider what counts as bad pleasure. Here are candidate replies: lowly, perverted, and false pleasures.

Lowly: In the *Philebus*, Plato seems to think of lowly pleasures as those that human beings share with animals (67b). Socrates asks what pleasure amounts to if very little cognitive activity is going on, as is presumably the case in some animals. His example is a sea-urchin. Its pleasures are lowly in the sense that they are barely registered and as such not pleasant in the way in which pleasure figures in a human life. Even if the sea-urchin were in constant pleasure, the word 'constant' would lack meaning: without memory, experience, anticipation of the future, one cannot find oneself in ongoing pleasure. Lowly pleasures, conceived along these lines, are not simply bodily. More fundamentally, they are pleasures that involve only a low level of complexity in cognitive activity. That may coincide with bodily pleasures, assuming, say, that cows enjoy activities like grazing. But the badness of lowly pleasures, insofar as hedonists concede it, hangs on something else, namely that we would not want them.[41] Even with respect to bodily pleasures, human beings prefer versions that are reflective of their cognitive abilities, involving memory, anticipation, and so on.[42]

---

40   Cf. *Philebus* 36c–38a.

41   'Moreover, due to lack of memory, it would be impossible for you to remember that you ever enjoyed yourself, and for any pleasure to survive from one moment to the next, since it would leave no memory. But, not possessing right *doxa*, you would not realize that you are enjoying yourself even while you do, and, being unable to calculate, you could not figure out any future pleasures for yourself. You would thus not live a human life but the life of a mollusk or of one of those creatures in shells that live in the sea.' (*Philebus* 21c1–8).

42   For a similar line of thought, cf. *Eudemian Ethics* I, 1215b301216a5 (tr. Inwood and Woolf 2013): 'Nor indeed would anyone who was not completely slavish prefer life merely for the pleasure of nourishment or of sex, if deprived of the other pleasures that knowledge of sight or any of the other senses provide people with. It is evident that whoever makes this choice might just as well have been born a beast as a human being. At any rate the ox in Egypt, which is worshipped as the god Apis, is lavished with a good deal more of those

Perverted: Republic VIII–IX offers an analysis of psychological decline that involves detailed engagement with perverted pleasures. Pleasures of addiction, pleasures taken in self-destructive and excessive activities, pleasures in activities that to others are unthinkably shameful, and so on, fall into this category. Arguably, hedonists share the view that such pleasures are not to be pursued. In choosing between pleasures, the hedonist is guided by prudence and prefers pleasures that leave intact sober reasoning.[43]

False: Plato's *Philebus* classifies bad pleasures as false. Though hedonists accept that there are pleasures which, via their object (that which the agent enjoys), are bad, they do not accept the identification of the bad and the false (36c–42c). Scholars have long puzzled over the precise interpretation of the notion of false pleasure.[44] What matters for my proposal is that the debate between hedonism and non-hedonism reaches an impasse. Non-hedonists can admit that there are lowly and perverted pleasures. They may reject the notion of false pleasures, but non-hedonists other than the Plato of the *Philebus* do not employ this notion either. The Bad Pleasure Problem does not settle the dispute.

7   The Nature of Pleasure Problem

The *Philebus's* discussion of pleasure starts with the observation that pleasure is manifold, ποικίλον (12c). According to Socrates, pleasure goes by one name, but comes in forms that are quite unlike each other.[45] In effect, it is not clear whether everything we ordinarily call pleasure falls under one genus; or whether on the contrary there is no unified notion of pleasure that captures all of them.[46] These considerations pose what I consider the hardest challenge for hedonism. It is an implicit premise of hedonism—and arguably of anti-hedonism—that pleasure is a sufficiently unified phenomenon for general claims about pleasure to make sense:

---

sorts of things than many monarchs. Similarly, one would not choose life just for the pleasure of sleeping. What is the difference between an uninterrupted sleep from first day till last, for ten thousand years of any period you like, and living as a plant?'.

43   Epicurus, *Letter to Menoeceus* 127–132.

44   Vogt (2016) contains discussion of recent trends in scholarship on this issue.

45   Socrates also admits that there are many forms of knowing (ἐπιστῆμαι). But he describes this in non-derogative terms as a plurality (πολλαί), while pleasure is characterized as manifold (ποικίλον), which for Plato is a negative term.

46   Fletcher 2014.

UNITY: Pleasure is a sufficiently unified phenomenon for there to be such a thing as the nature of pleasure.

A hedonist account of the nature of pleasure can accommodate distinctions between kinds of pleasure, as we saw earlier. But it insists that all pleasure is unified by the goodness of pleasure. However, if there is no such thing as the nature of pleasure, hedonism does not get off the ground. Today this objection is known as the heterogeneity objection. Theorists argue that, say, the pleasures of smelling the scent of a rose, solving a math problem, and hitting someone in anger, are too different to share one nature.[47] Accounts of the unity of pleasure are hard to come by, whether they are formulated by hedonists or other theorists interested in pleasure.[48] Does this mean that hedonism and anti-hedonism are untenable, for reasons that are more basic than debates about the value of pleasure and pain suggest?

In *NE* X.1–5, Aristotle offers a sideward step that may help both non-hedonism and hedonism. According to *NE* X.4, pleasure does not occur without activity and every activity is completed by pleasure.[49] Though this proposal is often called an account of pleasure, it is not. It is not an account of the nature of pleasure; it merely characterizes the relationship between pleasure and activities. Pleasure is said to be an accompaniment of activities, one that goes along with them, depends on them, and is generated by them.[50] On this picture, there

---

47 Cf. Feldman 1997.

48 One option is to just say that pleasure feels good; but one may wonder whether this goes beyond the claim that pleasure is pleasant. Another option is to ascribe a certain role in motivation/desire to pleasure; but that, like the *NE* X.4 proposal, is a proposal about a relation in which pleasure stands with something else, not an account of the nature of pleasure. Cf. Sidgwick 1907 for a combination of both: 'for my own part, when I reflect on the notion of pleasure,—using the term in the comprehensive sense which I have adopted, to include the most refined and subtle intellectual and emotional gratifications, no less than the coarser and more definite sensual enjoyments,—the only common quality that I can find in the feelings so designated seem to be that relation to desire and volition expressed by the general term 'desirable', in the sense previously explained. I propose therefore to define Pleasure—when we are considering its 'strict value' for purposes of quantitative comparison—as a feeling which, when experienced by intelligent beings, is at least implicitly apprehended as desirable or—in cases of comparison—preferable (book II, ch. II, s. II, pr. III, p. 127).

49 Aristotle, *NE* X.4, 1175a20–21: 'without activity, pleasure does not occur, and every activity is completed by pleasure' (ἄνευ τε γὰρ ἐνεργείας οὐ γίνεται ἡδονή, πᾶσάν τε ἐνέργειαν τελειοῖ ἡ ἡδονή).

50 Scholars often call this relation supervenience. I refrain from using this term here, because pleasure does not 'supervene' on activities in the sense in which philosophers today speak of supervenience; and Aristotle himself does not employ such a notion.

are as many pleasures as there are activities. This multitude is not surprising or perplexing—we consider it evident that there is a wide range of activities that people can engage in.[51] Nevertheless there is unity, namely, there is one kind of relation that obtains between activities and pleasure. The *NE* x proposal thus recognizes both the variety and unity of pleasure.[52]

By the standards that this debate sets up, this is a success. But for whom? In effect, Aristotle adapts a hedonist move. He shifts attention from pleasure to the activities that are being enjoyed. Pleasures differ, on his account, according to the ways in which activities differ. And this is a version of Protarchus's argument in the *Philebus*. Pleasures are bad, insofar as they are bad, by virtue of the object or cause of pleasure—and that is, the activity that is enjoyed—being bad. This leaves intact the positive valence of pleasure no matter how bad the activity that someone takes pleasure in. Does the *NE* x proposal concede too much to hedonism, in effect enabling the hedonist to account for bad pleasure? Or does its refusal to offer—or to even aim at—an account of the nature of pleasure undercut hedonism, because hedonism needs a more robust unity of pleasure? Either way, and this is what I hope to have established in this chapter, hedonism's presence in ancient ethics inspires some of the most subtle analyses of pleasure philosophers have formulated, with surprisingly much common ground between hedonists and non-hedonists.

So, by way of conclusion, what is hedonism? It is, or so I have argued, the claim that pleasure is the only non-derivative good. Qua pleasures, all pleasures are good. The positions that Plato and Aristotle develop in a whole range of texts are not the opposite of hedonism, and they are not the strongest rejection of hedonism that is conceivable. Plato and Aristotle admit good pleasures and both find a place for pleasure in good lives. The position that should be called anti-hedonism is genuinely different. It holds the opposite of hedonism, namely that all pleasure is bad. It has ancient proponents, among them the Stoics and a group of people Plato refers to as haters of pleasure.

---

51   Heinaman 2011 discusses what he calls a coarse versus a strict division of pleasures into kinds in Aristotle. According to the former, the pleasure of doing geometry, for example, is one kind of pleasure. According to the latter, proving one theorem goes along with one kind of pleasure, and proving another theorem with another kind of pleasure. Cf. Vogt 2014.

52   Shields 2011 and Heinaman 2011.

CHAPTER 7

Pleasure, Pain, and the Unity of the Soul in Plato's *Protagoras*

Wolfgang-Rainer Mann and Vanessa de Harven

1 A Few Preliminaries

The question of whether the hedonism Socrates introduces into the discussion at *Protagoras* 351 B is a position he means to endorse *in propria persona* or is rather part of a complicated dialectical maneuver he deploys against Protagoras has sharply divided interpreters of the dialogue for generations.[1] It seems, on the one hand, unbelievable that Socrates (whether the historical figure or Plato's character) would espouse such an ethically or philosophically 'lowbrow' view, as commentators tend to see it. On the other hand, many commentators have found it equally difficult to accept that Socrates would argue from (what are by his lights) false premises to a conclusion he endorses: the unity of virtue. Many of those who take Socrates to be a hedonist have tried, in various ways, to rehabilitate the thesis, or to deflate the commitment to pleasure, in order to avoid the apparent awkwardness.[2] Others attribute the view about pleasure to the historical Socrates, or regard it as a phase in Plato's intellectual development.[3] Those who deny that Socrates is a hedonist do so either

---

1 For the pro-hedonist position see e.g. Grote 1865, Adam and Adam 1893, Hackforth 1928, Vlastos 1956, Dodds 1959, Crombie 1962–63, C. C. W Taylor 1976, Gosling and Taylor 1982, Nussbaum 1986, Irwin 1995, Rudebusch 2002, Rowe 2003, and Moss 2014. For the anti-hedonist position see e.g. A. E. Taylor 1926, Grube 1933, Guthrie 1956, Sullivan 1961, O'Brien 1967, Vlastos 1969, Dyson 1976, Zeyl 1980, Annas 1999, Kahn 2003, Dimas 2008, and Shaw 2015.

2 For example, Crombie 1962–63, Gosling and Taylor 1982, Rudebusch 2002, and Moss 2014 take Socratic hedonism to be high-minded or enlightened, and so less offensive as a thesis; Nussbaum 1986 and Rowe 2003 minimize the commitment by making hedonism a placeholder or stalking horse for the good; and Irwin 1995 deflates the thesis by retaining the good as *motivationally* prior to pleasure (i.e. we pursue pleasure because we think it is good), which is a respectable order of priority, and taking pleasure to be *epistemologically* prior (i.e. we make judgments about pleasure before making judgments about goodness), which is a morally benign order of priority (since what we 'really' want is the good).

3 For example, Adam and Adam 1893, Hackforth 1928, C. C. W Taylor 1976, and Gosling and Taylor 1982 attribute the hedonism to the shortcomings of the historical Socrates; Vlastos

by, again, rehabilitating or deflating the view he 'really' commits himself to, so that it no longer counts as hedonism, or by divorcing hedonism from the argument for the unity of courage and wisdom, or, most commonly, by taking Socrates to endorse hedonism formally but to be ironic or insincere in his commitment to pleasure, so that readers (at least those 'in the know') are meant to understand an implicit disavowal or criticism of the thesis.[4] In what follows, we will argue that excellent sense can be made of the relevant passages, taken at face value, without maintaining that Socrates himself holds that pleasure is the good and therefore ought to be pursued.[5] We are thus 'anti-hedonists,' not by invoking irony or insincerity, but by following the letter of the text: a close

---

1956 and Gosling and Taylor 1982 take the character Socrates, and thus Plato, to be confused in the *Protagoras*.

4   Vlastos 1956, Kahn 2003, and Dimas 2008 deflate the Socratic commitment to pleasure being (a) good, but not *the* good, while Guthrie 1956 goes for high-minded hedonism. Vlastos 1969, changing his mind, takes the majority to be committed to full hedonism (where pleasure is identical to the good), while Socrates remains committed to the weaker thesis that pleasure is (a) good, but Vlastos now counts as an anti-hedonist insofar as he denies that either version of hedonism is relevant to the argument against the possibility of *akrasia* (lack of self-control, weakness of will, or incontinence); Shaw 2015 also argues that this argument of Socrates does not rely on the premise of hedonism; Dimas argues that Socrates is committed the weaker view that pleasure and the good are co-instantiated, which is compatible with but does not require hedonism. (NB: *Akrasia* is of course an Aristotelian term, not a Platonic one—whereas its opposite, *enkrateia* (self-control, strength of will, or continence) does occur in the *Republic*—but by now it has become standard to use both terms in discussions of Plato, a convention we too are following.) Grube 1933, Sullivan 1961, O'Brien 1967, Dyson 1976, Klosko 1980, and Zeyl 1980 all take the route of ascribing some kind of irony or insincerity to Socrates.

5   Present day philosophical discussions of hedonism often distinguish between a *psychological* or *descriptive* claim—people, as matter of psychological fact, are *motivated* to go for (what they take to be) pleasurable, and are motivated to avoid (what they take to be) painful—and some version of a *normative* claim. (See e.g. Katja Vogt's contribution to the present volume.) Such normative hedonism can either be of a straightforwardly *prescriptive* sort—people *ought to* go for what is pleasurable, and *ought to* avoid what is painful—or be of an *evaluative* sort—pleasure is the good, or is the highest good, or is the only thing that is good in its own right (with any other putative goods counting as good only if they are appropriately related to pleasure, e.g. by being somehow conducive to it). One could then get to either a descriptive or a prescriptive claim via a suitable version of the *sub specie boni* principle: if everything is pursued under the guise of the good, and if pleasure appears in the guise of the good, and vice versa, then everything will be pursued under the guise of pleasure (descriptive). On the other hand, if one ought to pursue everything under the guise of the good, and if pleasure appears in the guise of the good, and vice versa, then one ought to pursue everything under the guise of pleasure (prescriptive). Since Plato does not draw a sharp fact/value distinction, it may well be misguided (or anachronistic, see Gosling and Taylor 1982, 57) to seek to attribute to him either a purely descriptive claim about pleasure, or a purely normative one. We briefly return to this issue near the end of our paper (see n. 43, below).

reading of the *Protagoras* shows that Socrates, in the course of the discussion, never commits himself to any form of hedonism at all.

The status of hedonism in the *Protagoras* is, however, also of interest beyond the confines of interpreting the dialogue, or indeed even beyond the project of reading Plato. The view that pleasure (sometimes) is good, and that thus one (sometimes) ought to go for what is pleasant can seem like a commonplace thought, a piece of basic folk psychology. And near the beginning of both the *Nicomachean Ethics* and the *Eudemian Ethics*, Aristotle points out that people in general regard pleasure as (a) good, and that some—those he whom he calls, as certain of our translations have it, 'voluptuaries' (*apolaustikoi*)—pursue pleasure as that which makes for human happiness and flourishing. The way Aristotle discusses the voluptuaries' view suggests that he takes it to be a rather low or slavish position (cf. e.g. *NE* 1. 5. 1095b14–22 or *EE* 1. 5. 1215b30–1216a2). Somewhat 'better' people will go for something like honor. And those with certain intellectual pretensions 'proclaim that [happiness] is some great thing, beyond the comprehension of [most people]' (cf. *NE* 1. 4. 1095a26–27). Aristotle's discussion further suggests, though he does not quite come out and say so, that ordinary people are thoroughly familiar with the view that pleasure is what is best (and thus makes for a good, happy life), and indeed that this a view they themselves at times hold and even avow.

We bring this up here at the outset because a striking feature of the *Protagoras* is that ordinary people are presented as *disavowing* (or pretending to disavow) the claim that pleasure is (the) good. They are made to say, via their 'spokesman', Protagoras, that pleasure is *only* good if it arises from *kala* things or actions (i.e. those that are noble, fine, or honorable).[6] Yet it turns out that they cannot give content to this claim and so are forced to concede that they are in fact committed to what (they say) they disavow. The hedonism in the *Protagoras* thus serves to bring to light both a deep incoherence in how people ordinarily think of themselves, their motivations, and behavior, as well as a certain falsity inherent in popular morality.[7] This, even more than the 'discovery' that Protagoras is not competent to teach virtue, is a central lesson of the work.

---

6 Some commentators have taken this disavowal as the final word and thus see the majority as denying hedonism throughout the discussion, e.g. A. E. Taylor 1926, Hackforth 1928, Dyson 1976, Irwin 1995, and Annas 1999.

7 Shaw 2015 in nice fashion appropriates Orwell's expression 'doublethink' to speak of the confused and self-deceived way in which the many understand their values and moral commitments, resulting from the social pressure to hold but never avow that injustice is prudent, and, at once, to avow but never really hold that justice and virtue are good.

2   Some Background on the *Protagoras*

The *Protagoras* opens, as do several other Platonic dialogues, with a framing conversation that provides the dramatic setting for Socrates to recount the actual exchange, in this case to an unnamed friend (cf. e.g. 309 A 1–310 A 7 and 362 A 4). The central discussion, however, begins considerably later, with the question of what Protagoras will teach his pupils (316 B 8). This postponement of the main discussion and the particular question it seeks to address is occasioned by an *initial* exchange within the narrated dialogue, the one between Socrates and his young friend Hippocrates (310 B 3–314 C 2), and Hippocrates' inability there to tell Socrates what, substantively, he hopes to learn from Protagoras (312 E 5–6). (Hippocrates is so eager on becoming Protagoras' student that he barges in on Socrates before daybreak, in order to enlist his help in securing him a spot as one of Protagoras' students (310 A 8).) This inability in turn prompts Socrates to ask Protagoras about his teaching, as it were, on behalf of Hippocrates. After some back and forth, Protagoras explains that his teaching (*mathēma*) is:

> ... sound deliberation (*euboulia*), both in household matters (*ta oikeia*)—how best to manage one's own household, and in civic affairs (*ta tēs poleōs*)—how to be maximally effective (*dunatōtatos*) in civic affairs, both with respect to acting and (public) speaking. (318 E 5–319 A 2)[8]

Socrates immediately paraphrases this as *politikē technē*, i.e. 'the art of citizenship' or 'the art of running a city' (C. C. W. Taylor), which promises to make men into good citizens (*poiein andras agathous politas*) (319 A 3–5). Protagoras eagerly embraces this paraphrase, and Socrates proceeds to challenge him, offering reasons why one might very much doubt that this can be taught (319 A 10–320 C 1). These reasons rely on the idea that *democratic* Athens proceeds rightly in allowing *every* citizen to have a voice on questions of public policy. This shows, Socrates suggests, that the Athenians do not hold that there is any *special* expertise or wisdom in this sphere of human activity, which someone could teach to those who lack it. He thus puts Protagoras in the potentially awkward position of coming across as a member of an *anti-democratic* elite. For Protagoras cannot justify his fees by claiming (in Athens) that the Athenians have got it all wrong, that the *polis* in fact should not allow every citizen to have a voice on matters of public policy, but permit only those

---

8 Here and throughout the translations are by S. Lombardo and K. Bell 1992/1997, though often with changes of our own.

who have learned the art of citizenship (from him!) to speak in the Assembly, say. Protagoras' Great Speech (320 C 8–328 D 2) is, among other things, his attempt to answer or defuse Socrates' worries in line with the Athenians' democratic commitments.

Socrates, for his part, responds to the Great Speech by raising 'one small matter' (328 E 3; cf. 329 A 4, A 6, and B 6) he thinks Protagoras has not settled: is *virtue* or *excellence* a *single* thing, such that if someone possesses one of what are conventionally thought of as the virtues, she necessarily possesses them all (viz. by possessing that single thing)? Or are the *virtues* (note the plural) rather separate and distinct, so that someone could, for example, be courageous but not at all just (and so on)?[9] Via a series of further questions (329 C 6–330 B 6) Socrates sets out the agenda and method for the subsequent dialectical exchanges, which (despite various twists and turns) constitute the remainder of the narrated dialogue (330 B 6–362 A 3).

Protagoras is induced to adopt as his *thesis* the claim that the virtues are distinct (and the related claim that it thus *is* possible for someone to possess one virtue but lack another). Socrates, in his role as *questioner, attacks* that thesis, by putting a series of questions to Protagoras with the intent of inducing him to grant things *conflicting with* his thesis (or to deny things *following from* it). Protagoras, in his role as *answerer*, needs to *uphold* his thesis, that is, in order to 'escape' the question-and-answer exchange (the *elenchus*) unscathed, he must avoid granting (or denying) anything that is problematic in the way indicated.[10] Thus Socrates *indirectly* argues for the opposing thesis: the virtues are unified, i.e. virtue *is* a single thing; and he, likewise, in effect also argues for

---

9   It is worth pointing out that Plato's 'list' of the so-called cardinal virtues, both in the *Protagoras* and in other works, differs markedly from what the epigraphical evidence shows the Athenians took to be the most important virtues of someone who was of value to, or had benefited, the *democratic polis*. (See Whitehead 1993, where he speaks of 'democratic cardinal virtues' and develops further ideas initially presented in Whitehead 1983.) *Sōphrosunē* in particular seems to have retained 'oligarchic' overtones (Whitehead 1993, 70–72). For more on this virtue see also the extensive discussions in North 1966 and Rademaker 2005. Thus Plato may be seeking, already in the list of what virtue comprises, to exploit tensions between the professed democratic outlook of the Athenians and their *de facto* commitment to aristocratic values (a matter which surfaces at several points in the dialogue, for example, at 347 C–348 A). We are grateful to Elizabeth Scharffenberger for drawing our attention to Whitehead's important papers.

10   The terminology (*questioner, answerer, thesis*, and so on) used in the body of the text for Socratic-Platonic question-and-answer exchanges (i.e. dialectic and the *elenchus*) is drawn from Aristotle's discussion in the *Topics*; see Mann 1992, Mann 1998, and Reinhardt 2000, 61–67, as well as Mann 2003. On Plato's use of *dialektikē* and related expressions, Müri 1944 remains fundamental; and on dialectic in the Academy more generally, see Ryle 1965, Ryle 1968, Moraux 1968, and Brunschwig 1984–85. Lloyd 1979, 59–125 provides

the claim that this single thing must be knowledge or wisdom. However, crucially, given the dialectical context (viz. the method and its practitioners' goals as just described), it is not the explicit, or even, as far as the dramatic frames go, the implicit, objective of Socrates to establish *any* thesis or positive account. In short, Socrates is not arguing *for* anything, as is indeed customary in the so-called Socratic *elenchus*.[11] In this respect, then, we take the argument to be *ad hominem*: its goal is the negative one of showing that Protagoras' thesis is untenable—either because it is false, or because Protagoras lacks the resources for defending it adequately.

Here an important caveat is necessary. Taking the dialectic to be *ad hominem*, i.e. as being directed *at* the answerer, does not require ascribing insincerity, dishonesty, or the like to the questioner. We would like to emphasize this, because it is not uncommon for the expression '*ad hominem*' to be treated as interchangeable with terms like 'fallacious,' 'insincere,' and 'dishonest.' But in fact the *elenchus* may often proceed by means of false premises, namely those the interlocutor has committed himself to, without this requiring that we charge Socrates with insincerity, fallacy, or subterfuge; and Socrates is presumably always *in effect* arguing for an *intellectualist* view of our place in the world, so there should be nothing untoward about his arguments here leading to such results either.[12] Accordingly we agree with Michael J. O'Brien that this is a 'normal *elenchus*,' but we disagree with his further claim that Socrates is 'not being straightforward at all.'[13] Thus *for us*, to maintain that Socrates' argument is *ad hominem* is simply to say that it aims to examine critically Protagoras' claims to teach virtue, the picture of education he paints in the Great Speech, and his commitment to a popular conception of the virtues as separable and distinct.

3   The Immediate Context for Hedonism, and the Turn to *Akrasia*

By 349 A–D, after, again, some interruptions, Protagoras has been forced to concede that wisdom (*sophia*), moderation (*sōphrosunē*), justice (*dikaiosunē*),

---

additional, helpful background. The papers in Fink 2012 address a number of issues in 'the development of dialectic from Plato to Aristotle' (this is the volume's title).

11   Addressing the much-discussed issue of whether the Socratic *elenchus* can establish any positive results is beyond the scope of our present paper. The issue, fortunately, does not matter for the questions we are addressing.

12   By 'intellectualism' we here mean the view (which Plato's Socrates often avows) that 'the good life is a matter of *knowing* what is good,' (so Frede 1992, viii; emphasis added). In the *Protagoras*, as we will shortly see, Socrates correspondingly argues for an essentially *cognitive* picture of the emotions and other affective states: each such state turns out to be (for Socrates) a matter of *thinking* that something is good, or is bad.

13   O'Brien 1967, 138–139, our italics; cf. also Irwin 1995, 86.

and piety/holiness (*hosiotēs*) are 'reasonably close' to each other, but he insists that courage (*andreia*) is 'altogether different'. Socrates' immediate goal (at 349 E ff.) is thus to challenge this sub-thesis, i.e. to argue that courage, too, is to be identified with the other four virtues, in particular, with wisdom. His initial attempt at securing Protagoras' agreement to this identity *fails* (349 E 2–351 B 2). This failure leads Socrates to digress, in abrupt fashion, from their discussion of courage, changing the subject (or so it seems) by asking: 'Tell me, Protagoras, ... do some men live well (*eu zēn*), others badly (*kakōs*)?' (351 B 3).[14] And it is only here, in the context of exploring whether there is such a thing as living well, that talk of hedonism first surfaces in the dialogue: for Socrates will next go on to introduce the suggestion that pleasure is good, and pain bad.

Before turning to any of the details of that suggestion and its subsequent discussion, we can already note that hedonism appears very late in the dialogue. This would be an odd position to locate an allegedly central view of Socrates, especially since nothing in the earlier discussion can be thought of as preparing readers for its appearance. More importantly, we can see that hedonism appears as part of the immediate dialectical context or strategy; that is, Socrates brings it up as part of arguing towards the conclusion that courage is to be identified with wisdom. This, of course, does not suffice to show that Socrates does *not* endorse hedonism. But it suggests that the matter of whether or not he endorses it is irrelevant to the dialectical strategy, since it is Protagoras who is in the role of answerer (sometimes alongside 'the many'), and who thus is forced to take a stand on hedonism. Instead, we should rather ask: *how* do the claims about pleasure play the roles they are meant to play; *how* does hedonism contribute to Socrates' argument against Protagoras' assertion that courage is altogether different from the other virtues? If we can answer these questions, we will be well on our way towards answering the further question of *why* Socrates (i.e. Plato) introduces hedonism at this particular point in the work, and to *what extent*, if any, these roles require Socrates' own commitment to it. We might also hope to gain, concomitantly, a clearer sense of just what sort of hedonism is being considered here—a prescriptive thesis to the effect that everyone *ought to pursue* pleasure as the good (and *ought to avoid* pain as the bad), or rather a psychological thesis to the effect that everyone, in actual fact, *does pursue* pleasure as the good (and *does avoid* pain as the bad), or perhaps some sort of combination or conflation of the two.

∴

---

14   The abruptness here is sufficiently striking to have led C. C. W Taylor to posit a lacuna in the text in the original edition (1976) of his commentary; see Taylor 1991, 225, *ad* Taylor 1976, 162.

Now, some details about the part of the dialogue that is our main focus. At 351 C Socrates asks Protagoras whether living pleasantly is good (*to ... hēdeōs zēn agathon*), and living unpleasantly (sc. without pleasure (*aēdeōs*), or rather, in a painful manner) bad.[15] Protagoras wants to deny this: a pleasure is only good if it is also *kalon* (noble, honorable, or fine).[16] More generally: some pleasures are bad (and shameful); some pains are good (and honorable), or at least, not bad (and not shameful). At 351 E 1–3 Socrates sharpens the issue, by asking: are pleasurable things good, simply to the extent (*kath' hoson*) that they are pleasurable? Is pleasure itself (*hē hēdonē autē*) good? Protagoras is not prepared to accept this straightaway, and thus says that they need to investigate whether pleasure (*hēdu*) and good (*agathon*) are the same (*to auton*), or not (E 3–7).[17] That investigation follows.

First, however, there is a detour. Starting at 352 A, we encounter what seems to be an additional digression (from the more basic matter of whether or not courage is to be identified with the other virtues): about whether knowledge is something strong (*ischuron*), 'in charge' (*hēgemonikon*), and capable of ruling (*archikon*) in a person. This Socrates wants to affirm.[18] And about whether

---

15   We do not find Socrates making any commitment to hedonism here: the inference he makes here (*ara*) follows from what seems to Protagoras to be the case at 351 B 5–10; cf. A. E. Taylor 1926, 259 and Zeyl 1980, 253 for agreement on this point. Those who find Socrates committing himself to hedonism *in propria persona* at 351 C 1 include Hackforth 1928, 260, Sullivan 1961, 21–22, Crombie 1962, Vlastos 1969, Dyson 1976, Gosling and Taylor 1982, 47, C. C. W Taylor 1976, 164–166, Nussbaum 1986, 451, n. 56 (citing the emphatic *ego*—but against this, because it introduces a direct question, cf. Zeyl 1980, 255, n. 16), Irwin 1995, 82, 86, and Annas 1999, 168.

16   We doubt that this is a misunderstanding of Socrates' proposal on Protagoras' part, as Dyson 1976, 42 suggests; indeed, to the extent that the *Protagoras* is complimentary to the sophist, featuring him pushing back during the *elenchus* and artfully navigating his tangled web of commitments, we think it is more likely that Protagoras is mindful of speaking to public morality, false as it will be shown to be. Further, Protagoras' hedging language in 351 D 1–3 arguably shows that he, too, has the dialectical context in view: he says he is not sure it is 'fitting' (*apokriteon*) for him to endorse hedonism and that it would be 'safer' (*asphalesteron*) to answer otherwise (for the latter as a rhetorical term of art, cf. LSJ, *s.v. asphalēs*, I. 4–5). Thus we disagree with the thesis of Shaw 2015 that the sophists have absorbed and internalized the views of the many, as opposed to consciously exploiting and navigating them.

17   One could also construe the question as asking whether the same (thing) is both pleasure and (the) good, or is both pleasant and good. Contrast our view with the deflationary position of Denyer 2008, *ad loc.*: that Socrates is asking whether a person will count as having done well taking pleasure in living out a full human life, not whether pleasure is intrinsically good.

18   As does Protagoras, who of course is hardly in a position to deny that his wares are 'anything but the most powerful forces in human activity' (352 D 1–2).

there is such a thing, such an experience, as 'being overcome' by pleasure (or, implicitly, by *thumos*, pain, fear, erotic passion, or ... (cf. 352 B 5–8 and E 1–2)). This Socrates wants to deny. But he recognizes that he needs to explain *why* people are tempted to offer explanations of their behavior along these lines (353 A 2–6). Among those who are tempted to say such things are Medea in her great monologue (Euripides, *Medea*, 1021–86),[19] and Phaedra in her reflections on pleasure, shame, and knowing what one ought to do, but failing to do it (Euripides, *Hippolytus*, 373–90).[20] As Charles Kahn notes, given these two

---

19   Medea concludes her speech with these words: 'I understand what evils (*kaka*) I am about to do/ but my *thumos* is stronger than my *bouleumata* (*thumos de kreissōn tōn emōn bouleumatōn*)/—which [= this *thumos*] is the cause of the greatest evils for mortals' (1078–1080, tr. B. Seidensticker 1990, 90; Mastronarde 2002, *ad* 1078, offers 'harmful things' for *kaka* here). Matters are complicated by the fact that several scholars have challenged the authenticity of all or some of lines 1056–1080. The suggestion that these lines are interpolated goes back to Bergk 1884, 512 n. 140; and the case against them is argued vigorously by Reeve 1972. Diggle, in the 1984 OCT, brackets the lines. Defenders include Kovacs 1986 (who does, however, athetize 1056–1064), Rickert 1987, Seidensticker 1990, and Mastronarde 2002 (who does, however, excise 1062–1063 (a doublet of 1240–1241)); see also Mastronarde 2002, 343–346, *ad* 1078–1080. For an overview of earlier discussions along with copious references, see Seidensticker 1990 and Mastronarde 2002, 388–397. Additional complications arise from disagreements about how the two key words are to be understood. We follow those scholars who see *thumos* not as emotion or passion in some general way, but as amounting to an archaic/aristocratic sense of self-worth, involving self-assertion, pride, a commitment to honor and the avoidance of shame and humiliation, and so on, and who thus construe it as being very similar to what Plato, in the *Republic*, will likewise call *thumos* (or *to thumoeides*), i.e. the spirited part of the soul. (Cf. e.g. Rickert 1987, 99–101.) The word *bouleumata* is problematic for a different reason: earlier, Medea had used *bouleumata* to refer to her plans of wreaking vengeance on Jason (see 769 and 772); and by 1040–1048 it is clear that these plans include killing her children. Here, at the end of her speech, however, it is *thumos* that is pushing her to seek vengeance (and to do what is bad/harmful, *including* above all what is bad for/harmful to herself, viz. killing her children); thus the plans to be overcome by *thumos* can, in line 1079, no longer be the specific plans for revenge she had labeled *bouleumata* before. Lloyd-Jones 1980 urges that the term is 'colourless' as a way of evading the problem, whereas Mastronarde 2002, 395 suggests that Medea may be referring to all her deliberations, 'to the entire process of internal debate carried on in the monologue, not just to the one side or the other, so that Medea is almost acknowledging an impasse between the two sides but saying that her angry spirit makes this impasse and the process of debate irrelevant.' This points to two further, large questions, which we also cannot consider here. Is Euripides interested in the phenomenon of *akrasia*—situations where a non-rational, or at any rate, a not wholly rational force (here: *thumos*) conflicts with reason and its pronouncements (about what to do), and in fact 'overcomes' them? And might he be engaging with Socrates in doing so? (See, e.g. Snell 1948, Moline 1975, Irwin 1983, and Rickert 1987.)

20   Phaedra says that 'it is not on account of the nature of our minds (*kata gnōmēs phusin*)/ that we fare (or act) badly (*prassein kakion*), since thinking well (*eu phronein*) can be

notorious examples of *akrasia*, Socrates' denial of the phenomenon 'would seem just as implausible and paradoxical in Plato's day as in our own.'[21] (And this will seem so, even if we think that Euripides presents cases of motivational conflict rather than instances of *akrasia*, strictly speaking.[22]) Indeed, Plato's readership would very likely either itself be tempted to think and say that there is such a thing as 'being overcome' (by *thumos*, or pleasure, or ...), or at least it would be wholly familiar with thinking along these lines.

Protagoras, who in his role as expert and teacher needs to distance him-self from the majority (and who may even recognize the Scylla and Charybdis he is about to navigate), wonders why they should bother considering what most people say, since they are given to saying any chance thing (353 A 7–8; cf. 352 E 3–4). By way of response, Socrates indicates that he believes this issue 'is relevant to finding out' (*pros exheurein*) about courage and its relation to the other parts of virtue (353 B 1). Thus he flags explicitly what one would have suspected in any event, namely that all this *is*, somehow, in the service of the central project of arguing against Protagoras's initial thesis that the virtues are distinct. As noted above, given various points Protagoras has been forced to

---

found/ among many people. One ought rather to look at it like this:/ what we know and understand to be good-and-useful (*chrēsta*)/ we fail to follow through on—some [of us] because of laziness, / and some [of us] because they give precedence, not to the *kalon*, / but to some other pleasure (*hēdonē*)' (377–383). This passage, too, and especially the lines following it are subject to much controversy, which we cannot address here. (See, e.g. Segal 1970, Claus 1972, Solmsen 1973, and Kovacs 1980, whose construal of *hoi d' hēdonēn prothentes anti tou kalou/ allēn tin'* in 382–383 we are following. Snell 1948 and Irwin 1983 also consider this passage in connection with Socrates and Plato.) It may, however, be worth noting that Snell 1948, 128–129, sees here an allusion not just to the Socrates of Plato's early dialogues but also to thoughts along the lines of *Memorabilia*, 3, 9, 4, where Xenophon writes: 'He [sc. Socrates] did not distinguish between wisdom (*sophia*) and moderation (*sōphrosunē*). But if someone who knows which things are beautiful and good (*kala te k'agatha*) and acts in accord with them (*chrēsthai autois*), and knowing which things are base, avoids them, then he judged (*ekrine*) him to be both wise (*sophos*) and moderate (*sōphrōn*). When asked further if he thought that those who know what they ought to do but in fact do the opposite are simultaneously wise (*sophoi*) and un-self-controlled (*akrateis*), he said: "Not at all—they rather are unwise (*asophoi*) **and** un-self-controlled; for I think that all people choose, from among the possible options facing them (*ek tōn endechomenōn*), what they believe to be most beneficial (*sumphorōtata*) for themselves. And so I consider those who act wrongly (*mē orthōs*) to be neither wise (*sophoi*) nor moderate (*sōphrones*)."' Phaedra would thus seem to allow for something Socrates rules out: according to her, a person can be wise, but fail to act rightly, i.e. in accord with that wisdom, whereas for Socrates, the failure to act rightly—i.e. acting *mē orthōs* instead—simply shows that the person so acting is *not* wise.

21   Kahn 2003, 168.

22   See e.g. Rickert 1987, for an approach to Euripides along these lines.

concede, the only part of that initial thesis that still survives is the sub-thesis that courage is distinct from the other four virtues. Hence, the focus now is on *it*, and on the relation of courage to the other four. Allowing Protagoras to maintain, for the time being, his distance from the majority on both hedonism and *akrasia*, Socrates and Protagoras proceed to argue against the commitment the many have to the phenomenon of 'being overcome'. Along the way, Protagoras will endorse hedonism and will be forced to acknowledge that his sub-thesis falls prey to the same problems as the conception of *akrasia* which the many have (this, of course, is why the subject of being overcome is introduced into the discussion).

Though matters have not been spelled out fully at this point, Socrates relies on the following idea: getting clear about the nature of courage (and its relation to the other virtues, in particular, to wisdom) requires getting clear about what is *really* going on in cases where people speak of 'being overcome' (paradigmatically, by *pleasure* but in this case by *pain*, specifically *fear*) and accordingly saying that they are doing what they know, or believe, to be the *worse* thing to do.[23] (Or, in the case of cowardice, failing to do what they know, or believe, to be the *better* thing to do.) And getting clear about that in turn requires getting clear about what they think about *pleasure*, in particular, what they think about the relation of pleasure to the *good* and the *kalon* (the honorable, or noble, or fine). How is this meant to go?

4   *Akrasia*, the Unity of the Soul, and the Structure of Motivation

A naïve, everyday conception of *akrasia* requires what one might, with Jessica Moss and others, call *motivational pluralism*:[24] the sources of a person's motivation to act (or to refrain from acting) can differ; in particular, a person's *judgment* about what is good or noble (to do) can *conflict* with what she *desires*, with what is more pleasant (to do). And if there is such a conflict, one or the

---

23   Here we bypass a debate in the literature over whether the argument is meant to conclude that *only* knowledge (and not also belief) cannot be overcome. Anti-intellectualist and unitarian interpreters, e.g. Kahn 2003, restrict the argument to knowledge, so that Socrates is not denying the possibility of conflict but avowing the sovereignty of knowledge; others who restrict the argument to knowledge include Vlastos 1969 and Dyson 1976. We take Socrates to be arguing from the stronger intellectualist thesis that no one acts against what she *believes* to be best, in agreement with Frede 1992, xxix, and Moss 2014, 289, n. 9, and 305–308; but see Kamtekar 2018 for the view that Socrates is arguing not *from* but *to* this familiar Socratic thesis.

24   See Moss 2014, 300 and *passim*.

other of the two 'elements' involved can prove 'stronger'—or, as it may happen, 'weaker.' Thus one can further suppose on behalf of the naïve view that if, in the face of, say, a tempting pleasure (which, if pursued, would lead someone to refrain from doing what she judges is best (to do)), the person none the less does act in accord with the judgment, she is then being 'strong' (*enkratic*) and has 'mastered' the temptation (the pleasure). Correspondingly, if, in the face of that tempting pleasure she actually does pursue *it* (and thus refrains from doing what she judges is best (to do)), the agent is then being 'weak' (*akratic*) and has, by contrast, 'been mastered' by the temptation (the pleasure).

Now, first and foremost, Socrates' argument against the possibility of *akrasia*—i.e. against understanding the kind of behavior just described *as being a case of* akrasia *properly speaking*—is directed against motivational pluralism: the naïve, everyday way of describing and conceptualizing *akrasia* already involves the mistake of supposing that there could be more than one source of motivation (i.e. it denies the unity of the soul). If there is only a *single* source of motivation, there obviously cannot be any motivational conflicts of the sort that (supposedly) characterize the *akratic* agent (or, for that matter, the *enkratic* one); and without such motivational conflicts, there cannot be *any* cases of 'mastering' or 'being mastered,' strictly speaking. Thus the phenomenon, i.e. bad behavior of a certain sort, and the account of it need to be re-conceptualized and re-described.[25]

At this point, the dialectical context and strategy becomes highly relevant. If we simply encountered Socrates denying motivational pluralism while people in general endorsed it (at least implicitly), we might well be faced with a standoff. What speaks in favor of Socrates' view (and any proposed re-description he might offer) as opposed to the naïve view, which, after all, is likely to be *our*

---

25   Many interpreters of Plato hold that a major reason why Plato, in the *Republic*, divides the soul into *three* parts, and thus allows for three *distinct* sources of motivation, is precisely to make room for a different description and analysis of phenomena like *akrasia*—different, that is, from what he offers in the *Protagoras*. (See e.g. Frede 1992.) Indeed, Moss 2014 takes it to be a desideratum on interpreting the *Protagoras* that we find in it the seeds of the *Republic*'s tripartite psychology. We cannot here take up this kind of developmental claim, though we are sympathetic to the idea that the *Republic* responds to and departs from strict intellectualism (but not to the idea it does so by simply rejecting the premise of hedonism and thereby, automatically, intellectualism as a whole, conceived of as dependent on Socrates' own hedonism in *Protagoras*, as Moss 2014, 288 argues). We would like to stress that one should not read *back into* the *Protagoras* the *Republic*'s tripartite psychology and the motivational pluralism associated with it. Doing so makes it impossible to understand correctly either the arguments about pleasure, pain, and *akrasia*, or the claim that knowledge can be that which is 'in charge' in a person.

view as well?[26] Given how dialectical arguments work, it would be sufficient for breaking the impasse, if Socrates could successfully show that the many—despite their overt avowal of the existence of *akrasia*—are *also* (by their own, though as yet unavowed, hedonistic lights) committed to rejecting motivational pluralism (and thus to accepting the unity of the soul). That is, for 'success' in this argument, what matters is neither Socrates' own view, nor whatever speaks in its favor; rather, what matters are the views of his interlocutors and the commitments they involve. Here, these are officially the views of the many, but it turns out that they are *also* those of Protagoras, for his views are revealed to be not as different from those of ordinary people as he would like to say they are.[27] Whether Socrates himself is committed to hedonism or not is thus wholly beside the (dialectical) point, as indeed the medical pretense at 352 A serves to remind us.[28]

If the preceding remarks are along the right lines, it means that the premise of hedonism is strictly part of the argument against motivational pluralism. In one way, it is trivially easy to see why this is so: if, in fact, *all* behavior is motivated by the desire to obtain pleasure (and to avoid pain), then we simply and straightforwardly have *motivational monism*. The difficulty will be getting 'the many' to recognize that their embrace of the possibility of *akrasia* (as they describe and conceptualize it) and their motivational pluralism turn out to be two sides of one and the same mistake.

---

26   Note that the sentiments Euripides has Medea and Phaedra expressing sound completely banal and uncontroversial: our anger, sense of pride, or fear of humiliation can interfere with, and override, our rational deliberation and planning; likewise, plenty of people know what it would be right for them to do, yet for all that fail to act in accord with their knowledge (see notes 19 and 20 above).

27   That Protagoras stands with the many (and not Socrates) on the matter of motivational pluralism is something he has already revealed—as Jessica Moss nicely argues—in his exchange with Socrates, at 349 D–351 A, where he resisted Socrates' attempt to identify courage with knowledge. In particular, Protagoras there said that confidence (*tharsos*) arises from (*apo*) skill or craft (*technē*, viz. a kind of knowledge), but also from spirit (*thumos*) and insanity (*mania*), whereas courage (*andreia*) arises from nature (*phusis*) and the proper nurture of souls (*eutrophia tōn psuchōn*). (Protagoras had agreed with Socrates that those who are courageous are confident, but he had denied that those who are confident are therefore also courageous.) Protagoras thus in effect relies on the view that a certain kind of behavior can have a variety of motivational sources. See Moss 2014, 301.

28   Socrates suggests that he wants to examine the *mind* of Protagoras in the way in which a doctor examines the *body* of a patient. That is, the focus is to be on what *Protagoras* thinks (and is committed to), not on what *Socrates* himself holds.

5   The Many (and Protagoras) on What Makes Good Pleasures Good,
         and Bad Pleasures Bad

Socrates' route into the issue is somewhat indirect. Having affirmed their commitment to the phenomenon of 'being overcome' (353 C 5–7), he asks the many on what basis (if not on the basis of being unpleasant/painful) they deem so-called bad pleasures bad, and on what basis (if not on the basis of being pleasant/not painful) they deem good pains good. More precisely, he offers the many a suggestion for what this basis is: do *they* not call certain pleasures bad, not on account of those pleasures *themselves* (i.e. not account of them *qua* pleasures, or *qua* pleasant), but rather on account of various bad consequences which result down the line, 'diseases and poverty and many other things of that sort' (353 D 2–3)? And those consequences, in turn, merit the label 'bad' 'on account of nothing other than the fact that they result in troubles/griefs (*aniai*) and deprive us of other pleasures' (353 E 5–354 A1). Correspondingly, do *they* not call certain troublesome/grievous things (*aniara*) good—e.g. harsh military training and medical procedures such as having a wound cauterized—not on account of the pain itself (i.e. not on account of these things, *qua* painful), but rather on account of their *later* bringing about 'health and good condition of bodies and preservation of cities and power over others and wealth' (354 A 1–7)? And these later results, for their part, count as good only because they lead to pleasure and to the relief from and avoidance of pain (354 B 5–7). At this point, having offered the many this diagnosis of their condition, Socrates directly asks them the following question:

> 'Or do you [sc. the many] have some other end-or-result (*telos*) in view,
> other than pleasure and pain, in regard to which you would call these
> things 'good'? They say "no," I think.'
>
> 'Nor does it seem so to me,' Protagoras said. [Protagoras here commits
> himself to hedonism, alongside the majority.]29

29   We take Protagoras to be committing himself to hedonism here along with the majority
      based on Protagoras' saying '*oute dokei*,' which signals that he is engaged with the content
      of Socrates' question to the many, saying it does not seem to him either (in agreement with
      the majority) that there is any *telos* beside pleasure and pain. If Protagoras were merely
      agreeing with Socrates that the many would say 'no,' one would expect an affirmative
      response like '*sunedokei*,' as in the previous three answers (354 A 1, A 7, B 5). With Protagoras
      agreeing here to hedonism (cf. Sullivan 1961, 23), there is no problem at 358 B 3–6 or 360
      A 2–3 when Socrates takes the thesis as given, a matter which worries C. C. W Taylor,
      who thus takes those passages as evidence of Socratic hedonism (C. C. W. Taylor 1976,
      201, 208). Indeed, commentators have found here evidence for just about every possible
      way of attributing the hedonism to one or another of the parties (Socrates, Protagoras,

'So then you [sc. the many and, implicitly, Protagoras as well] pursue pleasure as being good, and avoid pain as bad?'[30]

'Yes.' [Protagoras is officially answering on behalf of the many here, but in effect also on his own behalf.]

'So this you regard as bad: pain. And pleasure you regard as good, since you call the very enjoying of something "bad" whenever it deprives us of greater pleasures than it itself provides, or brings about greater pains than the very pleasures inherent in it? Since if you call the very enjoying of something "bad" by looking to *some other* end-or-result (*telos*) than the one I am mentioning, you could tell us what it is; but you won't be able to.'

'I [sc. Protagoras] don't think they'll be able to do so either.' (354 C 1–E 2)

Socrates is thus claiming that the practices of the many, as far as their labeling certain painful things 'good' and certain pleasant things 'bad' is concerned, *reveal* that they are relying on the thought that pleasure is good, and pain, bad.[31] Why? Because by interpreting them as relying on this thought, we can best make sense of their practices. He is also offering the many a chance to distance themselves from the very thought he imputes to them; but, he says, they will not actually be able to do so. Now, one reason they might not be able

---

and the many): A. E. Taylor 1926, 259, thinks the many are committed to hedonism, but not Socrates and Protagoras; Hackforth 1928 takes Socrates to be a hedonist, but not Protagoras or the many; Grube 1933, from the ironic perspective, denies that Protagoras is *really* committed to hedonism, but sees his inability to provide an alternative as dialectical license for Socrates to *take* him as so committed; Dyson 1976 thinks the many do not commit themselves to hedonism here, whereas Socrates and Protagoras do; C. C. W Taylor 1976, 176, 209, takes all of Socrates, Protagoras, and the many to be committed to hedonism; Irwin 1995 holds that the many are not committed to hedonism, but that Socrates is; Annas 1999, 168 finds that the many do not commit themselves to hedonism, but is agnostic about Protagoras and Socrates; Moss 2014, 290 takes Socrates and the many to be hedonists, but not Protagoras; Kamtekar 2018 thinks Protagoras is a hedonist, and that the many are ethical but not psychological hedonists.

30   Kahn 2003 finds Socrates here avowing *in propria persona* what he calls 'quasi-hedonism,' the view that pleasure is *a* good, while Protagoras misunderstands, and Socrates allows Protagoras to misunderstand, the thesis as pure hedonism, viz. the claim that pleasure is *the* good. Our view is that Socrates avows nothing *in propria persona*, just as the dialectical context would suggest, and that the relevant thesis is indeed pure hedonism and not something weaker—notwithstanding the fact that Socrates does initially state the premise in its weaker form (351 C), while Protagoras reformulates it in the stronger form (351 E).

31   See Segvic 2000, 28, 38 for the thought that one's true preferences are revealed not by the reflective opinion one expresses but by one's actions: you are what you do.

to do so is that this is in fact the correct view (and one Socrates himself holds).[32] Yet it might also be the case that they are not able to do so because *they* lack the resources for formulating an alternative account (and Socrates knows this), even though it is in principle possible to formulate such an account.[33] This would explain why Socrates proceeds with such confidence. By itself, the passage does not settle the matter. *We* would like to emphasize that the dialectical context only requires the second, weaker claim.

∴

What Socrates goes on to say next confirms that he has the dialectical context clearly in view: he stresses that the many could *still* retract their claim (about the relation between pleasure and good, and pain and bad) and stand by their commitment to the possibility of 'being overcome.' Although Socrates is addressing the many here, Protagoras' hedonism remains established and, so to speak, in the bank; it is not the dialectical focus of this portion of the discussion because Protagoras has formally denied the possibility of *akrasia*, and this will prove to be the downfall of his final sub-thesis that courage is distinct from wisdom.

> Now, again, people, if you asked me: "Why are you going on about this at such length and in so much detail?" I would reply: "Forgive me. First of all, it's not easy to show what that which you call 'being weaker than pleasure' really is; and secondly, all the demonstrations depend on this." But even now it is still open to you to retract [sc. your claim],[34] if you are able to say that the good is anything other than pleasure, or that the bad is anything other than pain. Or are you satisfied (*arkei*) to live [sc. your] life pleasantly without pains (*to hēdeōs katabiōnai ton bion aneu lupōn*)? If you are satisfied [sc. with that] and are not able to say anything else than that the good and the bad are that which result in pleasure and pain, listen to this. (354 E 4–355 A 5)

---

32   In this case, there would be no alternative to it, in some strong, literal sense of 'no alternative.' See for example Grote 1865, Hackforth 1928, Dodds 1959, Gosling and Taylor 1982, 51, 53, Irwin 1995, and Moss 2014.

33   Sullivan 1961, 27 takes the fact that Socrates here envisages an alternative to hedonism as a big knowing wink that reveals Plato to be operating on two planes: Socrates' formal endorsement of hedonism, and what he really thinks. We agree that Socrates envisages an alternative to hedonism, and that the perceptive reader is invited to notice this, but we deny both that Socrates is formally committed to any form of hedonism and, therefore, that the reader must advert to irony to understand what is 'really' being said.

34   For this meaning of *anathesthai*, see LSJ, *s.v. anatithēmi*, B. II. 2.

The 'this' which Socrates is asking them to listen to is the famous argument against the possibility of *akrasia* (as that notion is understood by the many), in 355 A 5–356 A 1. The rather tricky details of that *reductio ad absurdum*, happily, do not matter for our purposes here.[35] One thing that does matter, however, is that Socrates, in the immediate aftermath of the argument (at 356 A 5), considers an objection based on the effects of temporal distance, or, as we might say, on the question of whether one should discount (or weigh more heavily) something good (pleasant), depending on whether it is present or nearby in the immediate future, as opposed to being far off, in some more distant future. (And likewise, *mutatis mutandis*, in the case of bad (painful) things.)

6   Pleasure, Pain, and an Art of Measurement

The comments marking the transition between the basic argument against the possibility of *akrasia* and this further issue (of temporal distance and its distorting effects) are of central importance to the rest of Socrates' argument. For he suggests that one crucial effect of equating the good with pleasure, and the bad with pain, is that that this will make it easy to *quantify* good and bad (thought of as *qualitatively* homogeneous and therefore commensurable), and so to *measure* the relative excess of pleasure over pain, and vice-versa.[36] While Socrates does not say so explicitly, a significant reason for introducing hedonism thus is to pave the way for the suggestion that *akratic* behavior, in essence, results from making a cognitive *mistake*—it is a matter of taking less to be more, or more to be less.

But such an unadorned claim about measurability invites an immediate, seemingly fatal objection: if good and bad are commensurable in this way, then *how could we ever be mistaken about how pleasant or how painful things are?* In particular, is it not always clear, whenever we compare something pleasant to something painful, which one 'wins,' and why? Considerations of temporal distance allow for cases where it is fairly easy to grasp what the relevant mistake might be, and how it could arise. Far from introducing qualitative distinctness, the notion of future pleasures and pains brings out their homogeneity without sacrificing the possibility of error. Socrates proposes that temporal distance instead gives rise to a kind of perspectival distortion (much in the way that

---

35   See Wolfsdorf 2006 for extensive bibliography and a perspicuous summary of the relevant range of interpretations of that argument.

36   See the language of esp. 356 A 3–5; see also Nussbaum 1986, who takes Socrates to introduce hedonism *in propria persona*, albeit *pro tempore*, entirely for the sake of securing the art of measurement.

spatial distance does in the case of items having spatial dimensions). Thus, to take an obvious sort of example, a present or near-at-hand pain (e.g. that of a tooth being extracted, or being about to be extracted) looms much larger than do the prospects of longer-term pains (e.g. of dental decay and disease, in the future). Accordingly, in the moment of choosing or acting, the person may seek to put off this 'good' pain (good, because it will result in greater pleasure, or less pain, over the long run), because she misjudges the *quantity* of pain: it *seems* as if the short-term pain is *greater* than the longer-term pain (or, alternatively, as if the longer-term pleasures will be too *few* to make up for the present pains). Hence, there is a straightforward sense in which the *akratic* agent is *not being irrational*; she is rather weighing or measuring pains *incorrectly*.[37] Socrates is able to get Protagoras to agree, on behalf of the many, that an art of measurement would 'save' us—most immediately from such mistakes, but more generally from leading any life that is less pleasant (or more painful) than how pleasant (or painful) a life would be—if we always *measured correctly* all (available) pleasure and (avoidable) pain (356 E–357 A).[38] This in turn prepares the way for Socrates' interim conclusion: what is needed is some kind of quantitative art, that is, some kind of *knowledge* (357 B 4; cf. B 4-C 6).

∴

Having agreed that an art of measurement is needed, Socrates sets aside the inquiry into just which art this will be, in order to summarize the results they

---

37   Socrates proceeds as if what matters is *total* pleasure (and *total* pain) over the course of a person's whole life. One could easily object that this is misguided, that there should be (room for) *some* discounting/privileging based on temporal distance and/or the likelihood of various future scenarios happening (or not). But Socrates' basic argument will go through—though it would need to be complicated considerably—even if we only allow that *some* cases of privileging the present over the future are irrational, and that it *sometimes* makes good sense to forego, say, an immediate pleasure for the sake of a (pleasant) longer-term goal, or to endure immediate pain or discomfort for the sake of less pain and greater comfort in the future. If people claim they do what they 'know' they ought not to do in such cases, because they 'are overcome' (by pleasure or pain, respectively), Socrates can still say that they are misidentifying the *relevant amount* of pleasure and pain involved, and thus that their 'being overcome' really is a matter of their *incorrectly* measuring or weighing (the pleasure and pain).

38   Nussbaum 1986, 111 holds that 357 A marks the spot where Socrates endorses hedonism *pro tempore*, although his interlocutors have assumed it of him all along. For considerations against taking the passage this way, see Zeyl 1980, 256. See C. C. W. Taylor 1976, 199 (but cf. all of 194–200) for the view that Socrates' argument against *akrasia* and the measurement analogy generally fail altogether because he argues fallaciously for his own conclusions.

have reached (357 B 6–E 8). A key point Socrates stresses is that the many, prior to having heard the argument he has just presented, would have laughed-off as ridiculous his suggestion that the experience (*pathēma*) which they call 'being overcome by pleasure' is really a matter of ignorance (*amathia*). But now that they have taken on board that argument and its conclusions, were they still to laugh, they would be laughing at themselves:

> For you agreed that those who make mistakes with regard to the choice of pleasures and pains (*peri tēn tōn hēdonōn hairesin kai lupōn*)—that is, with regard to good and bad things (*tauta de estin agatha te kai kaka*)—do so because of a lack of knowledge, and not merely a lack of knowledge, but a lack of that knowledge you agreed was measurement. (357 D 3–7)

Note that the explanatory aside—'that is, with regard to good and bad things'— explains what *the many* have taken on board; it says nothing about Socrates' *own* view of the matter. And what he immediately goes on to say should give us pause before holding that it *does* reflect his own thinking:

> So this is what 'being overcome by pleasure' is—ignorance of the greatest sort, and it is of this that Protagoras, and so too Prodicus and Hippias, says he is a physician (*iatros*) [sc. one who can *cure* that ignorance]. But you [sc. the many], thinking it to be something other than ignorance, neither go to the sophists yourselves, nor do you send your children to them for instruction, believing as you do that we are dealing with something unteachable. By worrying about your money and not giving it to them, you all do badly in both private and public life. (357 E 2–8)

Taken at face value, Socrates is here saying that *if* people in general believed that what they *call* 'being overcome by pleasure' were actually ignorance, one would expect them to seek instruction. Indeed, they *ought* to do so insofar as they ought to be trying to do *something* if they think that teaching and learning will be of value. Hence, going to the sophists would at least be a start, since they do profess to teach virtue. But the many are not even doing that. This clearly shows how far *they* are from holding that what they conceive of as 'being overcome by pleasure' is really a matter of ignorance. Note that there is nothing in the passage suggesting that Socrates himself recommends going to the sophists; he merely cites the majority's *not* going as evidence of their beliefs, i.e. as *revealing* that they do not think virtue is teachable. No doubt, passages like this are laden with additional significance and nuance. For example, Socrates is in effect renewing the challenge about the teachability of virtue he had raised near the opening of the dialogue. He is thereby also raising the stakes of the discussion for Protagoras (namely, the justification of his fees and his bold embrace of the title 'sophist'). And Plato is surprising us with the dissonance that Socrates, of all people, is pressing the option of turning to the sophists in order to gain knowledge of virtue.[39] All this, however, does not mean that Socrates is being ironical or disingenuous, since he is neither endorsing nor recommending hedonism of any kind (whether explicitly or implicitly).

Now, to the extent that Socrates does think that virtue is teachable, i.e. to the extent that he has equated the virtues with wisdom, one might object that Socrates is, after all, recommending that people should seek out the sophists. Or rather, is he not, by offering this suggestion, inviting the many (and us) to think through more carefully the kind of knowledge and ignorance that would have to be involved? In other words: presumably (Plato holds that) one *cannot* learn what one needs to learn from the sophists; hence, the knowledge or wisdom in question must be something other than what the sophists (can) provide. Thus we of course concur with those interpreters who hold that Plato is engaging with the readers *of* the dialogue in a way that differs from how Socrates and his interlocutors engage with one another *within* the dialogue. But, once again, acknowledging this point does not require that one view Socrates as being insincere, or engaging in trickery—openly avowing one thing, while (covertly) intending another.

7   The Unity of the Soul and Socratic Neutrality on Hedonism

There is still, however, one further passage that may seem to tell in favor of Socrates' endorsing hedonism. At 358 A 1, he turns to Protagoras, Hippias, and Prodicus, and asks them if they agree with what he has been saying:

> 'Now, I ask you, Hippias and Prodicus, as well as Protagoras—for let this *logos* be shared by all of you—to say whether you think what I say is true or false.' They all thought that what I said was marvelously true.
> '*So you agree that the pleasant is good, the painful bad.* I beg the indulgence of Prodicus who distinguishes among words; for whether you call it 'pleasant' or 'delightful' or 'enjoyable,' or whatever way or manner you

---

39   The issue of Plato's own attitude towards the sophists is more complex than it is often thought to be. For a strong argument that he may be far less hostile than most readers have assumed, see Blank 1985. But contrast Tell 2011, for a sophisticated restatement and defense of the more traditional view.

please to name this sort of thing, my excellent Prodicus, please respond to the intent of my question.' Prodicus, laughing, agreed, as did the others.

'Well, then, men, what about this? *Are not all actions leading toward living painlessly and pleasantly honorable?*[40] *And isn't honorable activity good and beneficial?*' They agreed. (358 A 1–B 6)[41]

In reporting how he addressed Prodicus and Hippias together with Protagoras, Socrates signals a return to the outer frame (viz. to the question Socrates had posed on Hippocrates' behalf). That is, the remark 'They all thought that what I said was marvelously true' is addressed to the unnamed friend from 309 A–310 A. It turns out that all these sophists agree with each other, and with ordinary people: hedonism holds, as a descriptive thesis. And if it holds as a descriptive thesis—or rather, if no intelligible alternative to it is on offer—then we can in addition ascribe to the sophists and to the many the following *quasi-prescriptive* claim: it is reasonable for a person who in fact acts as if pleasure is the good (and who offers no alternative besides pleasure as to what the good is) also to hold that she *ought to* pursue pleasure as the good.[42] Socrates here need be committed only to the relationships among the several claims, not to the core claim itself.[43]

Secondly, *if* hedonism holds, *then* there is no such thing as 'being overcome by pleasure,' Socrates can endorse this conditional without committing himself to the truth of the antecedent. In fact, in the context of motivational monism, one could substitute anything else (of a sort suited to a similar functional role) for pleasure, and the conditional would, *mutatis mutandis*, still be true. This

---

40   Deleting *kai ōphelimoi* in 358 B 5, with Schleiermacher; cf. Burnet 1903, *ap. crit. ad loc.*

41   This is yet another passage where some commentators locate Socratic hedonism, e.g. Kahn 2003 finds Socrates committing himself to the weaker and thus more palatable thesis that pleasure is *a* good; C. C. W. Taylor 1976, *ad loc.* finds Socrates, but somehow not Protagoras, being committed to hedonism. Those who find the majority and Protagoras represented here, as well as Socrates, include Grube 1933, Sullivan 1961, 23, and Zeyl 1980, 257, all of whom take Socrates' formal commitment as ironic, fallacious, or disingenuous, and who justify his moves by reference to the sophists' own moral shortcomings (so they deserve it), to the purity of his motives (so it is for their own good), or to the nature of the *elenchus* (so that is just how the (dialectical) cookie crumbles).

42   We are grateful to Matt Evans for discussion of this point.

43   Thus we have bypassed debates over the precise kind of hedonism in play, whether psychological, evaluative or prescriptive (see n. 5, above). We suspect that Gosling and Taylor 1982 are right that the psychological and evaluative thesis are one and the same for Plato, but we are also sympathetic to the prescriptive claims made by Dyson 1976 and Zeyl 1980, and to the evaluative claims made by Sullivan 1961 and Moss 2014; we disagree with C. C. W. Taylor 1976, 189–190, who thinks that 356 A 8–C 3 expresses evaluative but not descriptive hedonism.

fact helps shed light on the point of introducing hedonism at all: it serves as an *illustration*, and a particularly vivid and easy-to-grasp one at that, of motivational monism. For *any* monist, 'being overcome' will turn out to be ignorance. Hence, *a fortiori*, for a hedonist 'being overcome' just is ignorance. Or rather, by seeing how and why for someone who accepts hedonism, 'being overcome' is really a matter of ignorance, we can see how it would likewise be a matter of ignorance for anyone who accepts a structurally similar view. *This* is a point Socrates endorses; but it is one he can cheerfully endorse without taking any stance on the question of whether or not hedonism is true. And such indeed is the summary Socrates presents at 358 C:

> 'Then if the pleasant is the good, no one who knows or believes there is something else better than what he is doing, something possible, would then do what he is doing when he could be doing what is better. This being overcome by oneself (*to hēttō einai hautou*) is nothing other than ignorance, and to control oneself (*kreittō heautou*) is nothing other than wisdom.' It seemed so to all. (358 B 6–C 2)

What Socrates agrees to here, as one of the 'all,' is again explicitly conditional:

> *If* the pleasant is good,
> *then* (i) *akrasia* is impossible,
> *and* therefore, (ii) the phenomenon that people call 'being overcome' is better understood as ignorance (sc. of the art of measurement).[44]

Now, one might still worry that Socrates' commitment to the consequent of the conditional strongly suggests that he is committed to the antecedent as well, even if this does not strictly follow.[45] However, the dialectical context shows that the argument is designed to persuade the *majority* that it is *their* commitment to hedonism that reduces *akrasia* to absurdity and thus forces the phenomenon of 'being overcome' to be re-conceptualized as ignorance. Recall that at 355 A Socrates makes this explicit, offering the majority the chance to retract their hedonism or be subject to the *reductio* that follows.

More importantly: it is open to Socrates to endorse the entire conditional as well as the consequent, while continuing to reject the antecedent, because the truth of the conditional is secured by the fact that hedonism can be understood

---

44   Note that, *contra* Vlastos 1969 and Shaw 2015, this shows that hedonism really does play a
        role in the overall argument.
45   As e.g. Hackforth 1928, 42 and so many others hold.

as *an arbitrary instance of motivational monism*. Thus it is not the truth of hedonism *specifically* that secures the truth of the consequent—that *akrasia* is impossible and 'being overcome' is really a matter of ignorance. Rather, it is the truth of motivational monism *generically* that entails the familiar Socratic thesis that no one errs willingly. If there is only *one* good for which we aim, then—*whatever it turns out to be*—there can be no motivational conflict, and doing the 'wrong' things must always be due to ignorance. To be sure, hedonism is not a haphazardly chosen instance of monism. The thesis is, after all, diagnostic of the *actual* values and beliefs of the many and the sophists. Again, however, the work that it does in securing the consequent is *not* a function of hedonism specifically, but of its being the instance of the monism that the many reveal themselves as being committed to.[46]

Pleasure, therefore, proves to be an excellent placeholder for the good: it makes for, first of all, a *bona fide* species of motivational monism (albeit one that is, in reality, *false* as a description of human motivation); hence, it secures the truth of the conditional and consequent.[47] Secondly, the hedonist thesis amounts to a diagnosis of conventional morality, so it is dialectically well suited for engaging with the majority, as the frame requires. Thirdly, for the same reason, it is dialectically suited to Protagoras as well. And, finally, Socrates (and Plato) may well think that pleasure is genuinely worth considering as a *candidate* for the good.[48] But Socrates need not be endorsing hedonism in order to

---

46   We are thus in substantial agreement with Moss 2014 concerning motivational monism, with the crucial exception of how to construe Socrates' (use of) hedonism. Moss takes Socrates to posit and endorse hedonism in order to *secure* the monism and thus 'save' his account from attack (note that the dialectical context speaks against this saving aspect of the reconstruction, as it would place Socrates in the defensive position of arguing *for* something—a task for the answerer, not the questioner). We, on the other hand, take Socrates to be working *from* motivational monism, selecting hedonism as the instance relevant to his interlocutors, in order to generate the *reductio* of *akrasia*. But he could presumably just as well have selected a monistic commitment to honor or to knowledge in, say, addressing Aristotle's 'better' classes of person mentioned above in our preliminary remarks, as a way of closing off the threat of the divided soul, as Moss puts it.

47   *Contra* Gosling and Taylor 1982, 53–54, who take it that the falsity of the premise would yield no support for the consequent. Note that the respect in which we take hedonism as a placeholder is not the same sense in which Nussbaum 1986 and Rowe 2003 do, since they understand Socrates as endorsing hedonism *in propria persona*, even if only *pro tempore* or as a stalking horse for the good. We thus take the argument to depend on hedonism to the extent that *akrasia* is understood as a matter of being overcome by *pleasure* (and cowardice as a matter of being overcome by *pain*), but we do not take it that the denial of motivational conflict rests on hedonism specifically. Thus we disagree (twice over) with those who have sought to deal with Socrates' apparent hedonism by divorcing the argument from it, e.g. Vlastos 1969 and Shaw 2015.

48   As Grube 1933, 206, n. 3 has urged.

bring it to bear on his interlocutors, nor need he be ironic or disingenuous in saying that he takes the thesis seriously.

8   Hedonism and the Relation of Courage to the Other Virtues

The next phase of Socrates' argument secures the sub-thesis introduced at 349 E: that courage, too, is to be identified with the other four virtues, and with wisdom in particular. Having agreed with the sophists on the truth of the conditional (as stated above), and having agreed, further, to the claim that ignorance is 'to hold a false belief and to be deceived about matters of great importance' (358 C 3–5), Socrates next secures joint agreement to the descriptive thesis that 'no one willingly goes toward bad things or what they believe to be bad' (358 C 6–D 4). With the final premise that 'fear is the expectation of something bad' (358 D 5–E 1) in place, Socrates is at last in a position to draw the inferences required to establish that courage is wisdom. If no one goes toward what is bad, and if fear just is the expectation of something bad, then it follows that no one goes toward (or faces) what they fear—but going towards (or facing) what one fears, of course, *would have been* Protagoras' majority-style definition of courage. Indeed, as A. E. Taylor points out, on the conception of courage the many have, courage in fact *is* irrational, for it amounts to overcoming fear so as to go willingly toward what you *know* to be bad for you and thus have *good reason* to avoid.[49]

Here, again, the remaining mechanics of the argument do not matter to our central point. What is salient is that Socrates has established that, by Protagoras' own lights as a hedonist, the motivational pluralism underwriting his initial thesis of the virtues as distinct and separable is false. The conventional definition of courage as mastering one's fear, just like the naïve description of *akrasia* as being mastered by pleasure (or by *thumos*, pain, fear, erotic passion, or ...), rests on the mistaken assumption that there is, or could be, more than one source of motivation. In fact, it is precisely because the virtues are usually thought of in terms of motivational pluralism (as Protagoras urges in resisting Socrates' first argument for the identity of courage and wisdom) that, according to popular Greek thought, they are as likely to be the source of our downfall as of our salvation. Medea is destroyed by an excess of *thumos*. Phaedra, having first been overcome by pleasure, succumbs to an excess of shame. In addition, we might note that Hector is seen as having been destroyed by an excess of courage, in his case as well arising from *thumos* and a sense of shame (see

---

49   A. E. Taylor 1926, 249, n. 1.

Iliad 6, 441–445; cf. Andromache's remark about Hector's great strength being his undoing at 6, 407). But these diagnoses are mistaken: for whatever, exactly, the good turns out to be, success in life will be a function of measure; and *virtue*, since it is *ex hypothesi* a matter of getting things right, *cannot be subject to excess*. Thus Hector does not suffer from an excess of strength or courage; rather, he wrongly values the glory of battle.[50] Phaedra is not succumbing to an excess of shame, but is rather failing to understand correctly what her good is. And Medea's vengeance is not a case of being overcome by *thumos*, but of wrongly valuing honor more than her children.

∴

We are now prepared to specify the role of hedonism in establishing the identity of courage and wisdom. We suggested earlier that one crucial effect of equating the good with pleasure, and the bad with pain, is that this makes it easy (at least *in principle*, or so Socrates seems to think) to *quantify* good and bad, and thus also to *measure* the relative excess of pleasure over pain, or vice versa—which in turn paves the way for reconceiving *akrasia* as an error in measurement; that is, any supposed *akrasia* proves to be a wholly *cognitive* matter. Now, in the case of courage, hedonism makes it easy (again, at least in principle) to quantify *fear* as a kind of pain: the coward, by measuring wrongly, arrives at the result that the pain of standing one's ground exceeds the pain of fleeing; the brave person, by measuring correctly, arrives at the opposite result. Accordingly, courage has now been reconceived, in intellectualist terms, as cognitive success—a matter of *knowing* what is and is not to be feared—rather

---

50   At *Iliad* 7, 67–91 Hector fantasizes that the tomb (*sēma* and *tumbos*) at the mouth of the Hellespont of a Greek warrior (whom, after having challenged him to single combat (cf. *Il.* 7, 49–51 and 73–75), he will kill) will serve, for future generations, to inscribe on the landscape his own glory, and so to enhance it: "'This is the tomb (*sēma*) of a man who died long ago, / who was performing his *aristeia* when illustrious (*phaidimos*) Hector killed him.'/ That is what someone will say, *and my kleos will never perish*' (87–91, trans. Nagy 1979, 28). Finkelberg 2002 argues that this is a reference to the tomb of Protesilaos, on the Thracian side of the Hellespont. But Nagy 1979, 28–29 and 341 considers a more intriguing possibility, based on his conviction that 'the traditions of the *Iliad* and the *Odyssey* constitute a totality with the complementary distribution of their narratives' (21), namely that Hector's words are deeply ironical here and would be so heard by the epics' traditional audience. For at *Odyssey* 24, 72–84, we learn that the Greeks built the *final* tomb (*tumbos*, 80) for Patroclus *and Achilles* at the mouth of the Hellespont (cf. *Il.* 23, 243–257, esp. 245–246)—thus in the tradition, it is actually Achilles' tomb (*tumbos*) that will be a beacon to future generations (cf. *Od.* 24, 83–84), and it is a marker (*sēma*) of his *kleos* at exactly the spot where Hector, delusionally, imagined that his own *kleos*, having been made 'concrete' in the tomb of an *unnamed* Greek warrior, would be immortalized.

than as the ability to master a conflicting motivation. Courage thus turns out to be wisdom after all. One major consequence we can draw is that Protagoras must be ignorant of *how* to teach virtue, since he seems not to know *what* virtue is. Furthermore, according to Protagoras' definition of courage as mastery, it could not even *be* something teachable, precisely because mastery is *not* a cognitive achievement, and precisely because on such an account, which allows for the possibility of *akrasia*, knowledge is construed as something that does *not* 'rule' in a person's soul (as Hector, Medea, and Phaedra illustrate so vividly). Socrates introduces hedonism *en route* to arguing for the unity of courage with the other four virtues, and, as we have seen, he uses it as a way of identifying virtue with knowledge *because* hedonism is an instance of motivational monism and *because* pleasure is a prima facie very plausible candidate for a single source of motivation.

We can say, further, that Socrates introduces hedonism at exactly the point where he does, because Protagoras evinces a commitment to motivational pluralism in replying to Socrates' first argument (349 E–350 C) for the identity of courage and wisdom. Protagoras had resisted Socrates' conclusion by maintaining that '*confidence* (*tharsos*), like power, comes from skill (and from passionate emotion as well); *courage* (*andreia*) [comes] from nature and the proper nurture of soul' (351 A 7–B 2). This means that someone could be confident as a result of emotion, *without knowledge*, and fail to be courageous. If Socrates can show Protagoras, via hedonism, that emotion (so construed) is *never* a motivator, he will then have secured the premise that Protagoras resists in the first argument, namely that the confident are courageous. And this is exactly what he proceeds to do: hedonism, as an arbitrary instance of motivational monism, secures the consequent—that *akrasia* is impossible, and that 'being overcome' is actually ignorance (sc. of the art of measurement). Though he does not make this point explicitly, Socrates has thereby shown that confidence can, after all, be achieved *only* by knowledge, *not* by other means, like emotion.[51] And having established motivational monism, Socrates can return to identify courage and wisdom, just as originally proposed. To be sure, he does not pick up the structure of the original argument (nor does the second argument for the identity of courage and wisdom (359 A–360 E) proceed by the same means), but he now has the resources to do so if he wants to. As it is, by the end of the second argument Protagoras is no longer fighting back (360 E).

---

51   That he conceives of the art of measurement as yielding confidence can be seen when he says it 'would make appearance powerless (*akuron*) by showing us the truth, would give us peace of mind (*hēsuchia*) firmly rooted in the truth, and would be the salvation of life' (356 D 7–E 2).

9   Final Remarks

In closing, we should again recall that after Socrates has 'established' hedonism, the many ask him, 'Why are you going on about this at such length and in so much detail?' He replies that 'all the demonstrations depend on this (viz. hedonism)' (354 E). We can now see *how* this is so. The demonstration of the sub-thesis that courage is not distinct from the other virtues depends on hedonism to convince Protagoras and the many of the consequences of motivational monism. The teachability of virtue also follows from hedonism, since the art of measurement, as a kind of knowledge, is presumed to be teachable. However, the teachability of virtue follows from everything that Protagoras was at pains to *deny*, starting with hedonism. Hence, the implied negative answer to the question (from much earlier in the dialogue) of whether or not Hippocrates should seek Protagoras' tutelage, also depends on hedonism. This is so twice over: first, the role hedonism plays in the argument shows Protagoras does not know what he is talking about when he talks about virtue (and therefore presumably is unable teach it); and second in that Protagoras' own initial reluctance to agree to hedonism, especially when it is put so baldly, reflects the express views of the conventional majority—few Athenian families would be willing to pay large fees for their young men to learn the art of measuring pleasures!

The merits of our account, we submit, are that there is no need to find Socrates espousing hedonism, nor is there any need to puzzle over why Socrates argues from premises that are false by his lights to a conclusion he endorses. Our reading not only does no violence to the text, it simplifies the interpretative process by consistently taking Socrates at face value. By the letter of the text, Socrates at no point endorses hedonism *in propria persona*; and the dialectical context makes it clear that the offensive premise is introduced as a diagnosis of conventional psychology and morality, so there is also no need to engage in subtle machinations in order to isolate a palatable thesis weaker than pure hedonism to attribute to Socrates. By the same token, there is no need to take a stand on whether the *Protagoras* represents the historical Socrates, the character Socrates as Plato's pawn but not mouthpiece, or the character Socrates as Plato's *alter ego*. In addition, our thesis is wholly neutral on questions of Plato's development (and where, in that development, to locate the *Protagoras*), having shown that the *Protagoras* is no longer anomalous in ways that have exercised commentators for so long. If we are right, the dialogue is not only not anomalous, but can be seen as setting out the motivational monism that lies at the heart of Socrates' intellectualism. Of course, to the extent that one regards the *Republic* as introducing motivational pluralism and thus as retreating from strict intellectualism, our account is wholly compatible with, though does not in all details require, a familiar developmental narrative: the *Republic* is later than the *Protagoras*, and in it Plato offers a more complicated moral psychology (the tripartition of the soul) so as to be able to offer a 'more realistic' account of motivational conflict in general, and of *akrasia* in particular.

Further, Socrates can legitimately argue from a (false) premise he does not endorse, to a (true) conclusion he accepts, not only because hedonism is true for his interlocutors, but also because, as an instance of monism, it has a structure that entails the impossibility of motivational conflict. That the many and Protagoras need to be brought around from behind their false moralizing talk of 'bad pleasures' and 'good pains' does not at all undermine their (unvoiced) commitment to hedonism. It rather underlines the incoherence of their unreflective views: the actions of the many reveal their (unavowed) commitment to the premise, and give lie to the conventional pieties they do avow. Thus neither is there any need to accuse Socrates, 'Socrates,' or Plato of confusion, disingenuousness, or fallacy—our interpretation is in this regard maximally charitable. Nor, likewise, is there any need to introduce irony or subterfuge in order to understand the 'true' meaning that Plato wishes to convey—our interpretation is maximally simple. Nevertheless, the *Protagoras* is exceptionally rich in its multiple frames, layers of engagement, and the tangled web that its title character weaves, so that the simplicity of our interpretation on this one point (the role of pleasure and pain in the work) leaves ample room for conversations between Plato himself and perceptive readers. Indeed, we believe our analysis has cleared out interpretative clutter for the sake of clarity in the ongoing dialogue with Plato.*

---

*   In the course of working on this material—beginning in 2012, in connection with several sessions of the New York Colloquium in Ancient Philosophy devoted to the *Protagoras*—we have incurred several debts of gratitude which we are pleased to acknowledge here. Jessica Moss very kindly sent us a copy of her paper (Moss 2014) prior to its publication, at an early stage of our joint thinking about the dialogue; and while we disagree with her on the matter of Socrates' hedonism, we have learned much from her discussion and framing of the issues. The 2015 conference at Columbia provided us with a wonderful opportunity to present an ancestor of this paper; we are grateful to the participants for their provocative questions and challenging objections. Very special thanks also to Kate Meng Brassel for taking the time to write up her very helpful comments on the penultimate version our paper. (W.-R. M. would like in addition to thank Elizabeth Scharffenberger for ongoing conversations about Plato and the *Protagoras* over a span of, by now, many years.)

CHAPTER 8

Lucretian Pleasure

Elizabeth Asmis

Epicurean hedonism has always been much reviled. Epicurus' follower, Lucretius, tried his best to defend it, but he incurred a special opprobrium. In the prologue to book 2 of his poem, he gives a description of what has been called 'Lucretian pleasure'. This is the pleasure of gloating over the miseries of others, or *epichairekakia* (*Schadenfreude*). Here is the passage (2.1–13):

> Suave, mari magno turbantibus aequora ventis
> e terra magnum alterius spectare laborem;
> non quia vexari quemquamst iucunda voluptas,
> sed quibus ipse malis careas quia cernere suavest.
> suave etiam belli certamina magna tueri
> per campos instructa tua sine parte pericli;
> sed nihil dulcius est, bene quam munita tenere
> edita doctrina sapientum templa serena,
> despicere unde queas alios passimque videre
> errare atque viam palantis quaerere vitae,
> certare ingenio, contendere nobilitate,
> noctes atque dies niti praestante labore
> ad summas emergere opes rerumque potiri.

It is sweet, when the winds are buffeting the water on the great sea, to gaze from the land on the great toil of another; not because it is a sweet pleasure that anyone should be distressed, but because it is sweet to perceive from what evils you yourself are free. Sweet it is, too, to behold great contests of war marshaled over the plains, when you have no part in the danger. But nothing is more pleasant than to occupy the serene temples, well fortified, that have been erected by the teachings of the wise, from where one may look down on others and see them stray at random and seek a path of life in their wanderings, striving with their talents, contending in nobility of birth, day and night struggling with exceeding toil to reach the height of wealth and have power over affairs.

DOI:10.1163/9789004379503_009

Using the literary form of a priamel, Lucretius first cites two examples of what is pleasant, then presents a climax. The first two examples are traditional.[1] The third tops these examples with a depiction of the goal of life: nothing is more pleasant than to occupy the heights of wisdom, from which one can look down on the aimless wanderings of others.

This description has disturbed many readers. Is Lucretius introducing malice into the Epicurean goal of pleasure? Here are two modern responses, both tinged with amusement. The first is from an essay entitled 'The Superannuated Man' by Charles Lamb, written in 1825:

> I can interrupt the man of much occupation when he is busiest. I can insult over him with an invitation to take a day's pleasure with me to Windsor this fine May-morning. It is Lucretian pleasure to behold the poor drudges, whom I have left behind in the world, carking and caring; like horses in a mill, drudging on in the small eternal round—and what is it all for?[2]

Retired from the drudgery of working in the city, Lamb calls it 'Lucretian pleasure' to spend a delightful day in Windsor, mindful of others toiling at their jobs. He gloats about inviting one of these drudges to join him. In a more recent version, John Betjeman strips away the misery of others. His poem 'Summoned by Bells', published in 1960, includes a section entitled 'Lucretian Pleasure in a hot bath'. The relevant lines are as follows:

> Luxuriating backwards in the bath,
> I swish the warmer water round my leg
> Towards my shoulders, and the waves of heat
> Bring those five years of Marlborough through to me,
> In comfortable retrospect: 'Thank God
> I'll never have to go through them again'.[3]

Betjeman spent five unhappy years at Marlborough College, an elite boarding school, prior to going to Oxford at the age of 19. Aided by the pleasure of a hot bath, he takes comfort in his own escape from misery.

It is one thing to be relieved from one's misery, another to look on the misery of others. Lucretius' wise person does look upon the struggles of others. How

---

1   See Fowler 2002, 28–33 and 44–45.

2   Lamb 1895 [1825], 80–81. I owe the reference to Catherine Mardikes.

3   Betjeman 1960, 63 and 65. The passage is cited in Fowler 2002, 39 n. 3.

offensive is his pleasure? We may note, first of all, that Lucretius addresses this question immediately after introducing his first example in the first two lines of the prologue (2.3–4): it is not the case, he explains, that we take pleasure in the miseries of others; what delights us is our own freedom from misery. Further, Lucretius immediately follows up the priamel with an expression of pity for those who are trapped in misery. This section begins as follows (2.14–19):

> o miseras hominum mentes, o pectora caeca!
> qualibus in tenebris vitae quantisque periclis
> degitur hoc aevi quod cumquest! nonne videre
> nihil aliud sibi naturam latrare, nisi ut qui
> corpore seiunctus dolor absit, mente fruatur
> iucundo sensu cura semota metuque?

> Oh, miserable minds of men, blind hearts! In what darkness of life, in what great dangers, you spend this little span of years. To think that you should not see that nature cries out for nothing than that pain should be absent from the body, and that it should enjoy a mind with a feeling of pleasure, removed from care and fear?

Finally, Lucretius concludes his entire prologue by comparing the misery and blindness of humans to that of children terrorized by the darkness (2.55–61). He has pity for those who have not yet found a way as though they were children.

Despite the initial disclaimer and subsequent expression of pity, however, the lines tend to dismay even the most sympathetic readers. Cyril Bailey observes that they leave 'almost all readers' with 'an unpleasant taste of egoism and even of cruelty'. He imputes an 'almost cynical pleasure' to 'the Epicurean philosopher, secure in his own independence, gazing on the troubles and struggles of his fellow-men'; and he thinks that the lines cannot be 'wholly defended'.[4] Some readers defend Lucretius by taking him at his word. Philip Mitsis, for example, notes that the pleasure is none other than that of perceiving one's own freedom from suffering.[5] Nonetheless, one might object that, by positioning the wise man above others, Lucretius allows a feeling of contempt to seep into the attitude of the wise person. It is difficult, in any case, to separate out pity from contempt. By juxtaposing the pleasure of enlightenment with the misery of the unenlightened, Lucretius lays himself open to the charge of sullying the pleasure of the wise person.

---

4 Bailey 1947, II, 797.
5 Mitsis 1988, 82 n. 54.

I doubt whether the priamel can be defended 'wholly'. Yet I think that more can be said in defense of Lucretius. What I shall attempt to do here is to strengthen Lucretius' own disclaimer by putting the priamel in a pedagogic context. As I shall argue, the prologue to book 2 is a stage in a journey to enlightenment. Lucretius carefully crafts this journey by means of his prologues. At the beginning of book 1, Lucretius shows the reader that he needs to raise himself from the mass of humans who are downtrodden by fear of the gods. At the end of book 1, the reader has had a rigorous course of instruction on basic atomic theory. At this point, as Lucretius moves on to book 2, he offers an interlude, designed to motivate the student to continue his course of studies by offering him a glimpse of his goal. He now sets out for the first time the Epicurean goal of pleasure, whose height consists of freedom from pain. As presented by Lucretius, this is the pleasure of one who has found his way, through great personal effort, to escape from a condition that still besets others. Later, Lucretius will focus entirely on the student's own inner condition, without reference to others. This is the aim of the journey; and it is entirely independent of the state of progress of anyone else.

1   Getting Started

As a follower of Epicurus, Lucretius has a very different relationship to his reader than Epicurus has to his reader. Epicurus is the discoverer who seeks to impart his teachings to others. Lucretius is the convert who attempts to convert others just as he was previously converted. As an intermediary between Epicurus and his Roman audience, Lucretius does not simply pass on Epicurus' teachings just as Epicurus set them out. Even though he proclaims himself a totally faithful follower, what he passes on is his own understanding, framed into a journey of conversion.[6] Lucretius announces this journey in refrain that recurs four times throughout the poem as a kind of leitmotif:

> This terror and darkness of the mind must be dispelled, not by the rays of the sun and the luminous shafts of daylight, but by contemplation and reasoning about nature (*naturae species ratioque*).[7]

Lucretius announces a course of instruction on 'nature', or physics; but his physics is continuously intertwined with ethics. Throughout his poem, Lucretius

---

6   I develop these points further in an article in *Hermes* (Asmis 2017).

7   1.146–48, 2.59–61, 3.91–93 and 6.39–41.

fits his physical instruction within an ethical framework; the goal is not merely knowledge, but escape from misery. There is a continual tension between looking forward and backward. The reason is that one gets to the goal by putting misery behind and, having put it behind, keeping it away.

This much is commonly accepted. Where there is disagreement is on the details of the journey. As I have argued elsewhere,[8] Lucretius first leads the student to an initiation described in the prologue to book 3. The initiation consists in a revelation of what goes on in the universe as a whole. This revelation is then followed by further instruction, showing the human being his place in the world. This additional instruction, which continues to the end of the poem, is divided into two main parts: two books (3 and 4) on the nature of man and two books (5 and 6) on the relationship of the human being to the world in which he is situated. In this paper, I shall focus on the first part of the journey, culminating in the initiation, as the context in which 'Lucretian pleasure' is embedded. Just like the poem as a whole, this first part presents three main kinds of pleasure: the pleasure of the poet; the pleasure of poetry; and the pleasure of enlightenment. The first two kinds serve as a means of leading the student to his goal, the pleasure of enlightenment. Whereas the pleasures of the poet and poetry suffuse the text from beginning to end, the pleasure of enlightenment develops only gradually for the student. Lucretius first offers the student a preview of this pleasure in the prologue to book 2, then transforms it into a present experience of ecstasy in the prologue to book 3.

2   The Pleasures of the Poem

Most readers would agree, I think, that there is nothing more joyous in all of Lucretius' poem than his exultation as a poet. Inspired by love of the Muses, he sees himself roaming untrodden meadows, as he takes pleasure (as emphasized by the repetition of *iuvat* at 1.927–28) in drinking from untouched springs and plucking 'new flowers'. These flowers are his own poetry. He gives two reasons for his pleasure: one is that he teaches about great things and seeks to free people from the bonds of religion; the other is that he composes such 'luminous' (*lucida*, 1.933) verses about an abstruse subject matter.

His first reason concerns the subject matter of his poem; the second concerns the verbal form of his exposition. In the first respect, he follows Epicurus; in the second, he does something new. Epicurus wrote in prose and, it appears, rejected poetry as a means of teaching philosophy on the ground that it does

---

8   Asmis 2017.

not have sufficient clarity.[9] Lucretius offers an implicit defense for his use of poetic form: he writes 'luminous' (*lucida*) verses about an abstruse subject matter.[10] His verses, he claims, have the clarity of bringing Epicurus' doctrines to light. In this claim, he is in no way faulting Epicurus' writings for lacking clarity; far from it. Rather, he has in mind the receptivity of the hearer. He hopes that, just like honey smeared on a cup of bitter medicine, his use of poetry will induce the Romans, most of whom (that is the meaning of *vulgus* in line 1.945) recoil from philosophy as something abstruse, to become familiar with it. Poetry sheds light on a subject matter that would otherwise remain hidden from his Roman audience.

Using a traditional trope, Lucretius says that what inspires him is love of the Muses. On a deeper level, what inspires him is his love of Epicurus. Lucretius speaks of this love in the prologue to book 3. As author, Lucretius here stakes out a position of his own in relation to a predecessor: he does not emulate, but imitates Epicurus out of 'love' for him, like a swallow in relation to a swan, or a trembling young goat in relation to a valiant steed (3.5–8). In case anyone might think that he is trying to outdo Epicurus through his use of poetry, Lucretius declares his reverence for Epicurus' 'golden sayings' (with repetition of 'golden', *aurea*, at 3.12–13), which he says are 'most worthy of everlasting life'. We cull these flowers, Lucretius says, in the manner of bees. The real flowers are the sayings of Epicurus. Lucretius' 'new flowers' are but a feeble imitation, seeking to make Epicurus' discoveries accessible to the Romans through the use of poetry.

Lucretius speaks to his reader with a twofold pleasure: that of his own enlightenment by Epicurus, and that of composing poetry for the enlightenment of others. The reader shares in Lucretius' love of poetry; but to attain enlightenment, much more is needed. The reader must himself come to a recognition of the truth of Epicurus' pronouncements. For this purpose, it is not enough to have the doctrines laid out in luminous verses; the verses must illuminate his mind through his own efforts. Lucretius has, indeed a lofty goal. He compares himself to a doctor who smears the rim of a cup with honey in order to fool the sick child into drinking the bitter medicine, so that the child may 'gain health (*valescat*), restored (*recreata*) in this way' (1.942). In the same way, he proposes to use the honey of poetry 'in case I can keep your mind in this way on my verses, while you obtain a full view (*perspicis*) of how the nature of things is arranged' (1.948–50). The reader is to be captivated, not captured

---

9   See Asmis 1995 [1991], 21–22.
10   There is a voluminous literature on Lucretius' use of poetry, including his use of the term *lucida*; see esp. Classen, 1968, 99–117, Milanese 1989, and Gale 1994, 38–55.

(*deceptaque non capiatur*, 1.941), into giving attention to verses, so that he can obtain a full view of nature.

The process of philosophical healing, however, is not as simple as this. Paying attention to verses gives one a view of Epicurean doctrine; but mere inspection is not enough. As implied by Lucretius' repeated use of the phrase *naturae species ratioque*, contemplation entails argument; to really see how things are arranged, the reader must use his own powers of reasoning. Mental healing is not merely a matter of absorbing doctrines, like so many drugs. One might indeed be deluded by Lucretius' own comparison to the doctor into supposing so. But Lucretius himself makes clear throughout his poem that he does not think so. The verb *perspicis*, it turns out, has a double meaning: seeing and understanding. The recipe Lucretius offers in his medical analogy is something of a shortcut: it needs to be supplemented by the hard work of thinking out the argument for oneself.

As Diskin Clay has pointed out, Lucretius emphasizes throughout his poem that the student must recognize the truth for himself.[11] Like a hound on the tracks of a wild animal, the student is to 'see yourself by yourself (*per te tute ipse videre*) one thing after another' by 'winding your way into all the dark hiding-places and dragging forth the truth from there' (1.404–9). Lucretius calls upon the student to 'weigh fully' the arguments 'with astute judgment' as well as 'gird himself' against falsehoods (2.1040–3). Even though one has been imbued with false beliefs from childhood, this is no excuse for clinging to them. Thus Lucretius blames the student for 'deciding' wrongly 'yourself for yourself' (*tute tibi ... constitues*) that the gods are subject to anger (6.73–74). False beliefs are not only deeply entrenched; but there is the added difficulty that we delude ourselves into thinking that we have already got rid of them. We wear a mask (3.58), which is torn off in conditions of extreme stress.

3   Getting to the Top

Lucretius starts the journey with an image of extreme oppression: humans were trod underfoot by the monster of religion looming in the sky. Simultaneously, he shows a path to salvation: the monster was defeated by a new kind of hero, a Greek mortal, who broke through the walls of the world.

---

11   Clay 1983, 225; cf. Classen 1968, 95–100. For further details, see Asmis 2017. In contrast, Mitsis 1993, followed by Volk (2002, 80–81), has argued that Lucretius takes an authoritarian, condescending attitude to the reader, as though he were a stupid child rather than an equal. On the image of the child, see further below.

After traveling throughout the universe and discovering all there is, he came back to report his discoveries to mankind. As a result, the initial condition of mankind is reversed: religion is now trod underfoot and humans are raised to the sky (1.62–79).

From this starting-point, Lucretius devotes the first two books to taking the reader on the same journey beyond the walls of the world. In the first book, he sets out the constituents of the universe; in the second, he shows how they create all things. The conclusion, stated near the end of book 2, is:

> If you know this well and hold on to it, nature is seen right away free, rid of proud masters, doing all things spontaneously itself by itself, without any share by the gods.[12]

Meanwhile, however, Lucretius has surprised the reader with a prologue to book 2 that seems to have nothing to do with the content of the two books. He begins book 2 with a short course in ethics, preceded by the priamel that we have seen. What is the point?

By the time the reader gets to book 2, Lucretius has said nothing yet about the type of life that humans will lead as a result of Epicurus' victory over religion. Humans are raised to the sky. But what will this life be like? After addressing Venus in the first line of the poem as the 'pleasure of humans and gods' (*hominum divumque voluptas*), Lucretius associated her with the pleasures of procreation, of poetry, and of peace. But he has said nothing about the type of pleasure that humans will enjoy when freed from religious oppression. Instead, he turned his attention to the horrors of religious oppression, as illustrated by the slaughter of Iphigeneia. There followed a weighty course of instruction, presenting a relentless sequence of intricate reasoning. Throughout book one, Lucretius has been cajoling and pressing the student to keep going, like a hound (as cited earlier), who must seek out the truth for himself; and now there is another book of abstruse reasoning coming up. At this point, the student surely needs an incentive. What is it all for? Why should he go on doing the hard work of trying to figure out for himself the very strange arguments that Lucretius has kept flinging at him? Lucretius responds in the prologue to book 2 by treating the student to a vision of the reward that awaits him. Though detached from the physical content, the prologue to book 2 has everything to do with keeping the student on course.

---

12   2.1090–92: quae bene cognita si teneas, natura videtur / libera continuo dominis privata superbis / ipsa sua per se sponte omnia dis agere expers.

The priamel that introduces the prologue to book 2 is the first step in show-ing the student the reward of his labors. We already briefly noted Lucretius' disclaimer in lines 3 and 4. In addition, it is necessary to pay close attention to the wording of the priamel as a whole. The student is to 'hold' (*tenere*, 2.7) the fortifications of wisdom. To 'hold' is not simply to dwell there; it is to stay there, holding on firmly. Lucretius emphasizes the effort of staying by adding *bene munita*: a person must keep the fortress 'well fortified'. Just like a soldier, as Lucretius puts it in the prologue to book 6 (6.32), one needs to know how to sally out from the gates against invading forces.[13] This 'holding' of the fortress is what one takes pleasure in; and it is an abrupt change from the pleasure of the first two examples. There, following a literary tradition, Lucretius said that it is a pleasure to look upon the struggles of others. Turning to Epicurean pleasure, he now says it is a pleasure to hold the 'serene temples' (*templa serena*) of wisdom, 'from which one can (*queas*) look down' on the wanderings of others. What gives pleasure is one's serenity, not the act of look-ing down on others. One has the ability to look down on others; but the source of pleasure is not the misery of others, but one's own freedom from misery, just as Lucretius had pointed out in lines 3 and 4. This freedom from misery is the Epicurean goal of *ataraxia*, 'lack of mental disturbance', as signified by *serena*.[14]

Why, then, does Lucretius put others into the picture at all, instead of simply directing attention to one's own freedom from troubles? Part of the reason is that he is appealing to a familiar sentiment—taking comfort in being safe from the perils that engulf others—as a stepping stone toward an Epicurean con-cept. More generally, Lucretius is continuing the imagery of ascent with which he began his poem. We first saw Epicurus ascending beyond the walls of the world to topple the monster of religion and raise humans to the sky. This con-quest, however, still remains to be fulfilled by each student; at this stage, it is only a promise. Although Epicurus did all he could, his efforts are not enough: humans need to do their part to attain the place Epicurus won for them. Each must make a personal effort to detach himself from the downtrodden masses. In book 2, Lucretius shows the student the fruit of his efforts: he will occupy a height from which he can look down on others, who are still lost.

As Lucretius shows immediately after the priamel, the height attained by wisdom is directly opposed to the summit that those wandering humans are struggling to achieve.[15] What they try to reach is the summit of wealth and power (*ad summas emergere opes rerumque potiri*, 2.13). Lucretius tells us about

---

13   See Clay 1983, 186.
14   *Letter to Menoeceus* 128 and 131, Diogenes Laertius 10.136, and *De rerum natura* 2.19–20.
15   See Fowler 1989, 134–40.

the futility of this struggle later on in book 3, where he shows us Sisyphus forever straining to roll a stone uphill, as it keeps crashing back down again as soon as the top has been reached (3.995–1002). The traditional height of the rich and powerful is an illusion. Unlike the height of wisdom with its staying power (*tenere*), it dissipates as soon as one thinks one has got hold of it. In reality, it is an abyss of misery, where people wander without a goal, competing with another to no purpose. The height of wisdom engages people in a different kind of competition. Lucretius has been directing his attention to his Roman audience from the very first line, or rather first word (*Aeneadum*, 'descendants of Aeneas'), of his poem. Now, at the beginning of book 2, Lucretius makes clear to the Romans the particular suffering in which they are trapped. In contrast with the traditional competition for wealth and power, the Romans are to redirect their competitive impulses to the acquisition of wisdom. This type of competition is not a zero-sum game, where some must lose for others to reach the top. Anyone can reach the top; and the entire journey is marked by cooperation, not aggression.

Granted, then, that Lucretius is seeking to motivate his reader to raise himself above the unenlightened, does he nonetheless introduce a feeling of contempt? Here, it is necessary to keep in mind once again the reader whom Lucretius is addressing at this stage of instruction. Seeing himself lifted above the masses, it is possible that the novice student may succumb to a feeling of smugness, or even malice, toward the people below. The totally disengaged reader may likewise share this feeling. But this is not, in my view, the attitude of the teacher, Lucretius, at this stage of his teaching; nor is it a constituent part of the pleasure that is the goal of one's efforts. Lucretius tries to eliminate this suspicion in the first lines of the priamel by denying outright that there is any *Schadenfreude*. He provides further clarification in the lines that follow the priamel, to which we turn next.

There is unmistakable pity in the exclamation 'Oh, miserable minds of men, blind hearts!' (*o miseras hominum mentes, o pectora caeca*, 2.14). One might object that the term *miser* ranges in meaning from 'pitiable' to 'pitiful' and 'wretched', so as to invite contempt. Likewise, *despicere*, as used in the priamel, ranges from the literal meaning of 'looking down' to the sense of 'despising'. Further, blindness is not necessarily deserving of pity. One might have nothing but pity for those who are wholly innocent; but how innocent are those people who are grubbing for power and wealth? Commentators often cite Socrates' address to mankind in the pseudo-Platonic *Cleitophon* (407a–e) as a parallel. Speaking as though 'from a tragic hoist (*mêchanê*)', like a *deus ex machina*, Socrates exclaims: 'Where are you rushing, humans?' Then he denounces his hearers for neglecting their moral education and that of their children. Does

Lucretius likewise blame those below? In the prologue to book 1, Lucretius portrayed the whole of humanity as innocent victims of a cruel monster. In the prologue to book 2, he draws a distinction between those who have risen to the top and those who remain below. Does Lucretius continue to pity the people below; or does he now extend some blame, at least, to them?

After setting out in brief the Epicurean goal of pleasure (as quoted above, 2.17–19), Lucretius illustrates it by contrasting a life of luxury, as exemplified by a lavish banquet, to a simple life, as exemplified by a simple picnic with friends. Further (2.37–53), he explains in detail that serenity is not won by power or wealth, but by the 'power of reason' (*rationi' potestas*, 2.53). In this section, he addresses his reader repeatedly as 'you' in the singular (2.40, 41, 43, 44, 53). Behind 'you' is Memmius, the dedicatee of his poem, standing for the Roman elite in general. Lucretius tries to jolt his audience out of their preoccupation with battles and money-making by pointing out how ridiculous it is to suppose that this will chase away fear and worry. He adopts a bantering tone rather than one of blame. Lucretius concludes by elaborating the leitmotif of darkness and light that he introduced in the first prologue (at 1.146–48, as quoted above). He now adds another image, likening those who are trapped in terror and darkness to young children (2.55–58):

> nam vel uti pueri trepidant atque omnia caecis
> in tenebris metuunt, sic nos in luce timemus
> interdum, nihilo quae sunt metuenda magis quam
> quae pueri in tenebris pavitant finguntque futura.

> For just as children tremble and fear everything in the blind darkness, so we sometimes fear in the light things that are no more to be feared than what children dread in the dark and imagine for the future.

Lucretius now extends his view to 'us', including himself: 'we' are like children trembling in the dark. After introducing the image here, he adds it to the remaining two occurrences of the leitmotif later in the poem (at 3.91–93 and 6.39–41).

Lucretius frames his second prologue, then, by an initial view from the top together with a final view of the unenlightened as children, trapped in darkness. Within this frame, he shows what is wrong with 'us', humans as a whole and the Romans in particular, as seen from the height that we can attain. We are lost, not knowing in what direction to turn. What we need is a view of the goal toward which we should direct our strivings. Lucretius puts this goal out front, right at the beginning of the prologue, as a way of orienting those he is attempting to convert. Having reached the top, the student can finally see the full extent of the misery he has escaped. What the student sees is not just the misery of others, but his own misery, now left behind. The prologue as a whole is designed to show the audience a way out of their misery, not fault them for not yet having got out of it. This is a message of encouragement; and there is no place in it for a feeling of contempt for those who are yet to attain their goal. If there is a feeling of contempt, it lies outside Lucretius' purpose.

The third prologue follows up with another type of ascent. Here, the student breaks through the walls of the universe, just as Epicurus did, to obtain a view of the entire universe.[16] He is initiated, all at once, into the truth that he has been laboriously working out for himself in the previous two books. Epicurus now reappears in a new guise, as the hierophant who initiates the student into the light of truth. From heroic victor, Epicurus is recast as a sacred figure, uttering truths that arise from a 'divine mind' (3.15). Lucretius first calls upon him as one who 'had the power to raise so bright a light out of so great a darkness' (3.1–2). After an extended eulogy (as discussed above), he has him utter his revelations about the universe (3.14–30):

> nam simul ac ratio tua coepit vociferari
> naturam rerum divina mente coorta
> diffugiunt animi terrores, moenia mundi
> discedunt, totum video per inane geri res.
> apparet divum numen sedesque quietae,
> ...
> at contra nusquam apparent Acherusia templa,
> nec tellus obstat quin omnia dispiciantur,
> sub pedibus quaecumque infra per inane geruntur.
> his ibi me rebus quaedam divina voluptas
> percipit atque horror, quod sic natura tua vi
> tam manifesta patens ex omni parte retecta est.

For as soon as your reason, springing from a divine mind, begins to proclaim the nature of things, the terrors of the mind flee, the walls of the world part, and I see things happening through the entire void. The power of the gods appears and their calm seats ... By contrast, the Acherusian realm appears nowhere, nor is the earth an obstacle to catching a view of everything, whatever happens below in the void beneath

---

16   For further details, see Asmis 2017.

one's feet. At these things, a certain divine pleasure and shudder seize me, because nature has been uncovered by your power, opened up so clearly in every part.

Just like the hierophant at a religious initiation, Epicurus both shows and tells. The 'walls of the world', as others have noted, are those that he broke down as the conqueror of religion. At the same time, these walls have a physical analogue at the initiation: the doors of the initiation chamber open up to revel the sacred objects. Lucretius relives his own initiation, as shown by the shift to first person verb *video* (3.17). What 'I see', Lucretius tells the reader, is what goes in the entire universe, together with the brightly lit realm of the gods and the absence of any underworld. Like the initiate into the cult of Isis, as described by Apuleius, he comes to know all the elements and all the gods; in pointed contrast, he does not 'tread the threshold of Proserpine' or meet up with any gods below.[17] As is typical of a religious initiate, Lucretius is suddenly released from terror and darkness into a light that dispels ignorance and fear.

Lucretius feels himself seized by 'a certain divine pleasure (*voluptas*) and shudder (*horror*)'. The shudder is that of religious awe. The term 'pleasure' points to the Epicurean goal of pleasure. Lucretius' feeling, however, is not the same as the serenity that he set out briefly in the prologue to book 2. The Epicurean distinguished between two kinds of pleasure (as well as pain): kinetic and katastematic. The first consists in movement, the second in a condition; and the second is the height of pleasure, whereas the first merely varies the pleasure, without increasing it.[18] Serenity is a mental condition consisting in an absence of anxiety. As a feeling of ecstasy, Lucretius' pleasure is best classed as a type of kinetic pleasure, consisting of a momentary exultation.[19] It also

---

17 Apuleius, *Metamorphoses* 11.23: Accessi confinium mortis et calcato Proserpinae lumine per omnia uectus elementa remeaui, nocte media uidi solem candido coruscantem lumine, deos inferos et deos superos accessi coram et adoraui de proxumo. ('I approached the border of death. After treading the threshold of Proserpine and traveling through all the elements, I came back. At midnight I saw the sun flashing with a white light. I approached the gods below and the gods above with my presence and worshipped them in closest proximity').

18 *Principal Doctrines* 3, *Letter to Menoeceus* 130–1, and Diogenes Laertius 10.136. There is much controversy about the distinctions. For a clear overview, see Wolfsdorf 2013, 148–67.

19 More precisely, it may be classified as a type of *chara*, 'joy' (listed by Diogenes Laertius at 10.136). Ecstatic pleasure is attested for Epicurus' own time by Plutarch, who derides the "the bacchic howlings and shrieks of pleasure' whereby the Epicureans call each other 'imperishable and equal to the gods' (*Non posse* 1091b–c). An example is the occasion when Colotes fell to Epicurus' knees upon hearing Epicurus lecture on physics; Epicurus reciprocated by 'sanctifying' and 'revering' Colotes in turn (*adv. Col.* 1117b–c).

has a corporeal component, as the mental pleasure together with a feeling of awe, spreads as a kind of shudder throughout the body.[20] Bodily and mental feelings combine into a single overwhelming feeling of being transported to a condition of divine bliss.

The initiation, too, is a promise that Lucretius holds out to the student. Just a few will attain it; but it is a realistic goal, as Lucretius illustrates in his own person. Those have not yet attained it need to work harder at working out the doctrines for themselves. Those who have achieved initiation, too, have more work to do. The challenge for the initiate is to have not merely a momentary pleasure, but a lasting pleasure, consisting of freedom from mental pain, *ataraxia*. Lucretius will strive throughout the rest of the poem to help the reader acquire this pleasure. The initiation is merely a prelude to the task of putting in practice the insights that have been gained and acquiring further knowledge. In time, as we shall see, Lucretius gets to be bitter toward those who won't make the necessary effort; nonetheless he shows nothing but pity for those who are innocent or are trying.

4   Follow-up

Lucretius shows pity for mankind once more in his history of religion in book 5. 'O unfortunate human race' (*o genus infelix humanum*), he exclaims (5.1194), without any suggestion of blame. What makes humankind so 'unfortunate' (with an implicit rejection of the religious connotation of *infelix* as the target of divine anger) is that those who first formed opinions about the gods falsely attributed great power and anger to the gods; the result was great suffering 'for themselves', 'for us', and 'for our descendants' (5.1196–97). The error was born out of ignorance, together with a rational impulse to find a cause for the events in the heavens. In their initial reflections on the gods, humans naturally slipped into error, as well as hit upon some truths.[21] This was a hit-and-miss attempt at trying out their rational powers. Unfortunately, the initial error persisted, as reinforced by the priests (1.102–6). It is the ultimate source of the oppression described in the prologue to book 1. Even though Epicurus has

---

20   As Lucretius illustrates in detail, a strong mental feeling may involve the body in a sympathetic reaction. A strong fear, for example, may cause the body to collapse (3.152–60); fear of the power of the gods seizes the limbs with trembling (5.1218–25).

21   As Furley (1978, 22) points out, nature suggests 'both the right and the wrong idea about the gods'.

shown the way out, the oppression will continue. Lucretius' pity extends not merely to the past and the present, but also to future generations.

In book 5, Lucretius' pity for the religious oppression of humans stands in stark contrast with his immediately preceding attack on the quest for power and wealth. There, after emphasizing the envy that keeps toppling men from the height of power and wealth, he exclaims (5.1131–34): 'let them sweat blood', since they are content to listen to others rather than trust their own senses. He adds: 'This is no more now, nor will be later, than it was before' (5.1135). Just as fear of the gods will persist, so will the quest for power and wealth. But whereas religious oppression elicits Lucretius' pity, the relentless pursuit of power and wealth prompts nothing but scorn. This is an attack on traditional Roman values, passed on from one generation to another, with devastating consequences for Lucretius' own era. Lucretius demands that these values be examined critically, and consequently abandoned, by reference to one's own sensory experience. Lucretius wants people to confront the reality of their own unhappiness: they should realize, by looking into themselves, that they are not getting what they want. This is another case of needing to tear off the mask.

The image of 'sweating blood' for the sake of power and wealth is also in stark contrast with the image of people wandering aimlessly below the heights of wisdom in the prologue to book 2. There, too, people succumb to the lure of power and wealth; but they are shown as adrift, not knowing what to aim for. Lucretius has pity for these people as needing instruction; those he attacks in book 5 are impervious to instruction. At this point in his own course of instruction, Lucretius has come to draw a clear distinction between those who are receptive to instruction and those who are not; and the latter attract the full force of his scorn.

Pity and contempt thus lie at opposite ends of a range of emotions displayed by Lucretius. As every reader of Lucretius is aware, this range is amazingly complex. It is also in keeping with Epicurean pedagogy. It was a cornerstone of Epicurean pedagogy that a teacher should adapt his methods to the needs of the student. As illustrated by Philodemus in On Frankness (peri parrhêsias), teachers must adjust their own attitudes to the circumstances and needs of the student (including social standing, age, gender, personal toughness, and so on) of their students: they are gentle to some (col. 8b), and harsh to others (fr. 7); they are continually frank to those who do not listen (frs. 64–65); there is no need to be frank in every case (col. 2b); some people are incurable (fr. 84); and so on (I employ the numbering of Konstan et al. 1998).

Lucretius' own efforts as a teacher are unique in that he uses a poem to educate not just a particular individual, but the Romans (or Roman elite) in general. His starting point is the supposition that the mass of humans is oppressed by ignorance; and this condition elicits his pity. Accordingly, he arranges his poem into a step-by-journey from oppression to enlightenment. At the beginning of book 2, Lucretius has just begun to open up to his readers a view of the universe. At this point, it would be entirely inappropriate to denounce them for still clinging to their old ways; they continue to have Lucretius' pity. What they need at this stage is the motivation to continue the course of instruction; and this is what Lucretius tries to provide by showing them the reward that awaits them. He nudges gently, without any contempt. He follows up in the prologue to the third book with a celebration, which takes the form of an initiation. After this, he shows a great variety of emotions to particular individuals, including bitter contempt in book 5 for the willingly blind and self-destructive exertions of those who persist in a lust for power.

The view from the top thus admits of a variety of attitudes toward others, including pity and (when merited) contempt. But Lucretius shows no such contempt in the prologue to book 2; nor is it inherent in the Epicurean goal of pleasure.

5   Sequel

I shall end with a quotation from Francis Bacon. He paraphrases Lucretius' priamel and offers a correction:

> The poet, that beautified the sect that was otherwise inferior to the rest, saith yet excellently well: 'It is a pleasure, to stand upon the shore, and to see ships tossed upon the sea; a pleasure, to stand in the window of a castle, and to see a battle, and the adventures thereof below; but no pleasure is comparable to the standing upon the vantage ground of Truth ... and to see the errors, and wanderings, and mists, and tempests in the vale below; so always that this prospect be with pity, and not with swelling, or pride. Certainly, it is heaven upon earth, to have a man's mind move in charity, rest in providence, and turn upon the poles of truth.[22]

Bacon's correction consists in the admonition: the mind must 'move in charity, rest in providence, and turn about the poles of truth'. This is a Christian point of view. What Bacon advocates is humility, born of a recognition that there is a god who takes care of us. In Lucretius' lines, what we see are individuals who

---

22   Bacon 1996 [1625], 342.

have reached the height of happiness through their own efforts in mastering the teachings of Epicurus. This is an achievement that is worth being proud of. Humans take the place of god. The resulting pleasure may be viewed as egotistical, but it is hardly cruel. As Lucretius illustrates by his own pity for mankind, it is accompanied by a deep concern for others.

CHAPTER 9

Joy, Flow, and the Sage's Experience in Seneca[1]

Sam McVane

1 Introduction

Unlike Epicurus, Plato, and Aristotle, most Stoic sources do not seem to make pleasure of any sort an integral, still less an emphasized, part of the good life.[2] No sort of pleasure, good or bad, plays an essential role in making a Stoic life good. Only virtue and its enactment grant this. Yet the good life does involve certain sorts of pleasure. Sages—that is, wise people living a good life—still feel the sort of pleasure that naturally arises when, for example, we eat or drink. And, equally, just as we 'fools' (*phauloi* or *stulti*) take an active pleasure in what we deem good, so too can sages actively enjoy what they know is good. But neither this naturally arising pleasure nor its attendant joy affects the goodness or flourishing of the sage's life. Should sages, *per impossibile*, never feel natural pleasure or enjoy anything, they can still lead a good life. Indeed, incredibly, sages *can* still flourish even amidst intense pain.[3]

Whether as a sign of their philosophical interest or because of the vagaries of transmission, almost all extant Stoic sources spend little time discussing the sorts of pleasures available to the sage.[4] Seneca, as he often does, bucks this trend. In particular, he spends much of the *De vita beata* discussing the pleasure of the sage juxtaposed with the base and, as Seneca sees it, ultimately distressing pleasures of the Epicureans. This paper will explore the sage's pleasures

---

1 I should like to thank the participants in the Pain and Pleasure conference for their thought-provoking questions and comments. I also want to thank Giulia Bonasio for her offer to edit this paper's initial drafts and, especially, Katja Vogt for her numerous suggestions and objections and her generous guidance, without which this paper would certainly not be as it appears before you.

2 On the philosophical debate about 'pleasure', see Vogt in this volume, together with Mann and de Harven on Platonic notions of pleasure.

3 Importantly, this 'can' expresses mere possibility, not inevitability or necessity. Should pain preclude the sage's ability to lead a virtuous life, he is justified within Stoicism in committing suicide in order to preserve to the end his virtue (Cicero, *Fin.* 3.60–1; see also Englert 1994).

4 On why the Stoics might have introduced the sage's affective correlates to the fool's emotions, see Brennan 2002, 182–184, Cooper 2005, and Kamtekar 2005.

DOI:10.1163/9789004379503_010

and, in particular, his unique sorts of joy.[5] In part one of this paper, I shall argue that the sorts of joy that Seneca discusses in the *De vita beata* are not the standard 'good emotions' or *eupatheiai* of the sage that most modern accounts focus on, but rather the related but much less frequently mentioned joys that are 'accompaniments' or *epigennēmata* of virtue. Unlike the good emotion joy and its varieties, these accompanying joys are not voluntary impulses, which we might think of as actively and intentionally taking joy in some good state of affairs, but rather the affective side of the sage's thinking and actions in so far as they are virtuous. I am thus proposing a distinction that addresses a fundamental point about pleasure and pain: the distinction between emotions, which have intentional objects—that is, are *directed at* and *about* some specific object or state of affairs, such as some offense (anger) or someone's death (grief)—and moods or generalized states of mind that are not about anything in particular. My paper explores how these latter figure in the Stoic account of a good life. Beyond that, it aims to highlight the idea that positive and negative moods firmly belong in the domain of pleasure and pain, as reflected upon in ancient thought.

Seneca's account of joy raises certain questions of psychological plausibility. According to Seneca, sages are always in this state of joy, but, paradoxically, they may at the same time be enduring torture. Just as we may balk at the Stoic claim that someone can flourish even under torture, we may equally, if not more vehemently, reject Seneca's claim that the sage will or even can joyfully endure torture. To address this, in part two, I shall briefly consider what this joy is like and defend the plausibility of the sage's joy by drawing parallels to a psychological state much studied by modern psychologists called 'flow'.

2   The Two Types of *Gaudium*

In the opening sections of the *De vita beata* (§§ 3–5), Seneca provides a number of different but mutually reinforcing Stoic descriptions of happiness. After defining happiness in the more standard ways, such as 'living in accordance with one's own nature' and a knowledgeable and virtuous mind (3.3–4), he expands on the nature of this flourishing mind (4.1–3). It is upright, unfrightened, and stable. It considers only what is honorable, viz. virtue, as good, and,

---

5   While I favor the non-gendered plural where feasible, I use the generic 'he' or 'she' only for the sake of variation, vividness, and brevity—versus the more cumbersome 'he or she' or the sometimes implausible singular 'they'. I take what Seneca and the Stoics say (as, theoretically, they would too) to apply to all human beings.

hence, it recognizes that the various things society counts as good or bad in fact neither add nor subtract from the *summum bonum* that makes life good. And he continues:[6]

> It is necessary that, whether it wants it or not [*velit nolit*], a continuous cheerfulness [*hilaritas continua*] and a profound gladness [*laetitia alta*] that comes from deep within accompanies this mind that is grounded in this way [viz. holds only virtue as the good and so on], since it enjoys [*gaudeat*] its own things and does not desire anything more than what is in its own store ... Then that invaluable good will arise, the quiet of a mind that is posted in a safe place and a sublimity and, after error has been eliminated due to the grasping of the truth, a great and unshakable joy [*gaudium*] and kindness [*comitas*] and relaxation [*diffusio*] of the mind, which things please it not as goods but as what arises from its own good. (4.4.1–3 and 5.2–6)

Of interest here is Seneca's initial striking remark that the sage's continuous cheerfulness and gladness arise from the virtuous mind 'whether it wants it or not' (*velit nolit*, 4.4.1). This is striking for two reasons. First, it is an odd statement, for why would anyone not want perpetual cheerfulness and gladness? In my view, this is not a merely rhetorical aside, but rather a substantive point. And this point concerns the second reason *velit nolit* is striking, at least to readers who know much about Stoicism. Cheerfulness and gladness as most Stoic sources present them are precisely the sorts of mental conditions that *do* only arise when one wants them to. They are 'good emotions', which require assent to occur.[7] I suggest, then, that Seneca's remark identifies the cheerfulness and gladness that accompany virtue as, though good, *not* good emotions, but rather general affective states of mind that are not directed at anything in particular. Emotions, good or bad, involve assent, and assent is a mental act with an intentional object. A state of mind that is not directed at something particular thus cannot technically count as an emotion. But, first, why think *velit nolit* has anything to do with assent?

Scholars typically, and I think rightly, take what I am translating as 'cheerfulness' and 'gladness', *hilaritas* and *laetitia*, as Seneca's Latin equivalents of the Greek *terpsis* and *euphrosunē*.[8] Other Stoic sources applied these two Greek

---

6 All the Latin and numberings are from the edition of L. R. Reynolds (Oxford, 1977). Unless noted otherwise, all translations are my own.

7 On *eupatheiai*, see Brennan 1998 and Kamtekar 2005; cf. Cooper 2005.

8 See Grimal 1969, 37 and Asmis 1990, 232 n. 47.

terms to specific sorts or subspecies of joy, the standard translation of *chara* or *gaudium*, and Seneca's linking in the passage quoted above of *hilaritas* and *laetitia* with *gaudium* suggests that he similarly identifies them.[9] There was also a third subspecies of joy called 'tranquility' or *euthumia*, which, in the *De tranquillitate animi*, Seneca explicitly translates as *tranquillitas*.[10] And both here and later in the *De vita beata*, he relates *tranquillitas* to both *laetitia* and *gaudium*.[11] Yet the Stoics typically identify joy and its varieties as good emotions. The good emotion joy is a 'well-reasoned expansion' (*eulogos eparsis*)[12] of the soul, what Seneca in *Ep.* 59 calls an 'expansion of a mind confident in its own, true goods' (*animi elatio suis bonis verisque fidentis*, 2.3–4). It is an affective mental reaction, an impulse, to a particular present situation or object that arises only when the sage assents to or buys into the impression that this situation or object is good and appropriate to react to thusly.[13] Hence, as defined in our sources, joy in the form of gladness is being glad about, e.g., a particular virtuous action you or your wise friend performs.[14] Or, tranquility, which unfortunately does not translate well in this context, is rejoicing in the particular present course of one's life, which is permanently well-ordered due both to one's own virtue and to god's.[15]

Joy as a good emotion then stands as the virtuous counterpart to our vicious emotion (*pathos*) of pleasure (*hēdonē* or *voluptas*).[16] This pleasure is an 'irrational expansion' (*alogos eparsis*) of the soul and a reaction that stems from the fool's assent to an impression of some present putative good.[17] Yet this pleasure, like all emotions, is excessive and ephemeral.[18] Due to our ignorance and the instability of our minds, we flutter between taking pleasure in something

---

9   Diogenes Laertius 7.115 (= Long and Sedley 1987 65F, henceforth 'LS').

10   2.3.3.

11   *Tranq.* 2.4.3–4 and *V.B.* 15.2.3.

12   Diogenes Laertius 7.115 (= LS 65F).

13   Our sources clearly set out *eupatheiai* as the virtuous correlates to the emotions, both as impulses and judgments, but the formulaic content of the impression as described above is a widely accepted reconstruction.

14   Andronicus, *Peri Pathōn* 6 (= SVF 3.432): εὐφροσύνη δὲ χαρὰ ἐπὶ τοῖς τοῦ σώφρονος ἔργοις ('gladness is joy towards the deeds of the prudent man').

15   *Ibid.*: εὐθύμια δὲ χαρὰ ἐπὶ διαγωγῇ ἢ ἀνεπιζητησίᾳ παντός ('tranquility is joy at the course of life or not craving anything').

16   On *pathē*, see LS chapter 65, Inwood 1985, Frede 1986, Brennan 1998, Cooper 1998, and Graver 2007.

17   Andronicus, *Peri Pathōn* 1 (= LS 65B).

18   Stobaeus 2.88.8–90.6 (= LS 65A).

and being distressed about it, whether simultaneously or with the passing of time, to the detriment of the ideal 'smooth flow' of our lives.[19]

Assent is fundamental to both types of emotion, as Seneca makes clear in the *De ira*, where he uses the language of 'wanting' and 'not wanting' to discuss it. Assent is voluntary: it is one of the few things in the Stoic world that are truly 'up to us'. And while the psychic movements of emotions, whether good or bad, require assent, not every psychic movement we experience involves it. So, for example, 'pre-emotions' or *propatheiai* are movements of either the body or the mind, like the welling of tears or a jolt of surprise, over which we have no control and which occur in the ignorant and wise alike.[20] As Seneca writes, 'all these are motions of minds that do not want to be moved, not emotions but beginnings that are preludes to emotions' ('omnia ista motus sunt animorum moveri nolentium, nec adfectus sed principia proludentia adfectibus', *De ira* 2.2.5.7–8). These minds are not actively unwilling, at least not in the case of the sage, who would accept their inevitability. Rather, *nolentium* captures the fact that pre-emotions arise without our assent, which is the main point of Seneca's discussion. While Seneca does not use *velle* as an equivalent shorthand for 'to assent', he does use one of its cognates, *voluntas*, to denote assent.[21] Now, I am not suggesting that joy is a sort of pre-emotion (for these do not require a certain, viz. a perfected, state of mind to occur), only that *velle* and *nolle* are often the Senecan language of assent. And hence, I suggest that when Seneca declares that *laetitia* and *hilaritas* occur *velit nolit* (*V.B.* 4.4.1), he means that they do not depend directly on assent to occur and thus (implicitly) are not good emotions.[22]

But if these joys are not good emotions, what are they? Elizabeth Asmis was I think right to suggest that Seneca discusses the joy and its varieties that the

---

19   Zeno first identified *eudaimonia*, life's *telos*, as an *euroia biou* ('smooth flow of life') (Stobaeus 2.77.16–27 [= LS 63A]).

20   *De ira* 2.3–5. On *propaetheiai*, see Graver 2007 85–108, cf. Inwood 1993.

21   E.g. *De ira* 2.4.1.4. On the complexity of *voluntas* in Seneca, see Inwood 2000.

22   Cf. Asmis 1990 233 n. 50, who translates *velit nolit* as 'in any case', and takes this merely to mean that joy follows virtue in any circumstance, which she juxtaposes with a Stoic position outlined in *Ep.* 66 that she argues Seneca rejects, viz. that joy only follows in favorable circumstances. But, first, it is by no means clear that Seneca really does break from the Stoic position presented, for the remarks that suggest this are explicitly made hypothetically (49.1). And second, the *gaudium* of *Ep.* 66 must be some sort of affect other than the two sorts of *gaudium* under discussion here since it directly concerns indifferents (e.g. 15.1–3), and Seneca states that the virtue of this *gaudium* rests in its being undergone 'moderately' (*moderate*, 29.3), which makes no sense vis-à-vis an affect available only to the sage.

Stoics identify as *epigennēmata* or 'accompaniments' of virtue.[23] Although scholars have sometimes suggested otherwise, I maintain that accompanying joy is not the same thing as the good emotion.[24] In other words, a single sort of joy is not *both* an accompaniment *and* an impulse, but, rather, the latter are two different mental events or conditions, even though they are related enough to justify using the same term to identify both. Despite Stoicism's penchant for neologisms, this sort of polysemy often occurs.[25] As we will see, these accompanying joys are not reactions to particular situations or objects, like the good thing one just did, but general, mood-like affects that emerge from the virtuous functioning of the sage's mind.

We have already seen the distinction in assent between good emotions and accompaniments. In addition, our other source on this accompanying joy, Diogenes Laertius, implies their separateness. He writes:

> Likewise, the good is defined as 'the perfection in accordance with nature of the rational *qua* rational.' And that sort of thing is virtue, with the result that what participates [sc. in virtue], both actions in accordance with virtue and virtuous men are [also] such things, and the accompaniments [ἐπιγεννήματα, sc. of virtue], joy [χαράν], gladness [εὐφροσύνην], and the rest. Likewise, concerning what is bad, it is foolishness, cowardice, injustice, and the rest; and what participates in the vices, both actions in accordance with vice and vicious men; and the accompaniments [sc. of vice], discontentedness [δυσθυμίαν], sadness [δυσφροσύνην], and similar things. (7.94 = SVF 3.76)

Were Diogenes Laertius talking about the good emotions of joy, gladness, and so on, then when he comes to their vicious opposites, we would expect to read of pleasure and some of its subspecies, such as *Schadenfreude* and arrogance.[26] But instead we see the negative states of mind *dusthumia* and *dusphrosunē*, clearly the opposites of *euthumia* and *euphrosunē*, but not of the good emotion variety.

Moreover, later in the *Vita Beata*, Seneca seems, implicitly at least, to distinguish good emotions from accompanying joys. There, Seneca refutes his

23   Asmis 1990, 233. See also Grimal 1969, 75, who identifies them as accompaniments only at 15.1–3.

24   Cf. Haynes 1962, Long 1968, Rist 1969, Asmis 1990, Sorabji 2000, 51, and Evenepoel 2014, 55–57.

25   See, e.g., the different uses of *psuchē* (Sextus Empiricus, *Math.* 7.234 [= LS 53F]) and *hexis* (Diogenes Laertius 7.138–9 [= LS 47O]).

26   Stobaeus 2.90.19–91.9 (= LS 65E).

imaginary interlocutor's Aristotelian suggestion that the highest good is at the same time *qua* good, both ethically right and pleasing.[27] Seneca writes:

> Because a part of what is right [*honestum*] is not able to be so unless it is right, nor will the highest good retain its own purity, if it sees anything in itself that is unlike its better part. Not even joy, which arises from virtue, although it is a good, is yet a part of the complete good, no more than gladness [*laetitia*] and tranquility [*tranquillitas*], although they are born from the finest causes. For sure these are goods, but they accompany [*consequentia*] the highest good—they do not complete it [*consummantia*]. (15.1.3–2.5)[28]

This seems to contradict other Stoic accounts such as that of Stobaeus, who records in Aristotelian language that Stoic joy is a 'final' good, which 'completes' one's happiness.[29] And we may think that Seneca simply disagrees with this Stoic theory. That is not impossible, but it is an unnecessary conclusion here. For Stobaeus includes among such so-called final goods the other good emotions and virtuous impulses such as prudent walking. If, as I have suggested, the joys that attend virtue are not good emotions, and thus of a different type than the joy-cum-*eupatheia* under discussion in Stobaeus, then there is no inconsistency.

Lastly, as suggested to me by Katja Vogt, mood-like affective states such as joy and discontentedness fill an otherwise disconcerting gap in human life as described by Stoicism. The Stoics are psychological monists. Humans think and feel in the same part of the soul, the 'commanding faculty' (*hēgemonikon*), whose sole currency, so to speak, is 'thought' (*noēsis*).[30] As such, conceptual processing and affection are two aspects of the same cognitive activity, thinking. Put differently, thinking has an 'affective coloring'—thinking in a certain

---

27   See, e.g., Aristotle, *Eth. Nic.* 1153b.1–1154a.7 On this passage in the *De vita beata*, see Grimal 1967.

28   I take this to mean that virtue's goodness, unlike Aristotelian virtue, does not depend in part upon its being enjoyable. Hence, even if human psychology makes joy and virtue inseparable or, as I shall suggest, the former the experiential component of the former, this does not make joy a part of virtue *qua honestum*.

29   Stobaeus 2.71.15 (= SVF 3.106). See also Cicero, *Fin.* 3.55 and Diogenes Laertius 7.96 (= SVF 3.107).

30   'Thoughts' = 'rational impressions' (Diogenes Laertius 7.49–51 [= LS 39A]; see Frede 1987, 152–157). On Stoic monism, see Aetius 4.21.1–4 (= LS 53H), Aetius 4.23.1 (= LS 53M), and Stobaeus 1.368.12–20 (= LS 53K). Cf., e.g., Plato's psychology, where different sorts of feelings are spread across different faculties and rational thought occurs only in one faculty (e.g. *Rep.* 435–442).

way feels a certain way.[31] Consider again Seneca's discussion of *propatheiai* and emotion. A propathic agitated feeling (*agitatio animi, De ira* 2.3.5.1–2) occurs with being struck by the mere thought of being disrespected (*species iniuriae*, 2), while the full 'commotion of the mind' (*concitatio animi*; 5) in anger proper only arises with assent, viz. when thinking one is, in fact, disrespected (where disrespect is, in the thinker's view, a bad thing), and feels the subsequent impulse to seek revenge.[32] Seneca treats such feeling and thought as a unity (cf. *simplex*, 1.5.1): to have this thought is to feel this way. There is an affective phenomenology to thinking in a certain way.[33] And all cognitive activity has an affective dimension. Take a less obvious example like thinking through a logical puzzle whose premises we accept as sound though it leads to an unacceptable conclusion.[34] Our thoughts conflict, we recognize that something we have taken to be true cannot be true—we 'are in turmoil' (*tarassesthai*; e.g., Epictetus, *Diss.* 1.7.20.7). Confused and contradictory thinking itself does not feel good, a fact that logical puzzles, no less than conflicting motivation, reveal.[35] Thus, if Stoic emotions, both good and bad, are specific affective attitudes and reactions involving assent and a particular intentional object (i.e., something good or bad), then Stoic theory needs something more to identify the affective dimension of non-emotional thinking in general. The type of Stoic joy that accompanies and is the affective side of a virtuous state of mind falls into this category. Moreover, if we experience confused and disordered thinking as unpleasant, then it follows that we experience its opposite, which precisely constitutes Stoic virtue, as pleasant and enjoyable. As we shall see, Seneca recognizes this and identifies the experience with one type of *gaudium*.

---

31 I gratefully borrow this phrase from Katja Vogt.

32 On Senecan anger, see Vogt 2006, 70, where she rightly stresses the definitive feature of anger as the impulse to revenge, not the 'negative type of experience' of the accompanying indignant feeling.

33 Importantly, the nature of Stoic thoughts extends beyond their propositional content. So 'to have this thought' does not simply mean to have a thought with propositional content A, since one can have such a thought in different ways, e.g. as a perception versus a recollection (cf. Frede 1987). The affective coloring of thinking will thus depend on more than its propositional content.

34 On such 'sophisms', see Barnes 1982, Atherton 1993, 407–457, Bobzien 2005, and Burnyeat 1982.

35 It is not simply that we feel bad *about* being confused. Epictetus remarks that we are in turmoil 'because we do not recognize what follows' from the accepted premises (*Diss.* 1.7.20.7). Cf. the affective quality of the 'smooth movement' (*leion kinēma*) of a persuasive impression (Sextus Empiricus, *Math.* 7.242–6 [= LS 39G]). On the affective link between the conflict of 'pure' thinking and motivational thinking in Stoicism, see Vogt 2014.

3   The Nature of 'Accompanying' *Gaudium*

What does it mean for joy to be an affective state of mind, and what then should we make of this joy? In the first place, it is not the sort of pleasurable feeling or experience we often think of as pleasure. It is not pleasurable in the sense that drinking a glass of water is pleasurable after a long run or listening to a favorite song is pleasurable. As Seneca famously writes in *Ep.* 23:

> Believe me, real joy is a serious affair. Or do you think that someone with a relaxed and, as those playboys say, delighted expression thinks little of death, opens the door to poverty, keeps pleasures within rein, and mentally prepares for the endurance of pains? He who thinks on these things with a level head is in a state of great but not very pleasing [*parum blando*] joy. (4.1–6)

Yet, while joy is distinct from the sorts of pleasures the sage moderates, Seneca draws parallels between them because, I shall suggest, they are both types of affective coloring, described by the Stoics as 'accompaniments'.[36]

Sages will never take pleasure in something, for this is an emotion, but they will nonetheless experience certain actions and states as pleasurable. In the *De vita beata*, Seneca allows that virtuous action may well provide the experience of pleasure, but if it does, it is not for this sake that we do it. He writes as follows:

> Just as some flowers grow amidst a field that has been plowed for grain, such work was not undertaken for this little wildflower, although it pleases the eyes—the aim of sowing was something else, this supervened [*supervenit*]—thus pleasure is not the reward nor the reason for virtue but an accompaniment [*accessio*], and it [i.e. virtue] does not satisfy [*placet*] because it pleases, but, if it satisfies, it also pleases. (9.2.1–6)

Here Seneca expands upon the Stoic claim that there is a sort of pleasure, an 'accompaniment' or *epigennēma*, that may supervene when one 'seeks and obtains what is in harmony with [one's] constitution, in which manner animals

---

36   These moderated pleasures are the experiences of the sort of pleasure that the Stoics count, in various ways, among the indifferents (even as most fools mistake it as a good) and are thus available to the sage. As a preferable indifferent, see Seneca, *Ep.* 76.18, 87.29–35, 116.1 and *V.B.* 24.5; and Diogenes Laertius 7.102 [= LS 58A]; as indifferent, Gellius 9.5.5, Stobaeus 2.57 [= SVF 1.190], and Sextus Empiricus, *Math.* 11.73.

thrive and plants bloom'.[37] All this betrays an Aristotelian influence, and like Aristotelian pleasure, this pleasure seems to be not a distinct product but rather an affective feature of our doing or getting what befits our constitution.[38] Briefly, the idea is that, say, eating doesn't cause a separate process of pleasure or feeling pleasure, but rather that the very process of eating is itself pleasurable and an instance of pleasure. For the Stoics, I suggest, this experience of natural, accompanying pleasure is the affective facet, the coloring, of the cognitive activity—the impressions, cognitions, and impulses—that drives and arises from eating, i.e. seeking out, obtaining, and consuming food, in a way that is 'in harmony with [one's] constitution'.[39] There are, of course, ways of eating and engaging in other potentially pleasurable activities that are not constitutionally harmonious, such as at the wrong time, in the wrong way, or with the wrong objects, and are thus not pleasant or even painful. In this way we can make sense of Seneca's frequent talk of pleasures turning into pains as opposed to simply ceasing to exist, for it is, e.g., eating as a pleasure that becomes a pain when it is done to excess.[40]

Among these pleasures Seneca includes not only any pleasure of the senses but also the pleasures of the mind, such as study, contemplation, and solving puzzles, as well as mental relaxation.[41] Importantly, this pleasure arises without our direct assent and, thus, is not an emotion. In this, the Stoics pinpoint a crucial difference between, say, the pleasure that attends eating and the pleasure we may take in that same meal because we are happy to have it or delight in it for its deliciousness. And while the pleasure experienced in study and the pleasure of procreation certainly differ, they and their equivalents are pleasing in a way that serious joy, which may arise from forgoing these pleasures, is

---

37   Diogenes Laertius 7.85–6 (= LS 57A): ἐπιγέννημα γάρ φασιν, εἰ ἄρα ἔστιν, ἡδονὴν εἶναι
      ὅταν αὐτὴ καθ' αὑτὴν ἡ φύσις ἐπιζητήσασα τὰ ἐναρμόζοντα τῇ συστάσει ἀπολάβῃ, ὃν τρόπον
      ἀφιλαρύνεται τὰ ζῷα καὶ θάλλει τὰ φυτά.

38   On Aristotelian pleasure as an *epigennēma*, see *Eth. Nic.* 10. On Aristotelian pleasure,
      see also Cheng in this volume. On Aristotelian pleasure as a feature, see Dow 2011,
      69–74. Unlike the Stoic counterpart, pleasure for Aristotle involves a non-rational part of
      the soul.

39   Some such pleasures may reasonably be called 'bodily' (cf. *corpusculi motibus*; Seneca,
      V.B. 4.4.5), but only in so far as reference to the body is necessary to fully account for
      them. Sensation (*aisthēsis*) occurs in the mind (Aetius 4.23.1 [= LS 53M]; Hierocles 1.5–33,
      4.38–53 [= LS 53B]; Calcidius 220 [= LS 53G]). Thus, e.g., it is with the mental awareness
      of the physical process of satiation that we experience pleasure. Cf. Dyson's different yet
      still perhaps compatible formulation of this pleasure (2009, 136).

40   See, e.g., *Ep.* 27.2, 51.8, 77.16, 90.34, 91.5, and *V.B.* 7.4, 14.1.

41   See *Ep.* 50.9 (on the *voluptas* of philosophy), 78.22, 84.11, *Ben.* 5.12.2 (puzzles), and *De Otio*
      7. On mental relaxation, see *Tranq.* 17.6.

not. Beyond any difference in their, as it were, feel, this accompanying pleasure arises only from particular and inevitably intermittent activities, and while this mode of accompaniment serves as a useful parallel to that of joy, it is essential that joy accompanies *all* of the sage's activities. In this aspect the sage's joy most clearly represents a sort of mood or generalized, affective state of mind.

Although Seneca remarks on this sort of pleasure in *De vita beata* 9.2.1–6 (just quoted), that passage equally concerns joy. He responds to the objection that even one who seeks virtue as the good hopes for pleasure. This objection addresses Seneca's previous claim at 8.1–2 that the virtuous life includes accompanying pleasure as an ally and not as a leader (8.1.4–5). But the objection also stems from Seneca's immediately preceding description at 8.5–6 of the harmony of the sage's mind, which lacks contradictory beliefs and desires. Three sections later at 12.1.1–3, the interlocutor uses precisely such mental discord to argue that those who indiscriminately and successfully pursue pleasure are nonetheless distressed and disquieted. Hence, I suggest, the objection alludes both to the sort of pleasures that attend certain activities and the pleasure that accompanies a well-ordered, virtuous mind, which Seneca identifies as the sage's joy. And although Seneca uses the term *voluptas* throughout 9.2.1–6, as this is the language of the interlocutor's objection, Seneca's rejoinder actually makes better sense if he has joy in mind.

This passage, without any qualification, suggests that pleasure accompanies virtue or virtuous action in so far as it is virtuous. But, if we are talking about accompanying *pleasure*, then this is not quite right, for vicious men also experience this pleasure. And while the 'aim' (*propositum*, 9.2.4) discussed here is ostensibly virtue itself, the aim that pleasure attends is not virtue but the performance, virtuous or otherwise, of some action or the obtaining of some other object or state. It is important to recognize that, for the Stoics, virtue consists in perfect reasoning, particularly about what to select and pursue.[42] Like the rest of us, sages will usually seek to stay healthy, avoid poverty, and actively engage in society. And as with the rest of us, when they do these things and eat, exercise, make a living, and help their fellow man, these activities may be pleasurable.[43] But unlike us, they will not take pleasure in them: that is, the affective coloring of their cognitive activity may be pleasant, but they will not undergo the emotion of pleasure in response to them.[44] The unwise pursue

---

42   On Stoic 'selection' (*eklogē*), see White 2010 and the works he cites in n. 4.

43   On the pleasure of benefaction, see *Ben.* 2.24.2, 3.17.3, 4.13.2, and 5.42.2.

44   *V.B.* 12.2: 'But on the other hand, the pleasures of the sage are calm, measured, almost faint and restrained, and scarcely noticeable [*remissae ... et modestae ac paene languidae ... compressaeque et vix notabiles*], since they arise unsought [*neque accersitae*] and,

and take pleasure in all this because they think they are good and essential to their happiness, and, often, because they are pleasurable. But the wise seek all these things not because they are what make life good, but because they are valuable, useful to living a good life, and, all things considered, the wise prefer them, even if they can lead a good life without them.[45] The key point is that the wise and virtuous will do what they do for its own sake as what is right, not with an eye to the pleasure it might bring.

But elsewhere Seneca uses *propositum* to translate the Greek word *telos*, which marks the goal to which all human life is ideally referred.[46] For the Stoics, this is virtue.[47] And a certain sort of pleasure broadly speaking does accompany virtue itself as a *propositum*, namely joy. While sages do not act virtuously for the sake of joy, it emerges from and colors their activity regardless. From this angle, Seneca's final remark in *V.B.* 9.2.1–6 that virtue does not satisfy because it pleases but rather pleases because it satisfies, is far more persuasive and precise. A sage's action satisfies her because it was her desire to act virtuously for its own sake, and part of the virtue of the action lies in this very desire for virtue itself. And only as an additional feature is the action enjoyable and a joy.

But we need to be careful in identifying the breadth and nature of virtuous activity that joy accompanies, for the passage in *De vita beata* risks obscuring it. The key lies in determining how virtue functions as a *propositum*, together with recognizing the accompanying joy as affective coloration. Sages do not aim for virtue in the same way as they aim for, say, health. Virtue is the disposition of a mind that has assented only to what is true and coheres perfectly with whatever else the mind has assented to.[48] In this condition, a virtuous mind thinks in a perfectly smooth, seamless way without various commitments

---

although they occur on their own [*per se accesserint*], they are neither held in honor nor received with any joy by those experiencing them [*percipientium*].'

45   On the vital Stoic distinction between goodness and value and its relationship to action, see esp. Diogenes Laertius 7.101–3 (= LS 58A); Stobaeus 2.83.10–84.2 (= LS 58D); Stobaeus 2.84.18–85.11 (= LS 58E); Cicero, *Fin.* 3.50 (= LS 58I); and Stobaeus 2.76.9–15 (= LS 58K). See also Vogt 2014 and Brennan 2003, 279–292.

46   See, e.g., *De Otio* 3.1.1, 7.2.2; *Tranq.* 2.6.2; *Ep.* 5.4.4, 55.5.6, 66.41.4, and 71.2.

47   On the Stoic *telos*, see LS chapters 63 and 64.

48   Plutarch, *Virt. Mort.* 440E–441D (= LS 61B); Cicero, *Acad.* 1.41–2 (= LS 41B); Plutarch, *St. Rep.* 1056E–F (= LS 41E); and Seneca, *Ep.* 31.8, 113.2, and esp. 66.6. In Stoic epistemology, only a body of true commitments can be entirely coherent (cf. together Sextus Empiricus, *Pyr.* 2.81–3 [= LS 33P]; Diogenes Laertius 7.46 [= LS 40C]; and Sextus Empiricus, *Math.* 7.151–157 [= LS 41C]).

contradicting each other and the mental turbulence of doubt and vacillation.[49] Virtuous action is a type of this virtuous thinking in the form of a selection of what to pursue, which is a movement of the mind—an impulse—towards that.[50] Two points thus arise: (1) sages 'aim' at virtue by selecting whatever they think appropriate to pursue or do. They achieve their goal of virtue necessarily, since their selection and pursuit are the results of perfect reasoning. The virtue of an action lies in the virtuous nature of the cognitive activity that underlies it. Hence (2), joy emerges from any cognitive activity of the virtuous mind (cf. *V.B.* 4.4.1–3, quoted above, p. 158), not simply its impulses, on which the passage in 9.2.1–6 focuses. So joy accompanies not only the sage's prudent, steady impulses but also her 'mere' thinking, such as her un-conflicted deliberation on what to do and her clear-minded consideration of some matter before her.[51] In other words, joy is the affective coloring of *all* virtuous cognitive activity as a result of its virtue.[52] Joy is the experience of virtue as a 'smooth flow of life'. Recall Seneca's remark in *Ep.* 23.4, quoted above, that the sage is in a state of joy 'when he thinks with a level head' (*apud se versat*, 5–6 [this = level head?]).[53] In the opening sections of the *De tranquillitate animi*, Seneca writes:

> Thus we seek how the mind may always move in a level and favorable way [*aequali secundoque cursu eat*, cf. *aequali et concordi cursu fluentia, Const.* 8.2.5] and may be well-disposed towards itself and may look upon its own affairs gladly and have this joy be uninterrupted, but remain in a calm state never exciting nor depressing itself: this will be tranquility. (2.4.1–6)

---

49   Sages may of course weigh their options and consider competing impressions, but unlike the fool, they will not assent until it is clear that they ought to, with the result that their assents are not liable to change due to further consideration on the same question. On this doubt and vacillation, see *Tranq.* 1–2 and Cicero, *Tusc.* 4.29.34–5 (= LS 61O).

50   See, e.g., Stobaeus 2.88.2–6 (= LS 33I).

51   There is a difference between the impulse that underlies the sage's, say, investigating the cosmos and the thinking (i.e. the consideration of and assenting to the impressions that arise in his mind) that constitutes this investigation.

52   Note that this does not rule out the sage experiencing both joy and pleasure (of the accompaniment variety). I see no reason why mental activity can't be variously affectively colored, such that, say, as the sage sates his hunger he isn't both joyous and experiencing the pleasure of eating.

53   Cf. *Ep.* 23.7.1–3, where Seneca writes that *gaudium* arises 'from a good conscience, right decisions, proper actions, disdain for what chance brings, and from the calm and steady course of a life that holds to one path' ('ex bona conscientia, ex honestis consiliis, ex rectis actionibus, ex contempt fortuitorum, ex placido vitae et continuo tenore unam prementis viam'). For *apud se* as 'with a level head' or 'sanely', see, e.g., *Tranq.* 17.11.5.

Here Seneca identifies tranquility, a form of joy, directly with level-headedness-cum-virtue, rather than alongside it, as in *Ep.* 23, or as arising from it, as in *V.B.* 4.5.2–6. But this descriptive ambiguity is to be expected for the sort of affective coloring and accompaniment we have seen joy and pleasure to be.[54] In the framework of Stoic monism, the affective experience of a mode of thought such as the smooth flow of virtuous thinking is only distinct in the abstract. We talk equally of eating being pleasurable and a pleasure. Similarly, the state of virtue is both enjoyable and a joy.[55]

4   *Gaudium* as Flow

The passage from *De tranquillitate animi* 2.4.1–6 helps us imagine what the experience of joy, or at least one type, tranquility, is like, but I think we can do better. In this part of the paper, I will describe a state of mind that we should be able to recognize in order to understand better what the sage's joy would be like. This state is called 'flow', a name coined by Mihaly Csikszentmihalyi, the leading scholar of this phenomenon.[56] Flow, according to him, is 'the state in which people are so involved in an activity that nothing else seems to matter; the experience itself is so enjoyable that people will do it even at great cost, for the sheer sake of doing it'.[57] 'Flow', he says, 'is the way people describe their state of mind when consciousness is harmoniously ordered, and they want to pursue whatever they are doing for its own sake'.[58] This is the state of being so absorbed in some book that we lose track of time or being so immersed in a workout that we fully embrace the deep burn in our muscles. In studies on flow conducted around the world, researchers have found both that flow is a universal human experience and that the experience itself is regularly described in similar ways, regardless of the variety of activities in which people find it. Indeed this is why Csikszentmihalyi calls this state 'flow', for people regularly describe it as enjoyable activity that smoothly and effortlessly flows

---

54   Cf. the variation in Aristotle's description of pleasure as 'an unimpeded activity of our natural state' (bk. 7: 1153a.14–15) or as 'a completion [τέλος] and accompaniment [ἐπιγινόμενόν] of an activity' (bk. 10: 1174b.31–33).

55   Cf. *V.B.* 3.3.3–4, where Seneca says that *perpetua tranquillitas* follows from the *vita beata* (= virtue), yet at *Ep.* 92.3, he says that the *vita beata* is *securitas et perpetua tranquillitas*.

56   On 'flow' in general, see Csikszentmihalyi 1990, 1997 and Csikszentmihalyi and Csikszentmihalyi 1992, 15–35. For a more current overview of flow research (which still largely follows Csikszentmihalyi), see Engeser and Schiepe-Tiska 2012.

57   Csikszentmihalyi 1990, 4.

58   Csikszentmihalyi 1990, 6.

from action to action without the disruptive doubts, self-consciousness, and self-criticism that characterize much if not most of our day-to-day life.[59]

Flow arises from an ordering of the mind that lacks conflicting thoughts and impulses. This ordering comes about through the focusing of attention. But our attention is limited. We can only pay attention to so many things at one time. Thus, how we direct our limited attention controls what we are aware of and what intentions or desires we have: an awareness of hunger leads to the desire for food, whereas an awareness of one's goal to lose weight leads to the opposing intention to disregard one's hunger.[60] And it is within or through the process of attention, in Csikszentmihalyi's account, that we evaluate what we become aware of as either positive or negative, depending on whether it supports or threatens our goals.[61] Cognitive distress and disorder, what he calls 'psychic entropy', arise when particular contents of our attention conflict with, threaten, or distract us from our current goals. The greater the conflict, the greater the distress, since we must divert our attention and mental energy to deal with something besides our current goal.[62] The opposite state, what Csikszentmihalyi calls 'optimal experience', occurs when everything that comes to our attention and to which we direct our attention coheres with our goals, and thus our mental energy flows smoothly in a unified direction, which is to say, in a state of flow.[63]

In drawing upon this theory in modern psychology, I am not suggesting that we can find in Stoic works precise parallels to all the details of the modern concept of flow, or that the Stoics describe flow in precisely the same way as Csikszentmihalyi.[64] But there is good reason to see it as an apt and illuminating *comparandum* for Stoic joy. One may object that researchers of flow study not emotion but a particular state of mind that consists in a certain directing of attention, and thus, even if being in flow is experienced positively, it is incommensurate with Stoic joy. Yet if I am right that the 'accompaniment' joy is *not* an emotion, but rather the affective experience of being virtuous, then flow

---

59   Csikszentmihalyi 1990, 39–40.

60   Csikszentmihalyi 1990, 27.

61   Csikszentmihalyi 1990, 30–31.

62   Csikszentmihalyi 1990, 36–39.

63   Csikszentmihalyi 1990, 39–41.

64   For instance, Csikszentmihalyi 1990 distinguishes what he calls 'pleasure', which 'is a feeling of contentment that one achieves whenever information in consciousness says that expectations set by biological programs or by social conditioning have been met' (p. 45), from 'enjoyment', an affection that attends flow, which 'occur[s] when a person has not only met some prior expectation or satisfied a need or a desire but also gone beyond what he or she has been programmed to do and achieved something unexpected, perhaps something even unimagined before' (p. 46).

actually helps clarify the phenomenological relationship between virtue and joy. Our enjoyment during flow is not a reaction to flow but a dimension of it, in the same way I have suggested joy is the affective dimension of virtue.[65] Thus, flow offers a more familiar avatar of the enigmatic affective and cognitive unity of Stoic psychology. There are, however, two fundamental, substantive differences between flow and Stoic joy that are worth noting. (1) Flow is amoral.[66] Immoral activities can be performed in flow just as readily as good ones, since none of the conditions necessary for flow involve morality. And, relatedly, (2) flow does not require any special epistemic state, which is to say we fools undergo flow. But Stoic joy cannot exist apart from virtue, goodness, and wisdom. Neither difference, however, negates the comparison's appropriateness, but rather qualifies the sort of flow we may liken to Stoic joy as a flow state that is, as it were, perfect in its quality and continuity and that accompanies ethically good activities (in the eyes of the Stoics).

Three key components facilitate a state of flow during an activity (whether physical, like running, or entirely mental, like solving riddles).[67] One is that the activity has explicit goals that allow clear feedback on whether one is reaching those goals. Two: that the activity is just challenging enough to require our full attention. Too challenging and we become anxious due to thoughts of inadequacy. Not challenging enough and we become bored and distracted. And three: that the agent is intrinsically motivated to perform the activity. In a state of flow the agent performs the activity and strives to perform it well because the activity itself is rewarding.

This brings me then to my last point concerning the psychological plausibility of joy, viz. the simultaneous presence of great pain, a condition Seneca allows the sage.[68] Joy as flow offers a possible explanation. Pain plays an interesting role in flow.[69] On the one hand, pain is particularly distracting and distressing and thus inhibitory of flow. But, on the other hand, in a state of flow, pain may recede into the background of our awareness or even provide necessary feedback concerning the performance of an activity. As such, pain neither rules flow out nor must it necessarily be eliminated or overshadowed by more positive feelings to allow flow. In fact, warfare can be an immensely

---

65   Cf. flow researchers' distinction between the emotional reaction of 'happiness' resulting
      from flow experiences and the 'positive affect' of enjoyment that is a component of flow
      (Landhäußer and Keller 2012, 74).
66   Schüler 2012 and Csikszentmihalyi 1990, 70.
67   Csikszentmihalyi 1990, 71–93. On 'the flow of thought' see Csikszentmihalyi 117–142. Cf.
      the discussion above of the affective side of logical puzzles in Stoicism.
68   See, e.g., *Constant.* 9, *Ep.* 72.4–6, and *Ep.* 76.27–29.
69   Csikszentmihalyi 1990, 192–201.

painful experience, but researchers have found that soldiers routinely describe it as a particularly flow-inducing activity.[70] Taking, then, a particularly Senecan example, consider a sage who finds himself captured and being beaten in the enemy's camp. And say he decides to endure it, which will, as a wise decision, be the right one. Of course he prefers to escape it, and this preference underlies his decision to endure and, let's say, try to escape the camp. He will turn all his attention to this task, and, importantly, every moment of effort to endure his beating is worthwhile for its own sake as a virtuous act, for this and the choice (to endure and escape) that underlies the effort is what the sage holds as truly good. In its virtue, this will be clear to him, and he will neither waver nor hesitate in his decisions. In this, then, the sage will proceed virtuously in a state of flow, which is to say that he will be in a state of Stoic joy. Of course this is not a pleasurable experience, but taking into account the sage's great strength of mind, it is conceivable that he should be able to remain calmly committed and focused on enduring the pain of the beating, never despairing in his ability or situation nor feeling distressed by the pain. Even in great pain, his endurance will be a smooth flow of mental and physical activity in the form of, for example, keeping his composure, remaining uncowed, and perhaps even doing what Seneca finds particularly admirable—taunting his captors.[71] These activities will be satisfying not in the sense of thinking 'job well done', but in the sense that they lack any doubt, hesitation, or mental discord. And it is this feature of the sage's action, this flow that accompanies the expression of his virtue, that qualifies even the endurance of great pain as, in its own way, enjoyable.

5   Conclusion

In closing, the Stoics, and Seneca in particular, identify a sort of pleasure, the sage's emergent, accompanying joy, that avoids the standard pain-pleasure

---

70   E.g. Csikszentmihalyi 1997, 139, Schüler 2012, 132–135, and esp. Harari 2008. As researchers recognize, warfare is a good example of the amorality of flow. One may act rightly in a state of flow in warfare, but equally the single-mindedness of flow may deny soldiers relevant ethical considerations and involve conflict with their other goals and values or the enjoyment involved may lead to a desire to fight simply for the sake of fighting. The sage is at risk for neither of these situations, as his flow in battle would arise precisely from the coherency of his evaluative worldview, and, as we have seen, he would only choose to fight because it is right, not because it may be enjoyable.

71   See, e.g., *Ep.* 78.18–19.

dichotomy. Pleasure typically stands as the opposite of pain.[72] They are mutually exclusive, at least in respect to the same activity. One may experience both pleasure and pain, say, during a massage, but the pain is in the muscle twinge while the pleasure is in the resulting relaxation. But, as I have described, it seems possible to experience joy in the Stoic sense from the very thing that is painful.[73] This is not masochism; the sage does not enjoy the pain itself. But it also is not simply pleasure in one thing and pain in another, for the sage's joy emerges from or in doing what is also and at the same time painful. And at least according to Seneca, this joy is far preferable to any sort of mere pleasure or lack of pain.

---

[72]   This is especially so in Epicureanism, where pain simply is the absence of pleasure and vice versa.

[73]   Cf. *Ep.* 99.19–28, where Seneca discusses a certain *voluptas* that accompanies the pain of grief (*tristia*) and denies that the Epicureans, despite their insistence, can coherently make sense of this.

CHAPTER 10

Alexander of Aphrodisias on Pleasure and Pain in Aristotle[1]

Wei Cheng

1 Introduction

The nature of pleasure and its role in human psychology and ethics attracted many early Greek philosophers such as Prodicus and Democritus, and then engaged almost all of the best minds of the Platonic Academy, sparking a series of intense intra-school debates. In these debates Aristotle's understanding of pleasure has a particularly noteworthy and extraordinary status. In contrast to Plato, subsequent Platonists, and the early Greek tradition as a whole, which associate pleasure with a restorative process, the satisfaction of desire, or the quality of our positive affect,[2] Aristotle offers an *energeia*-based definition of pleasure, which connects pleasure with the exercise (*energeia*) of our natural faculty in its good condition, a goal-immanent and self-realized activity.

There are, however, two distinct treatments of pleasure in the *Nicomachean Ethics*, each of which seems to describe the way in which pleasure is connected with *energeia* differently. While according to Book VII, pleasure is the unimpeded activity of the natural state (ἐνέργειαν τῆς κατὰ φύσιν ἕξεως, *EN* VII.12, 1153a14), in Book X Aristotle maintains the following:

> Pleasure completes the activity. But the way in which pleasure completes the activity is not the way in which the perceptible object and the perceptual capacity complete it when they are both excellent—just as

---

1 I would like to thank audiences at the Humboldt-Universität zu Berlin and Columbia University. For the comments on earlier drafts, I am indebted to Philip van der Eijk, David Merry, Tianqin Ge, Oliver Overwien, and Elizabeth Asmis. I owe special thanks to William Harris for his invaluable proof-reading, advice, and critical remarks. Finally, I am grateful for the support of the Alexander von Humboldt-Stiftung (van der Eijk's research programme: 'Medicine of the Mind, Philosophy of the Body—Discourses of Health and Well-Being in the Ancient World') that supported me to accomplish my research in Berlin.
2 Here I follow the traditional interpretation of Plato's concept of pleasure, cf. Frede 1997; van Riel 2000, 7–43; Evans 2008; Carpenter 2011. For its reception in later medical tradition, in particular in Galen, see Boudon-Millot in this volume.

health and the doctor are not the cause of being healthy in the same way
[...]. Pleasure completes the activity not in the same way the state does
by being present [in the activity], but as a sort of supervenient end, like
maturity on the prime of life.

EN 1174b24–26, b31–33[3]

The account of pleasure in *EN* X seems to differ from that in *EN* VII in one
substantial respect, inasmuch as the latter *identifies* pleasure with a particular
activity while the former implies that pleasure and activity are *distinct* via some
sort of supervenience relation (ἐπιγινόμενον).[4] Many scholars believe that these
two accounts in principle are incompatible.[5] Moreover, although the majority
of scholars are inclined to hold that *EN* X offers a philosophically more promising account of pleasure, what persists is widespread disagreement about how
to understand the so-called supervenience of pleasure on activity.

In contemporary Aristotelian scholarship we can roughly divide the interpretations of supervenience into two groups. Let us call one the Extrinsic
Reading and the other the Intrinsic Reading. The former treats pleasure as an
epiphenomenon or a by-product[6]—something that is generated by an activity,
but does not exert reciprocal influence on the activity in question.[7] Inwood,
for instance, claims that 'in the *Nicomachean Ethics* pleasure is not constitutive of the activity which is happiness, but reliably accompanies it. What

---

3 τελειοῖ δὲ τὴν ἐνέργειαν ἡ ἡδονή. οὐ τὸν αὐτὸν δὲ τρόπον ἥ τε ἡδονὴ τελειοῖ καὶ τὸ αἰσθητόν τε καὶ
ἡ αἴσθησις, σπουδαῖα ὄντα, ὥσπερ οὐδ' ἡ ὑγίεια καὶ ὁ ἰατρὸς ὁμοίως αἰτία ἐστὶ τοῦ ὑγιαίνειν. [...]
τελειοῖ δὲ τὴν ἐνέργειαν ἡ ἡδονὴ οὐχ ὡς ἡ ἕξις ἐνυπάρχουσα, ἀλλ' ὡς ἐπιγινόμενόν τι τέλος, οἷον τοῖς
ἀκμαίοις ἡ ὥρα. The translation is based on Irwin, but modified. With respect to the sense of
the simile—οἷον τοῖς ἀκμαίοις ἡ ὥρα, I follow Hadreas 1997. For a more detailed discussion, see
Cheng 2015, 332–3. For a recent defence of the traditional reading 'like the bloom on youths',
see Warren 2016.

4 Following the custom of Aristotelian scholarship, I use supervenience and its cognates to
refer to the particular relationship between pleasure and activity (*energeia*), which can be
traced back to the Latin translation of ἐπιγινόμενόν τι τέλος (*EN* X 4.1174b33) as '*superveniens
quidam finis*' by Robert Grosseteste (cf. Hadreas 1997, 372). Although it is an open question
how to specify this relation in Aristotle (cf. Vogt in this volume), certainly it cannot be confused with the term 'supervenience' which is commonly used to characterize a particular
dependence of mind on body in contemporary philosophy of mind (cf. Kim 1991). For a discussion of supervenience in Aristotle's philosophy of mind, see Caston 1993.

5 Alexander, *PE* 143.13–146.12; Festugière 1936; Dirlmeier 1964, 567, 580–1; Lieberg 1958, 7–15;
Ricken 1976, 115–17; Gosling and Taylor 1982, 250–4; Wolf 2002, 191, 205; Irwin 2007, 169, n35;
Rapp 2009, 222; Heinaman 2011; Shields 2011; Salim 2012; Harte 2014.

6 For the ancient concept of epiphenomenalism see Caston 1997; for this concept in contemporary philosophy see Robinson 2015.

7 Van Riel 1999; 2000, 43–78.

motivates us is the drive to activity in accordance with our characteristic rational excellence'.[8] The Intrinsic Reading, on the contrary, understands pleasure
as the *perfection* of the activity upon which it supervenes. As such, pleasure
is constitutive of, and intrinsic to, the activity with which it is connected.
Proponents of this reading, however, are not unanimous about how to specify
the way in which pleasure makes the activity perfect. Does pleasure function
as a final cause,[9] a formal cause,[10] the passive dimension of an activity,[11] or the
overall interplay of all excellent aspects?[12] While the Extrinsic Reading justifies
the priority of activity over pleasure by appealing to the ontological dependence of pleasure on activity, which allows for the completeness or perfectness
of the activity in question as well as a fixed hierarchy between pleasure and
activity, the Intrinsic Reading highlights the constitutive role of pleasure by
emphasizing its particular contribution to the perfection of activity.

The dispute between these two readings is still in progress, and perhaps
will not end. In what follows, however, I do not want to broach this point
of contention directly. Instead, I aim to draw attention to a similar, yet basi-
cally ignored debate in antiquity over the obscure relation of supervenience
between pleasure and activity in which both Alexander of Aphrodisias and
other interpreters of Aristotle, probably his colleagues, students, and even some
of his predecessors, took part.[13] This exegetic debate is hidden in Alexander's

---

8   Inwood 2014, 40.

9   Cf. Gauthier and Jolif 1958–9 (vol. II.2), 839–42.

10   Gosling and Taylor 1982, 241–54. Taylor (2008, 263) has changed his mind, admitting that
     his early suggestion of pleasure as a formal cause is 'less plausible'. Shields (2011, 207–8)
     suggests that pleasure is first of all an efficient cause, but that it is also a formal and final
     cause.

11   Salim 2012.

12   Strohl 2011. Strictly speaking, Strohl's position stands somewhere between the Intrinsic
     and Extrinsic Reading. For he denies that pleasure can function as any of Aristotle's four
     causes, and qualifies it as a perfect aspect of a well-operative activity. Pleasure is intrinsic
     to the activity only insofar as it is an ingredient of the *excellence* of the activity. The excel-
     lence of activity x, however, seems to be *extrinsic* to x inasmuch as it is *added* to form x
     rather than being an integral part of form x. As the contrast drawn between the minimal
     condition and the perfection of x shows, Strohl understands the form of something as
     the bottom line of what this thing is, a set of basic features shared by all the individuals
     subordinated to this universal. Yet it is doubtful whether this understanding would be
     well received by Aristotle, who might be more inclined to take the form of something as
     an excellent realization of its intrinsic power in a teleological context.

13   This hypothesis does not necessarily commit us to believe that the debates in question
     happened between Alexander and his opponents in an established institution (as the
     hedonistic debates among the Academics in the Academy), because (due to the fact that
     there is no information about any of his immediate pupils) whether and in what sense
     Alexander had a school is still an open question (cf. Sharples 1990b). Rather, I simply want

theoretical criticism of some anonymous 'hedonists' in the *Problemata Ethica (PE)*—a collection of short and unsystematic notes about ethical issues.[14] I shall argue that Alexander develops his anti-hedonistic argument mainly based on the Extrinsic Reading of Aristotle's supervenience-based interpretation of pleasure, whereas the 'hedonists' criticized by him are those who advocate a pleasure-friendly and an Intrinsic Reading of the supervenience in question, or those who try to verify the goodness of pleasure by appealing to Aristotle in this way. In light of this dialogic situation, many of Alexander's argumentative moves are presumably reactions to, and influenced by, the proposal of his opponents who base their theories likewise on a reading of Aristotle.

The reconstruction of this forgotten debate within the Peripatetic tradition is of significance in three respects. First, it provides us a new way to understand Alexander's particular motivation and arguments in his account of Aristotle's pleasure, and in particular several extraordinary features of his interpretation. For instance, it is unusual that Alexander, unlike most Aristotelian scholars, expends so much effort on the clarification and classification of different kinds of pain. Arguably, one motivation for him to flesh out the conception and evaluation of pain is that his anti-hedonistic concern in determining the nature of pleasure—which is presumably initiated by some pleasure-friendly interpretations of Aristotle's theory—leads to a correspondingly friendlier attitude to pain, an opposite of pleasure in his account. This understanding of pain is, however, in tension with the negative evaluation of pain dominant in Aristotle.[15] Second, since there are only a few incomplete commentaries on Aristotle's *Ethics* surviving from antiquity,[16] a reconstruction of this debate

---

to argue that the main target at which Alexander aimed was the Aristotelian tradition. For my detailed discussion, see below.

14   For discussions of this collection, see Madigan 1987; Sharples 1990a. The collection edited by M. Bonelli: *Aristotele e Alessandro di Afrodisia (Questioni etiche e Mantissa): Metodo e oggetto dell'etica peripatetica* (Naples, 2015) awaits further examination given that it was published after I finished the main part of my manuscript. As a remedy, I have added a few footnotes to reflect some of the discussions that arose in that volume, in particular the contributions of L. Castelli and C. Natali.

15   Cf. *Top.* 119a39–b1; *EE* 1225a16; 1227a40; *EN* 1113b1–2; 1385b13–14; *Rhet.* 1386a7–9.

16   That is the commentary of Aspasius—who is supposed to have lived in the first half of the second century AD—on *EN* I–IV and on a larger part of *EN* VII–VIII (in CAG 19.1 ed. by Heylbut). For discussions of this commentary, see Moraux 1984, 226–93; Barnes 1999. A surviving anonymous commentary on *EN* II–V (CAG 20, 122–255, ed. by G. Heylbut) is sometimes believed to have been written later than Aspasius but before Alexander's works (the last quarter of the second century AD according to Moraux 1984, 325; Mercken 1990, 408; or about the late 170s according to Eliasson 2013, 200). The author of this text is taken by Kenny (1978, 37) to be Adrastus of Aphrodisias, a Peripatetic active in the

will provide a valuable slice of the history of the reception of Aristotle's practical philosophy in the ancient commentary tradition, which was overshadowed by extensive works on Aristotle's theoretical philosophy. In particular, it offers us a typical example of the dominant way of doing philosophy from the first century BC onwards, which connects the solution of problems with textual exegesis.[17] In other words, by virtue of this instance we can see how ancient commentators approach ethics in terms of Aristotelian exegesis, and conversely, how their textual interpretations are deeply influenced by the presupposed philosophical positions.[18] Finally, as indicated above, the ancient debate between Alexander and other Aristotelians actually foreshadowed the divergence in modern disputes on Aristotle's theory of pleasure. The parallel not only reflects the tension and potential of Aristotle's account itself, but also urges us to reconsider the hermeneutic situation with which we are now faced. If we are not to fall into the stalemate which beset the ancients, Aristotle's notion of supervenience needs to be approached by an alternative proposal which overcomes the opposition between the Intrinsic and Extrinsic Readings.

The structure of my article is the following: to begin with, I show how Alexander interprets Aristotle's doctrines about pleasure, and how his interpretation of these doctrines leads to a particular understanding of pain. After that, I argue that Alexander uses his interpretation of Aristotle to serve his own anti-hedonistic purposes. The hedonism he was most worried about here, however, is neither a vulgar hedonism nor Epicureanism but a pleasure-friendly trend within the Peripatetic tradition, which interprets Aristotle's doctrines of pleasure in such a way as to pave the way for a Peripatetic variety of hedonism. Finally, I shall briefly review the merits and disadvantages of Alexander' approach.

2   Defining Pleasure

Alexander's discussions of Aristotelian pleasure and pain are chiefly preserved in the so-called *Problemata Ethica*, a collection of short treatises probably

---

second century AD, yet it is more likely a compilation that in part depends on Adrastus' work *On Historical and Literary Questions in the Nicomachean Ethics of Aristotle* (cf. Moraux 1984, 323–9, Mercken 1990, 421–2; also see Barnes 1999, 15–18). For a rehabilitation of its philosophical relevance see Eliasson 2013.

17   E.g. Gottschalk 1987; Sedley 1997.

18   Natali (2015) has recently offered an excellent summary of how Alexander interprets Aristotle's concepts of pleasure and pain by appealing to the principle of *Aristoteles ex Aristotele*, and to what extent his interpretation is indebted to Aspasius. Nevertheless, the *philosophical* implication of Alexander's approach is not adequately explored.

based on his lecture notes, as its subtitle—'school-discussion problems and so-lutions on ethics'[19]—indicates.[20] Although *PE* is formally structured, like other works in the genre of *problemata* literature,[21] by '(question(s) and answer(s)' or by 'thesis and analysis', it is easy to discern that almost all the problems treated here arise from a reading of Aristotle's *EN*, and so the treatises express a strong interest in textual interpretation. The selection of topics in the collec-tion, however, is centered around the pair ἡδονή and ἀρετή, while neglecting many significant subjects in Aristotle's *Ethics*—which shows the influence of Hellenistic and later philosophical taste.[22]

In accordance with the contemporary mainstream interpretation, Alexander sees no substantial divergence between the two accounts of pleasure in *EN* VII and X,[23] but the cornerstone of his understanding of pleasure is *EN* X,[24] according to which pleasure is something that supervenes on a perfect activity (*energeia*) and completes it.[25] Alexander paraphrases the thought as follows:

---

19   σχολικῶν ἠθικῶν ἀποριῶν καὶ λύσεων κεφάλαια.

20   We have no compelling reason to deprive Alexander of the authorship of this text, see Sharples 1990b, 1–7.

21   For this genre see Pfeiffer 1968, 69–70; Oikonomopoulou 2013; Taub 2015.

22   The logical and dialectical interests of this text have been correctly highlighted by Sharples (1990a) and Castelli (2015). However, it seems to me exaggerated to claim that in this collection, Alexander's 'interest lies primarily in the theoretical or logical issues rather than in their ethical content as such' (Castelli 2015: 42). It is undeniable that Alexander here is interested in relations of contrariety, predication, and genus/spe-cies, and addresses them more frequently than Aristotle did in his ethics, yet this does not mean that 'the domain of ethical concepts becomes a privileged domain for test-ing and developing formal distinctions' (*ibid.*). In this study I aim to show that with respects to pleasure and pain, Alexander's approach and his strategy are essentially moti-vated by *ethical* interest and serve *ethical* proposes, so that many of his arguments cannot be properly understood without his *ethical* concerns.

23   Cf. Alexander *in APr.* 302. 5–6, 8–10; *in Top.* 164. 16–17. A central concern of Problem §23 ('If pleasure is unimpeded activity of the natural state according to Aristotle, how will happiness too not be pleasure?, 143.10) is how to reconcile the apparent incon-sistence of two different understandings of pleasure in *EN* VII and X, cf. *PE* 143. 25–144. 4. Alexander points out that pleasure is regarded as activity *because* it al-ways supervenes on activity. This answer suggests that he takes the definition in the *EN* VII as incautious yet compatible with *EN* X.

24   Pace Natali (2015, 79), according to whom *EN* VII plays a more important role in Alexander's interpretation.

25   Cf. *EN* 1174b23; 31–33; 1175a15, 21, 29–30; 35–36; 1175b30–35. In speaking of the dependence of pleasure on activity, Alexander interchangeably uses ἐπιγίγνεσθαι, γίγνεσθαι plus ἐπί, or only the preposition ἐπί. No matter whether Alexander provides a plausible interpreta-tion of Aristotle, I maintain the term 'supervenience' in order to show that Alexander's discussions are substantially based on Aristotle's view in *EN* X.

Pleasure follows activities and is in a way a part or an end of them, and it is from them that it has its [worthiness] to be chosen or avoided; for the [pleasures] that [supervene] on activities that are to be chosen are [themselves] to be chosen, and those that [supervene] on those that are not like this are to be avoided.

PE 127.11–13[26]

Readers who are familiar with Aristotle might expect Alexander to specify the supervenience relation between pleasure and activity (*energeia*). He does not, however, attempt to do this, but seems happy to loosely use different words—following (*hepomenē*), somehow a part (*meros*), and an end (*telos*)—to describe this relation at the outset. More surprisingly, he never returns to the whole-part or the process-end relation indicated at the beginning of this passage, but uses the supervenience relation to underline the overall dependence of pleasure on activity. This indicates that Alexander is not so much concerned to clarify the exact nature of the puzzling supervenience, but to justify the ontological priority of activity over pleasure—not only in this passage, but also in this whole collection—by appealing to such a relation. As a result, we cannot recover Alexander's view, if he had one, on how Aristotle thought pleasure played the role of perfection-maker. Alexander's basic idea can be roughly understood as follows:

Given that x supervenes upon y, any character of x is determined by a corresponding character of y, but not conversely.

In this model, as we have indicated, Alexander's purpose is to foreground the ontological and causal priority of activity over pleasure. As a result, pleasure turns out to be epiphenomenal insofar as the reciprocal contribution of pleasure to the activity with which it is connected is deliberately dismissed. On the basis of this ontological relation, Alexander establishes a corresponding *value* supervenience, to which he attaches the most weight. According to this, given that a pleasure supervenes on an activity, the pleasure will have the same value as the activity. The pleasure's value is determined by the activity's, but not *vice versa*.[27]

---

26   ἡ ἡδονὴ ταῖς ἐνεργείαις ἑπομένη καὶ μέρος πως ἢ τέλος οὖσα αὐτῶν παρ' ἐκείνων ἔχει τὸ αἱρετόν
      τε καὶ φευκτόν (αἱρεταὶ μὲν γὰρ αἱ ἐπὶ ταῖς αἱρεταῖς ἐνεργείαις, φευκταὶ δ' αἱ ἐπὶ ταῖς μὴ τοιαύ-
      ταις. Trans. by Sharples (1990a), modified.
27   *PE* 120.11–16; 120.24–31; 124.9–11; 18–21; 133.20–23; 134.12–14; 137.1–5; 137.25–27; 137.33–36;
      146.1–7.

This relation explains why some pleasures are good and others bad, by making their value dependent on the value of the activities they depend on. For according to this model, since activities can be good, bad, or neutral, the same goes with their associated pleasures.[28] It is therefore obvious that neither pleasure *as a whole*, nor pleasure in the absence of qualifying expression can be qualified as *the good* or *something good*.[29] This conclusion is lucidly expressed by the title of Problem §5 that 'if pleasure in general is a genus, it seems neither a good nor an evil nor something intermediate'.[30] As a consequence, it is categorically illegitimate to attribute any evaluative property to pleasure if pleasure is not determined by a quantifying expression.

It is remarkable that Alexander keeps silent about the fact that the activity in question is characterized by Aristotle as perfect or excellent (*EN* 1174b16–20). That is, according to Aristotle, pleasure is not simply causally determined by a random activity, but seems to be supervenient upon the activity as long as it is somehow functioning well. Pleasure does not only concur with a good activity, but also shares the same or at least similar characteristics of this activity. It is noteworthy that this extraordinary understanding of pleasure is put forward and gradually fleshed out in a dialectical context in which Aristotle takes issue with his opponents, in particular, the Academics, who define pleasure as a *kinēsis* or something like *kinēsis*, which is essentially *imperfect* according to Aristotle's conceptual schema. Thus, the concept of *energeia* should be adequately understood in reference to *kinēsis*, and their relation is the key for Aristotle in his attempt to defend the value of pleasure. Alexander, however, diluted the dialectical background in Aristotle's account,[31] and left the significant opposition between *kinēsis* and *energeia* unmentioned. In doing so, he underplayed (if not completely dismissed) Aristotle's normative motivations in making pleasure supervene on the *perfect* activity, so that he can ignore Aristotle's emphasis on pleasure as the perfection of the activity. A dramatic contrast between the ways in which Aristotle and Alexander utilize the supervenience is that whereas this relation is initially invoked by Aristotle to verify the value of pleasure, Alexander is mainly concerned to resist hedonism in

---

28   *EN* 1175a22, 27–28; 1175b1; 1175b36; cf. Alexander *PE* §3, § 13, § 17; §19.
29   For discussion about the distinction between the propositions with quantifying expression and those without it in Aristotle, see Malink 2015, 273–285.
30   ἡ κοινὴ ἡδονὴ ἡ ὡς γένος λαμβανομένη οὔτ᾽ ἀγαθόν ἐστιν οὔτε κακὸν οὔτ᾽ ἀδιάφορον, *PE* 124.1–2.
31   This aspect is properly emphasized by Natali (2015, 67 and 80). Yet he seems to go too far in claiming that Alexander's approach is thus scientific rather than dialectical ('un' indagine scientifica e non dialettica' (2015, 67).

appealing to the same concept of supervenience, which, then, also leads him to an extraordinary understanding of pain.[32]

It is well known that there is no systematic account of pain available in Aristotle's extant corpus. But sometimes he seems to presuppose that pain is a kind of mirror image of pleasure, so that its nature can be inferred from the nature of pleasure. This procedure can be called the 'mirroring method',[33] which also plays a significant role in Alexander's struggle to evaluate pain: 'for [pleasure] comes about by its affinity to them (sc. *energeiai*), like a sort of end for them; but pain[34] is a sign of alienation from the [activities] on which it supervenes' (*PE* 124.29–31).[35] As in his discussion of pleasure, Alexander does

---

32   It is extraordinary in the sense that pain, in parallel with pleasure, is understood by a particular supervenience relation between the affect and an *energeia* (for my more detailed discussion, see below). Ancient mainstream views on pain, however, were dominated by medical thought, in particular, the Hippocratic tradition, according to which pain amounts to some kind of imbalanced state of the body caused by unnatural and violent change (Scullin 2012, also cf. Harris and Boudon-Millot in this volume).

      Pace Castelli (2015, 42), who seems to suggest that Alexander's interest in the relations between the pairs pleasure/pain and good/bad is determined by his interest in the oppositions of contrariety. I think, on the contrary, that Alexander here addresses these pairs, not because they can be used to illustrate the relations of contraries, but because, in order to offer a proper evaluation of pleasure and pain, he feels it is necessary to struggle with problems concerning different kinds of contraries.

33   The name is owed to Frede (2006, 263).

34   Sharples 1990a consistently translates λύπη as distress and πόνος as pain in this collection, which seems to suggest that Alexander more or less follows the Stoic theory of emotion. Although Alexander is doubtless influenced by Stoics in this regard, this choice, however, does not work well for the whole collection for three reasons. First, a main target of Alexander's engagement with pain is to interpret Aristotle. Aristotle does not use λύπη as exclusively emotional, but every kind of pain as well as pain in general or the concept of pain *per se*. If we follow Sharples, the exegetic feature of Alexander would be obscured. Second, two main concerns of Alexander's handling of this topic are to explain (1) which kind of pain is opposed to pleasure (ἡδονή), (2) in what sense pain is opposed to pleasure. He does not distinguish between χαρά and ἡδονή in a Stoic way, but is more concerned about the relationship between pleasure and pain as such. Hence even if he draws the distinction between λύπη and πόνος in a Stoic way, his motivation is still to solve problems around pain. Finally, and most importantly, Alexander does not have a unified distinction between λύπη and πόνος. In *PE* 126.7–11, he seems to provide a Stoicism-like distinction between λύπη and πόνος by referring the former to a contraction of the soul (ψυχικὴν συστολήν), and the latter to some affliction (θλῖψιν) of the body. Nevertheless, in *PE* 125.32–35, λύπη becomes the general concept of pain, whereas πόνος counts as its part. This relation, however, is discussed in *PE* 127.8–10, in which πόνος is taken to be wider than λύπη.

35   κατ' οἰκειότητα γὰρ τὴν πρὸς αὐτὰς ἐγίνετο καὶ ὡς τέλος τι ἦν αὐτῶν, ἡ δὲ λύπη ἀλλοτριότητός ἐστι σημεῖον τοῖς ἐφ' οἷς γίνεται. Trans. by Sharples (1990a), modified.

not elaborate on the supervenience of pain, but aims to establish a reversed supervenience of value on this basis:

> Similarly it is reasonable to suppose that pains, too, supervening on certain activities, themselves derive from these their worthiness to be chosen or avoided, in the opposite way to the pleasures. For those that supervene on noble activities are to be avoided, those that [supervene] on shameful [activities] are to be chosen.
>
> PE 127.13–17[36]

As we can see from this passage, the crucial step for Alexander towards reconstructing an Aristotelian understanding of pain is that pain, in analogy to pleasure, is equally determined as something that supervenes upon *energeia*. This is by no means a self-evident move, not only because, intuitively, several kinds of pain—for instance, a headache—do not seem to presuppose that I am using my brain,[37] but also because Aristotle does not explicitly state that the supervenience between pleasure and *energeia* can be transferred into pain and *energeia*.[38]

Alexander seem to be aware of these problems. By appealing to the distinction between voluntary, involuntary, and non-voluntary actions in *EN* III.2, he tries to find concrete examples in Aristotle which show that pain not only supervenes upon *energeia*, but also does so in an opposite way to the supervenience of pleasure. For according to Aristotle, if someone's bad activity caused by ignorance is afterwards accompanied by pain and regret, this action should be assessed as better than the same action without pain. Pain, then, functions

---

36   οὕτως εὔλογον καὶ τὰς λύπας ὑπολαμβάνειν ἐπὶ ἐνεργείαις τισὶ γινομένας παρ' ἐκείνων καὶ αὐτὰς
       ἔχειν τὸ αἱρετόν τε καὶ φευκτὸν ἔμπαλιν τῶν ἡδονῶν. τὰς μὲν γὰρ ἐπὶ ταῖς καλαῖς γινομένας
       ἐνεργείαις φευκτὰς εἶναι, τὰς δ' ἐπὶ ταῖς αἰσχραῖς αἱρετάς. Trans. by Sharples (1990a), modified.
37   Pain of this kind seems to be well explained by ancient medical tradition (cf. Harris
       and Boudon-Millot in this volume). I leave open whether the same goes with pleasure.
       Aristotle at least believes that all kinds of pleasure required corresponding activities, but
       he does not explicitly apply the same thought to pain.
38   Usually Aristotle either takes pain as a hindrance of an on-going *energeia* (cf. *EN* 1153b3)
       or some sort of unnatural change (cf. *Resp.* 479b26–30; *Metaph.* 1022b15–21). In *DA*
       III.7.431a9–11, however, he seems to classify pain, in parallel with pleasure, under the category of *energeia*. 'Whenever there is something pleasant or painful, it [the soul] by, so to
       speak, affirming or denying, pursues or avoids. And it is the case that being pleased and
       being pained are the actualizations (τὸ ἥδεσθαι καὶ λυπεῖσθαι τὸ ἐνεργεῖν) of the mean of
       the perceptual faculty in relation to what is good or bad insofar as they are such' (trans.
       Shields 2016). For a detailed discussion about the sense in which pain can be regarded as
       an *energeia*, cf. Cheng 2015, 364–371.

as a meta-evaluative criterion in distinguishing between *in*voluntary and *non*-voluntary activities (cf. *EN* 1110b19–24; 1111a19–21). Leaving aside whether what Aristotle is saying here instantiates the supervenience in question, if this case represents the supervenience Alexander is focusing on, it would undermine his determination of pleasure and pain as epiphenomena, because the pain seems to be impacting the evaluation of the action rather than the other way round. Whether Alexander is aware of this problem or not, what is more important for him is to find a concrete example in Aristotle which can evidence the reversed supervenience of pain, extrapolated via the mirroring method mentioned above. This relation, contrasted to the label of the supervenience of pleasure as affinity (*oikeiotēs*) (*PE* 124.29–36),[39] is called by Alexander an 'alienation' (*allotriotēs*), according to which pains which accompany good activities are bad, pains which accompany bad activities are good, and pains which accompany indifferent activities (*epi tais adiaphorois*) are indifferent (124.24–26). Based on the notion of pain as an alien supervenience, Alexander establishes a converse value-supervenience of pain, which can be summarized as follows:

> Given that a pain supervenes on an activity, the pain will have the opposite value as the activity. The pain's value is determined by the activity's, but not *vice versa*.

It is remarkable that, just as in the case of pleasure, Alexander does not elaborate how pain supervenes upon activity in an alien way. He is more concerned to establish a systematic evaluation of pain by means of such alien supervenience, which functions perfectly as a counterpart of the supervenience relation between pleasure and activity. Although Aristotle also touches upon alienation, he does not determine pain as an alien *supervenience*, but only mentions that pleasure derived from activity x would become painful for someone who is doing y if x is alien to y (cf. *EN* x.5, 1175b1–24). No matter whether and

---

39 The Stoic terms are striking here (cf. Sharples 1990a, 27 n.55). Cf. Chrysippus fr.229a: οὐ μὴν ἀκολουθεῖ γε ταῦτα τοῖς Χρυσίππου δόγμασιν, ὥσπερ οὐδὲ τῷ μηδεμίαν οἰκείωσιν εἶναι φύσει πρὸς ἡδονὴν ἢ ἀλλοτρίωσιν πρὸς πόνον. On the Stoic *Oikeiosislehre*, see Pembroke 1971, 112–49; Engberg-Pedersen 1990; Bees 2004; Forschner 2008. Although it is intricate and controversial how the *Oikeiosislehre* of the Stoics is related to the Peripatetic tradition (cf. Brink 1956, Szaif 2012, 229–63), it is certain that some early Peripatetics (e.g. Theophrastus, Dicaearchus) propounded some Peripatetic versions of *oikeiōsis*, which, though impacted by Stoics to varying degrees, can also be somehow traced back to Aristotle's own teaching, cf. *EN* 1153a20–22; 1175a34–36; 1175b22–23; 1175b16–17; 1175b30–31; 1178a5.

to what extent Alexander does justice to Aristotle, his approaches have significant consequences.

First, hedonism is false, not because pleasure is bad, but because pleasure and pain cannot provide any non-derived reason or value for actions and choices. Second, even though they relate to activity in opposite ways, pleasure and pain are similar in that pleasures and pains as a whole are *essentially indeterminate* with respect to their evaluation.[40] In other words, neither of them is more prone to be good or to be bad. Pleasure as a whole is thus no better than pain as a whole. Third, a broad space is created for the evaluation of pain. This fits well with the Peripatetic preference of proper emotions in which certain kinds of pleasure and pain are blended, yet it is in tension with Aristotle's use in several arguments of the premise that pain is something bad.[41] The solution of this *aporia* thus becomes a main task in Alexander's treatment of the nature of pain.[42]

3   Alexander and the Aristotelian Forms of Hedonism

Alexander addresses the supervenience relation between pleasure and activity as part of a case *against hedonism*. Aristotle, in contrast, develops the theory of pleasure as standing in a supervenience relation to activity as part of a dialectical *defense of the value* of pleasure. *Prima facie* it appears unclear why Alexander, in contrast to Aristotle, is so worried about hedonism. It is reasonable to assume that this feature reflects a widespread hostility towards Epicureanism, which had been a commonplace since the Hellenistic period. Under closer scrutiny, however, Alexander seems to have had a different concern. For what he strives to do is not simply to refute hedonism from a theoretical point of view, but also to 'purify' Aristotle's theory of even the slightest hedonistic *hint*.

---

40   Note that the thesis that the value of x is indeterminate is not equivalent to the thesis that the value of x is intermediate between good and evil. Rather, it is another way to formulate the thought in Pr. §5 that pleasure as a genus seems 'neither a good nor an evil nor something intermediate' (*PE* 124. 1–2).

41   *EE* 1225a16; 1227a40; *EN* 1113b1–2; *Rhet.* 1385b13–14; 1386a7–9; *Top.* 119a39–b1.

42   Pace Natali (2015), who believes that Alexander's main concern in the *PE* is to verify the thesis that every pain is a bad, yet not every pleasure is a good. This characterization is too simplistic: it fails to pay due attention to the richness and complexity of Alexander's engagement, in particular his struggle with the problem concerning classification and evaluation of pain in terms of the supervenience.

Like other opponents of Alexander in the *PE*, the friends of pleasure also remain anonymous in his account. It is worth looking at how Alexander characterizes the hedonists in question:

> They (sc. the hedonists) are vulgar either because they locate happiness in bodily enjoyments, as do also slaves and cattle, <or> because, according to those, pleasure alone is to be chosen and pain is to be avoided on its own account.
>
> *PE* 138.8–10[43]

In this passage, the hedonists in question are divided into two groups: those who 'locate happiness in bodily enjoyment' and those who take pleasure and pain as the things to be chosen or avoided for their own sake. The former seems to represent a folk hedonism, according to which *bodily* pleasure is the ultimate good. The position of the latter, in contrast, alludes to a theoretical interest on the estimation of pleasure and pain in activities. It is thus not astonishing that the second group is Alexander's main target in his struggle against hedonism. In another passage, he reports their position in more detail:

> For [someone might] say both [1] that only pleasures are to be chosen on their own account, and that each of the other things that are to be chosen [deserves to be chosen] to the extent that it contributes something to pleasure, and also [2] that, while what is noble is to be chosen because it produces pleasure, what is shameful is not also to be chosen because of the pleasure brought about by it.
>
> *PE* 145.21–25[44]

In this outline of hedonism, we can discern few special Epicurean features. For it is not exclusively Epicurean to think that pleasure is worth choosing on its own account. There is little reason on this basis alone to suppose that the Epicureans were the unique target in Alexander's polemic. We should note that the pleasure-friendly tradition was so influential that it is by no means limited to Epicureanism, but was popular in ordinary thinking, and was even endorsed,

---

43   Ἡ διότι τὴν εὐδαιμονίαν ἐν ταῖς σωματικαῖς ἀπολαύσεσι τίθενται, ἐν αἷς καὶ τὰ ἀνδράποδα καὶ τὰ βοσκήματα, εἰσὶ φορτικοί, <ἢ> διότι καθ᾿ οὓς ἡ μόνη ἡδονὴ αἱρετὴ καὶ ὁ πόνος δι᾿ αὐτὸν φευκτός. Trans. by Sharples (1990a), modified.

44   τὸ γὰρ ὁμοῦ μὲν λέγειν τὰς ἡδονὰς μόνας εἶναι δι᾿ αὐτὰς αἱρετάς, τῶν δ᾿ ἄλλων αἱρετῶν ἕκαστον ἐφ᾿ ὅσον εἰς ἡδονήν τι συντελεῖ, ἐπὶ τοσοῦτον καὶ τὸ αἱρετὸν ἔχειν, ὁμοῦ δὲ τὸ μὲν καλὸν αἱρετὸν εἶναι λέγειν ὡς ποιητικὸν ἡδονῆς, μηκέτι δὲ καὶ τὸ αἰσχρὸν φάσκειν αἱρετὸν γίνεσθαι διὰ τὴν γινομένην ἡδονὴν ὑπ᾿ αὐτοῦ. Trans. by Sharples (1990a), modified.

to varying degrees, by several philosophers in other traditions, including Stoics and Peripatetics, who are supposed to have held a serious attitude towards pleasure.[45] This fact opens up the need to reconsider the complexity of the hedonistic tradition and their argumentative strategies,[46] which becomes more urgent if we take a look at Alexander's further account of his opponents:

> [This person might indeed] say that the pleasures that supervene on noble activities are pure and free from mixture with the opposite pains, and that on this account the activities that produce them, too, are to be chosen; while those [pleasures] that [supervene] on shameful [activities] possess little that gives enjoyment and much and more that produces pains, for which reason such activities too are not to be chosen, being productive of pain rather than of pleasure.
>
> *PE* 145.28–33[47]

It is striking at first glance that Aristotelian jargon and thought can be found in this report, which suggests that Alexander's opponents seem also to be interpreting Aristotle or philosophizing within an Aristotelian framework.[48] To put it more precisely, they follow Aristotle at least on four points. (1) They understand pleasure as something that supervenes upon activity. (2) They believe that pleasure resembles the activity it accompanies. Concretely speaking, good pleasure always supervenes on good activity, whereas pleasure that accompanies bad activity is shameful, mixed with pains, and thus undesirable.

---

45   For the traditional image of Stoics as typical anti-hedonists see Vogt elsewhere in this volume. In the intra-school debate, however, Poseidonius and Panaetius are believed to argue against the pleasure-hostile trend of the Stoic tradition by their attempts to defend the value of pleasure, and to incorporate it into the life according to nature (Pohlenz 1940, 6–7). The friends of pleasure among the Peripatetics include Lyco and many others. For my detailed discussion, see below.

46   For a systematic overview of ancient anti-hedonistic arguments, see Vogt in this volume.

47   τὸ γὰρ λέγειν τὰς μὲν ἐπὶ ταῖς καλαῖς ἐνεργείαις γινομένας ἡδονὰς εἰλικρινεῖς τε εἶναι καὶ ἀμίκτους ταῖς ἐναντίαις λύπαις, καὶ διὰ τοῦτο καὶ τὰς ποιητικὰς αὐτῶν ἐνεργείας ἔχειν τὸ αἱρετόν, τὰς δ᾽ ἐπὶ ταῖς αἰσχραῖς ὀλίγον ἐχούσας τὸ τέρπον πολλὰ ἔχειν καὶ πλείω τὰ λυποῦντα, διὸ μηδὲ τὰς ἐνεργείας εἶναι τὰς τοιαύτας αἱρετὰς οὔσας ποιητικὰς λύπης μᾶλλον ἢ ἡδονῆς. trans. by Sharples (1990a), modified.

48   With respect to the syncretic tendency of different philosophical schools from the Hellenistic time onward, it is of course possible that Alexander engages the view of his opponents in his own (i.e. Aristotelian) terms, so that the Aristotelian features of the hedonists in his report might stem from Alexander himself. It is, however, unlikely in our case, because, as I shall show, the resemblances between the hedonists and Aristotle's account of pleasure are so systematic that it cannot be explained only in terms of the contamination in terminology.

(3) The pleasure that originates from perfect activity is described by them as pure and removed from mixture with pain, which seems to correspond to Aristotle's concept of pleasure without qualification (*haplōs*). (4) They not only oppose pleasure to pain, but also hold that bad pleasure would give rise to a corresponding pain. This kind of pleasure seems to belong to pleasure *per accidens* according to Aristotle.[49] So far, Alexander's opponents appear very Aristotelian.[50]

Why was Alexander so annoyed by this doctrine that he thought it necessary to refute it? The central anxiety of Alexander is that these people are confused about the hierarchy of pleasure and activity, because according to the theory quoted above, Alexander complains, pleasure would not be worth choosing because of activity, but activity would be valuable because of pleasure. This critique appears a bit odd, since these hedonists seem to agree with Alexander that pleasure and pain *supervene upon* activities and thus their natures are somehow *determined by* the activities accompanied by them. For this reason, they do not necessarily belong among the hedonists who believe that only pleasure offers the ultimate or the non-derived reason for motivations and actions. The disparity between Alexander and his opponents is rather that the latter have in mind a different kind of supervenience between pleasure and activity, or that they interpret the Aristotelian supervenience in a different way. Alexander believes that the goodness of pleasure is determined by the goodness of activity, yet he does not think that a good activity must entail pleasure, nor that the concurrent pleasure constitutes the goodness of the activity. According to the 'hedonists,' on the contrary, the activity upon which pleasure supervenes ought to be good in a certain sense. Pleasure is not only causally effective, but also *constitutes* the value of the activity to which it is connected. Accordingly, Alexander holds that it is possible for pain to supervene upon any kind of activity, whereas the 'hedonists' seem to think that pain only supervenes upon incomplete or bad activities. Presumably they would justify this view by insisting that it is incoherent to claim that pain can supervene upon a perfect activity, because the coexistence of pain must have harmed the activity accompanied and thus undermined its perfection.

If we recall Aristotle's theory of pleasure in *EN* x—that pleasure is something that supervenes upon an activity and makes it perfect—it is clear that

---

49   About Aristotle's distinction between pleasure without qualification and *per accidens*, see *EN* 1152b27–31; 1153b2 ἁπλῶς ἢ τῷ πῇ; 1152b8–9: οὔτε καθ' αὑτὸ οὔτε κατὰ συμβεβηκός, also cf. 1153a29–30, 1154b15–20.

50   Sharples' conjecture (1990a, 45–6, n.142) that they are 'right-thinking people in general, to which some Aristotelians could belong. His suggestion seems to me too broad to grasp the character of these hedonists.

Alexander takes the asymmetrical relation entailed in the supervenience as the central lesson of Aristotle's definition of pleasure, whereas for the 'hedonists' what is more significant is the role of pleasure as a perfection-maker of a perfect activity. Since the theory of the 'hedonists' operates within Aristotelian philosophy, it is plausible to assume that the 'hedonists' criticized by Alexander are first of all those who stand for another line of interpreting Aristotle's theory of pleasure, or at least those who attempt to defend a pleasure-friendly position in an Aristotelian way. We should not forget that in contemporary Aristotle scholarship there are those who frankly acknowledge the close relation between Aristotle and the hedonistic traditions in later generations.[51] It is of course possible that a similar reading of Aristotle emerged preceding and contemporary to Alexander. In this sense, as anticipated above, the debate between Alexander and the 'hedonists' not only concerns the problem of whether hedonism is theoretically tenable, but is motivated by the question of which reading is *a more authentic interpretation* of Aristotle. This result fits well with the general character of the *PE*, which exhibits strong interest in textual exegesis.

Our hypothesis is in accordance with Sharples' general characterization of Alexander's approach—'Alexander's discussions of pleasure, a major concern of the *Ethical Problems*, are concerned with problems raised by Aristotelian doctrine rather than with specifically anti-Epicurean polemic'[52]—and it can also gain support from a broader historical point of view. Intra-school debates were not unusual within Greek philosophical schools, perhaps in particular among Peripatetics.[53] Hahm, for instance, has shown how Critolaus of Phaselis (c. 200–c. 118 BC), a Peripatetic philosopher and orator, argues against the technicity of rhetoric in favor of the relevance of philosophy to political education, whereas his younger colleague, Aristo of Cos, conversely insists that rhetoric is a science by appealing both to Aristotle and the Academics.[54] In tune with this tendency, Alexander also has no qualms about criticizing his Peripatetic predecessors such as Andronicus (cf. *In APr.* 161.1), Sotion (cf. *In Top.* 434.2), and Xenarchus (cf. *Mantissa* 151. 3–11, Simplicius *in Cael.* 21. 33),[55] although he does not always refer to the critical targets by name.[56]

---

51   E.g., Merlan 1960; Hardie 1968, 295; Rorty 1974, 482; van Riel 2000, 46; Wolfsdorf 2009.

52   Sharples 1990b, 95.

53   Cf. Sedley 1989, 99.

54   Hahm 2007, 54–60.

55   For Alexander's relations to his predecessors, see Sharples 1990b, 89–90.

56   In *Mantissa* 106.20–23, for instance, Alexander argues against a literal interpretation of the potential intellect as matter without mentioning Xenarchus, the Aristotelian who is supposed to hold this view (cf. Falcon 2012: 135–138). Sharples (1990b: 88) also assumes

It is especially telling that there was a divergence between pleasure-friendly and pleasure-hostile trends within the Peripatetic school prior to Alexander. Lyco of Troas (c. 299–c. 225 BC), who was the head of the school after Strato c. 269 BC for more than forty years, is representative of the former attitude, because he defines *eudaimonia* as true pleasure (*chara*) of the soul accompanying the noble (*epi tois kalois*, fr. 10 Wehrli).[57] By contrast, Critolaus, who famously rejects the idea that pleasure can be constitutive for the goal of activities and degrades it as something bad (fr. 23 Wehrli), belongs to the latter group.[58] The parting of ways among the Peripatetics happened not only for theoretical reasons, but was also probably motivated by issues in the exegesis of Aristotle.[59] Stephen White has convincingly argued that Lyco's theory comes into dialogue with Stoicism and Epicureanism,[60] whereas Inwood adds, with good reason, that what Lyco represents is presumably 'a more hedonistic interpretation of Aristotelian ethics.'[61] Remarkably, the phrase *epi tois kalois* is resonant with the frequent occurrence of the same phrase in Alexander,[62] in particular his use of the preposition '*epi*' as a shorthand to refer to the supervenience relation in Aristotle's theory of pleasure.[63] It is not impossible that Lyco

---

that in *PE* §11, Alexander might adopt Aspasius' discussion of the involuntary and voluntary actions (Apasius 59. 2–11), and that it contains a critical reply to Adrastus if the anonymous commentary uses Adrastus' materials on this topic. In any case, Aspasius and Adrastus are not mentioned here.

57   Cf. White 2004, 389–94.

58   For discussions of Critolaus' ethics in historical context, see White 1992, 86–90; Russell 2010, 160–71; Hahm 2007, 62–81; Szaif 2012, 156–67, 184–86.

59   Even if the interpretation of Aristotle did not take pride of place among the earlier Peripatetics as it had done since Antiochus or since the publication of Andronicus' edition, we cannot exclude it from the activities of the Hellenistic Peripatetics (cf. Lefebvre 2016, 28–30). Barnes (1997) has shown that the stories around the revival of Aristotle due to the rediscovery of his 'esoteric works' are more or less exaggerated. For a recent discussion about the reception of Aristotle's ethics in the Hellenistic period, see Nielsen 2015.

60   White 2002, 76–9.

61   Inwood 2014, 39. Although Inwood correctly, in my view, highlights the exegetical context of Lyco's hedonism, I suspect that he goes astray in regarding Lyco's position as 'an attempt to unify Aristotle's two accounts of pleasure and its relationship to happiness' (Inwood 2014, 41). This claim presupposes, indeed as Inwood himself believes, that the accounts in *EN* VII and X are actually incompatible, and that the former is advantageous for hedonism, whereas the latter is anti-hedonistic. As Aspasius, Alexander, and many others show, that ancient critics usually do not take the two accounts as contradictory in this way. The Aristotelian hedonists recorded by Alexander are not exceptional. We unambiguously see them freely using *EN* X to support their hedonism rather than exclusively insisting on *EN* VII.

62   Cf. *PE* 146.1; 152.21.

63   E.g., *PE* 126.1, 127.12–13, 137.3–4, 137.7–9, 152.20–23.

interprets the Aristotelian supervenience relation as if true pleasure is something that is so closely connected with the noble things that it must constitute *eudaimonia* as its central ingredient. If so, what we encounter is just a hedonistic interpretation of Aristotle's classical theory of pleasure, which resembles the hedonism criticized by Alexander.

This assumption can be further buttressed by another of Alexander's texts, namely a treatise in the collection *Mantissa* with the title 'From [the teachings of] Aristotle concerning the first appropriate thing' (*Mantissa* §17, 150–153).[64] Although there have been several studies of this text, most of them center on the Stoic elements in the Peripatetic arguments,[65] whereas none of them attaches due weight to the philosophical importance of the intra-school debates over the nature of pleasure implied here. In fact, just as in the *PE*, Alexander also takes this opportunity to attack hedonism in the *Mantissa*. Yet, unlike in the former case in which Alexander's opponents remain anonymous, here the polemic is unambiguously directed at the hedonists who defend their attitude by appealing to Aristotelian doctrines.[66] Alexander reports the first group as follows:

> Others say that, according to Aristotle (κατὰ Ἀριστοτέλη), the primary object of attachment (τὸ πρῶτον οἰκεῖον) is pleasure; they too are inspired (κινούμενοι) by what he says in the *Nicomachean Ethics*. For he says that

---

64   I follow the suggestion of Sharples 2004, 149 n. 507. Different translations of the title Τῶν παρὰ Ἀριστοτέλους περὶ τοῦ πρώτου οἰκείου are 'The Views of the Aristotelians about the Primary Object of Attachment' (Inwood 2014, 118), '[Selections] from Aristotle concerning the first appropriate thing' (Falcon 2012, 142); 'From the Aristotelian tradition concerning the first appropriate thing' (Sharples 2004, 149; 2008, 206). It is important to see that the phrase παρὰ Ἀριστοτέλους is ambiguous: it can refer to the views *derived from* Aristotle, or those *found in* Aristotle. For a discussion of this phrase, see Falcon 2012, 47–8.

65   Cf. Philippson 1932, 460–4; Striker 1997, 282–4; Sharples 2004. 149–59; 2010, 152–4; Falcon 2012, 145–57; Inwood 2014, 118–25.

66   At the beginning of this treatise, the followers of Epicurus (τοῖς δὲ περὶ Ἐπίκουρον 150.33) are mentioned, according to whom the primary object of attachment is pleasure (ἡδονὴ τὸ πρῶτον οἰκεῖον, 150.33). Alexander, however, does not return to Epicurus and his followers, but only addresses two different kinds of hedonistic arguments that are mainly based on Aristotle's theories (151.11–27). Although the 'Aristotelian' hedonists seem to agree with Epicurus in believing that pleasure is the first natural attachment, they do not think that pleasure is differentiated into two kinds: kinetic and katastematic (=freedom from pain) (cf. 150.34). Alexander's move from the Epicureans to the Aristotelian hedonists corresponds to, and is in parallel with, his shift from the Stoics (150.28–33) to the Stoicized Peripatetics Xenarchus and Boethus (151.3–11) in the same treatise. As in the *PE*, the main interest of this treatise is the intra-school debates, although the question itself—what is the primary object of attachment—manifests a Stoic influence.

there are three objects of desire (τὰ ὀρεκτά): the fine (τὸ καλόν), the advantageous, and the pleasant. And an object of desire is something to which we have an attachment (οἰκειώμεθα). But we come to grasp the noble and the advantageous as we get older, but we grasp the pleasant immediately (εὐθύς). So if these are the only objects of desire and attachment, and if the first of these is the pleasant, then this would be the primary object of attachment.

   Mant. 151.18–24[67]

In this passage, some Aristotelians attempt to justify their hedonism by arguing that pleasure is the primary object of desire, the ultimate end of life. This argumentative strategy is obviously influenced by the Stoic theory of *oikeiōsis*, yet, as a philosophical fashion since Hellenistic times, the use of this concept is by no means limited to Stoicism but spread widely among different philosophical schools.[68] In the so-called *divisio Carneadea*,[69] for instance, different attitudes towards three natural objects of desire—pleasure, freedom from pain, and the primary natural object (*prima naturalia*)—function as a guideline for classifying ethical theories.[70] Of nine different views on the ultimate good listed, the Peripatetics have diverged from each other, holding at least four different positions.[71] A pleasure-friendly view is espoused by Calliphon and Deinomachus,[72] who argue that the highest good is a combination of virtues with pleasure, whereas the others opt for the freedom from pain (Hieronymus), the combination of virtue with freedom from pain (Diodorus), and the primary natural object (anonymous). Although the details of the reasons for their divergence cannot be restored, the intellectual milieu has sufficiently manifested the flexibility and multiplicity of the Peripatetic tradition.

  In accordance with the para-Stoic tendency, the Aristotelian 'hedonists' in *Mantissa* 151.18–24 follow the same tactic in their attempt to verify the primacy of pleasure by demonstrating it to be the primary object of desire, yet it is uncertain whether their purpose, as with Calliphon and Deinomachus, was to make pleasure and virtue compatible by integrating both into a unifying concept of the ultimate end, or whether they go further, drawing out a more ambitious hedonistic consequence. It is of course dubious how far these Aristotelians can be taken as 'loyal' to Aristotle. For in their arguments,

---

67 Trans. by Inwood (2014), modified.
68 Cf. Trapp 2007, n. 43, with references.
69 For this table see Algra 1997; Leonhardt 1999, 135–212; Annas 2007.
70 It is reported by Antiochus through Piso in Cicero's *de Fin.* v 16–21.
71 According to Cicero, three of them are only theoretical possibilities, held by nobody.
72 Wehrli et al. 2004, 629; White 2002, 90.

not only are the Aristotelian terms *haireta* (*Top.* 118b28; 105a27) and *haireseis* (*EN* 1104b30) replaced by the Stoic term *orekta*,[73] but the hedonistic argument based on taking pleasure as the *direct* (*euthus*) attachment also echoes the classical Stoic strategy in their explanation of the significance of self-preservation as rooted in the primary *oikeiōsis*.[74] In spite of being tinged by Stoic vocabulary and conception, it is Aristotle who is explicitly invoked by the 'hedonists' as their authority, perhaps not only his classification of the good into the fine, the advantageous, and the pleasant,[75] but also his ranking of different kinds of ends in *EN* I. 7–8. It is remarkable that Aristotle claims on one occasion that the good is something of our own (*oikeion ti*) and hard to take from us (*EN* 1095b25–27), and he also praises Eudoxus' argument in favor of pleasure as something divine (*EN* 1101b27–31). Those 'hedonists' seem to read such scattered evidence through the prism of Stoicism, fashioning it into a coherent argument in favor of their pleasure-friendly position. Perhaps it is for this reason that Alexander underlines their approach as *inspired* (κινούμενοι) by Aristotle, which may insinuate some sort of reservation.

This hedonistic argument is not the only 'Aristotelian' argument for hedonism in Alexander's report. More revealingly, he goes on to discuss another hedonistic argument, which is obviously based on more solid evidence in Aristotle (his account of pleasure in *EN* VII and X) than his tripartition of the ends adduced by the first group, in which the nature of pleasure does not take pride of place:

> Verginius Rufus and before him Sosicrates said that each person desires perfection (ὀρέγεσθαι τῆς τελειότητος), i.e., being in activity (τοῦ ἐνεργείᾳ εἶναι), obviously being active with no impediment (ἀνεμποδίστως). That is why he says that for us too being in activity is desirable, and this is being alive and the activities dependent on life, which are pleasant. For this kind of natural activity is, as long as it is unimpeded, pleasant. But for each thing its perfection is a good. [...] By desiring to be in activity, one would desire one's own proper perfection. And this is a good for each, so that we desire it. It is consistent for those who postulate that the primary object of attachment (πρῶτον οἰκεῖον) is being and living in activity to

---

73   Cf. ἡ ὄρεξις in the pseudo-Aristotle's *Divisiones* 46.

74   Cf. οἰκειούμεθα πρὸς αὐτοὺς <u>εὐθὺς</u> γενόμενοι, Chrysippus SVF III.179; Hierocles: τὸ ζῷον <u>εὐθὺς</u> ἅμα τῶι γενέσθαι αἰσθάνεται ἑαυτοῦ, col. 1.38; <u>εὐθὺς</u> ὠικειώθη πρὸς ἑαυτὸ καὶ τὴν ἑαυτοῦ σύστασιν, col. 6.51–53; cf. 5.52, 6.7–8, 6.42–43.

75   *Top.* 118b28; 105a27; *EN* 1104b31, 1105a1; cf. *SE* 102b16–18, [*Div.*] 46. It is remarkable that this classification of the good is also admitted by Alexander himself, see *Fat.*15.185.21–28, *Mant.* 174.17–24. Cf. Sharples 2004, 155 n. 526.

say that the primary object of attachment and the good (τὸ ἀγαθόν) is pleasure.

Mant. 151.30–152.1, 3–6

At stake is obviously a hybrid account of Aristotle's understanding of pleasure. It is hybrid, not only because these hedonists,[76] like the first group of Aristotelians, align the Stoic discourse on the proper object of desire with Aristotle's theories, but also because they blend the two accounts of pleasure in *EN* VII and X into a coherent foundation for their pro-hedonistic view. Pleasure as a perfection, as mentioned above, is the key lesson from *EN* X, whereas the association of pleasure with an unimpeded activity apparently stems from *EN* VII. By identifying the unimpeded activity with the perfection (*teleiotēs*) of the nature of a subject, these hedonists establish a close link between pleasure, goodness, and activity. Just like Alexander, they are not puzzled by the supervenience relation in *EN* X, but are content with the vague affinity between pleasure and activity; it is thus also unclear in what sense pleasure and activity are identical with or different from each other. It is presumably in part for this reason that they have enough wiggle room to accommodate the accounts of both *EN* VII and X. In any case, it is not inconsistent if they, on the one hand, speak of the unimpeded *energeia* in *EN* VII, and on the other argue for hedonism by drafting the theory of *EN* X as an ally when necessary. Although Alexander is unsatisfied with their hedonistic implication, their treatment of Aristotle is irreproachable insofar as it fits well into the way Aspasius, Alexander, and other ancient commentators combine his two accounts of pleasure in their compatibilist readings.

4   Alexander Reconsidered

Alexander's criticism of the hedonists in the *Mantissa* appears less decisive than that in the *PE*. Either he has not found a proper way to meet the challenge from the Aristotelian hedonists (if this treatise was written earlier), or the Stoic framework of *Mantissa* §17 seems to constrain his argument, so that he cannot

---

76   It is not clear whether or in what sense Verginius Rufus and Sosicrates belong to the *Peripatos*. Verginius Rufus might be the consul of 63 AD who was the guardian of the younger Pliny. Sosicrates, according to Lautner (1997: 304–305), might either be Sosicrates from Rhodes, the author of *Successions* (διατριβῶν) in DL 2.84, 6.80 and 7.163 or a student of Carneades mentioned in Philiodemus' *Index Academicocum* XXIV. 8. The former can be Peripatetic, while the latter might be an Academic. cf. Sharples 2004, 155 n.527; Falcon 2012, 155.

develop his criticism at length by providing his more 'authentic' interpretation of Aristotle. In the *Mantissa*, he launches his attack on the Aristotelians from a 'Stoic' point of view, namely by disclosing their failure to grasp what the end actually is. He finds fault with the first group of hedonists in that they do not distinguish between two kinds of ends, confusing goodness for someone with goodness without qualification (*Mant.* 151.27–29). After that, he applies a similar criticism to the second group, pointing out that they fail to distinguish between the apparent good (= pleasure) and the true good (cf. 152.20–35). It is unexpected, however, that Alexander seems hesitant about whether this argument is sufficient to refute the second group of hedonists, perhaps because they appear to be able to gain more support from Aristotle's official account of pleasure. So he abruptly withdraws his criticism at 152.35, and turns to another convoluted argument (152.35–153.27), the gist of which is unfortunately difficult to tease out. No matter how we assess this elusive shift, what is more significant for our purposes is to note that Alexander's 'new' argument seems to be an embryonic form of his central anti-hedonistic strategy in the *PE*.

One has *not* made pleasure *the goal* of one's appetition (σκοπὸν τῆς ὀρέξεως), but has this as *accompanying* (ἐπομένην) the activity. For everything which is in accordance with nature is pleasant. It is not the case that, having first enjoyed pleasure, one then *on this basis* has appetition for that through which he enjoyed pleasure.

> *Mant.* 153.14–17[77]

Alexander distinguishes between the proper end and something that accompanies the end, which is equivalent to a distinction between the *energeia* as the end and pleasure as its concomitant. Based on this distinction, he replies to the hedonists that although all activities are pleasant if they are in accordance with nature, that does not mean that pleasure is thereby *the* reason or *the* end of one's appetite, because pleasure—due to its dependence on activity—does not have a non-derived status an intrinsic goal is supposed to possess. This argument, despite still being in a 'para-Stoic' fashion, accords in principle with the argument in the *PE* based on the supervenience-relation between pleasure and activity.

In this light, Alexander's debate with the hedonists (especially with the second group in *Mant.* §17) seems to foreshadow the conflict between Alexander and the anonymous anti-hedonists in the *PE*. The hedonists in the *Mantissa* (Verginius Rufus and Sosicrates) and the hedonists in the *PE* are in agreement that they champion the *intrinsic connection* of pleasure and activity based on

---

77   Trans. by Sharples 2004, my italics.

their reading of Aristotle. If we recall the aforementioned distinction between the Extrinsic and Intrinsic Readings of the Aristotelian definition of pleasure in contemporary Aristotelian scholarship, then the debate between Alexander and the Aristotelian hedonists foreshadows the classical debate over Aristotle's pleasure as supervenience in contemporary academia. According to the hedonistic Aristotelians, the intrinsic relation between pleasure and activity means that as long as an activity is perfect, pleasure occurs naturally as integral to this activity, sharing its central properties. For Alexander, however, the link between activity and pleasure is rather external. Alexander underlines how the value of pleasure is determined by that of its corresponding activity, and ignores or suppresses the reciprocal contribution of pleasure to the activity in question. He also emphasizes how pleasure can emerge indiscriminately from all kinds of activities, and is no more intimately bound up with the activity if it is unimpeded or in an excellent condition.

The discrepancy between Alexander and the 'hedonists' also extends to pain. Admittedly, both agree that pleasure is opposed to pain, and both use the mirroring method, trying to infer the properties of pain from its opposite pleasure. Nonetheless their findings are quite distinct. For the 'hedonists,' pain is connected with the incompleteness of activity, so that as long as an activity is bad, the corresponding pain occurs naturally. This also explains why shameful activity is not desirable. In this sense, pleasure and pain indicate respectively the properties of the activity they accompany as differentiating signs. By contrast, Alexander points out emphatically that 'pleasures supervene *no less* on shameful activities [*than* on noble ones]' (*PE* 145.20–21),[78] which shows that, in his view, pleasure is neither immanent in perfect activities nor does it (even partly) constitute these activities. Accordingly, there is no intrinsic relation between pain and bad activities.

Alexander argues against both the intrinsic connection between pleasure and good activity and the causal contribution of pleasure to activity, because he believes that these relationships pave the path towards hedonism, a view from which any true Aristotelian should distance himself.

> For it is not possible to say that nobility and pleasure are the same thing in the cases where they co-exist and exist at the same time as each other. For if their essence were the same, it would be necessary for them to be convertible with each other, so that everything that was noble would, in

---

78   τῷ μηδὲν ἔλαττον [...] τὰς ἡδονὰς γινομένας ἐπ' αἰσχραῖς ἐνεργείαις.

being noble, also possess the quality of being pleasant, and everything that was pleasant would simultaneously be both pleasant and noble.

PE 145.14–18[79]

In his view, the foundation of this hedonism is fragile because the hedonist point of view boils down to a dilemma from an Aristotelian point of view:

Either one must deny that certain pleasures supervene also on shameful actions, [saying that they supervene] only on noble ones; or else what is shameful will truly deserve to be chosen in the same way as what is noble, if it is the pleasure that they produce that is the cause of their being chosen.

PE 145.5–8[80]

The *aporia* Alexander raises is that either the 'hedonists' think that pleasure supervenes *only* on noble activities, or that they must permit that shameful activities are also worth choosing. If they choose the first alternative, Alexander would object that this does not square with common sense; if they opt for the latter, they would fall into self-contradiction because they also explicitly reject the pursuit of shameful activity, albeit for different reasons (*PE* 145.31–33).

In the debate with the hedonists, the criterion used by Alexander to distinguish between different kinds of activity is no doubt ethically oriented. So instead of predications of *good* and *bad*, he more frequently talks of *noble* (*kalon*) and *shameful* (*aischron*) activity.[81] By contrast, although what is determined as the perfect activity in Aristotle is not independent of ethical connotation, the key aspect is predominantly functional in a broader sense. A perfect activity, according to Aristotle, is one in which the subject, its object, and their relation are all in an excellent state for carrying out their functions.[82] Since both animals and the gods are included in Aristotle's account of pleasure, it

---

79   οὐ γὰρ δὴ ταὐτὸν οἷόν τε λέγειν εἶναι τὸ καλόν τε καὶ τὴν ἡδονήν, ἐφ' ὧν συνυπάρχει τε καὶ ἅμα ἐστὶν ἀλλήλοις. εἰ γὰρ εἴη ταὐτὸν αὐτοῖς τὸ εἶναι, καὶ ἀντιστρέφειν αὐτὰ ἀλλήλοις ἀνάγκη, ὡς πᾶν τὸ καλὸν ἐν τῷ καλὸν εἶναι καὶ τὸ ἡδὺ εἶναι ἔχειν καὶ πᾶν τὸ ἡδὺ ἅμα τε ἡδὺ εἶναι καὶ καλόν.

80   ἢ γὰρ οὐ χρὴ λέγειν γίνεσθαί τινας καὶ ἐπ' αἰσχραῖς πράξεσιν ἡδονάς, ἀλλ' ἐπ μόναις ταῖς καλαῖς, ἢ εἰ μὴ τοῦτο, ἀληθῶς αἱρετὸν ἔσται καὶ τὸ αἰσχρὸν ὁμοίως τῷ καλῷ, εἰ ἡ γινομένη ὑπ' αὐτῶν ἡδονὴ τῆς αἱρέσεως αὐτῶν αἰτία.

81   *PE* 127.16–18; 134. 20–22, 25–27; 138.10–11, 14–28; 139.3–14; 144.10–17; 144.33–145.11; 145.18–21, 23–24, 28–34; 146.1–7; 12–13.

82   *EN* x.4.1174b14–23, 28–31.

definitely demonstrates that the values in question are beyond moral good and evil.[83] If we bear this aspect in mind, the hedonists are in fact not so helpless when confronted with the dilemma raised by Alexander. To be sure, they will not deny the empirical fact that pleasures are present not merely in noble activities but also in shameful ones. But they can question what is meant by the so-called *noble* activity upon which pleasure supervenes. If the claim that pleasure supervenes merely upon the noble activity means that pure pleasures, namely the pleasures which are not mixed with any pain, must supervene upon the perfect activity and constitute this activity, the hedonists are willing to embrace this opinion without hesitation. And obviously, *this* kind of pleasure could not accompany shameful actions. But if the noble activity is understood in an ethical sense, they would reply that what they are chiefly concerned with is not limited to ethical value, but the overall function of a living organism or its part.

As we have seen, Alexander understands the supervenience relation between pleasure and activity as pleasure's being somehow a part of the activity or its end.[84] But, presumably in order to avoid any hedonistic implication to which such characterizations might lead, he does not address these options again. In fact, his final doctrine is not even compatible with them. For it is inconceivable that pleasure, if it is a part or an end of an activity, is causally inert. Although Alexander bases his anti-hedonistic argument on Aristotle's official doctrine that pleasure supervenes upon activity, his epiphenomenalist reading of this theory renders him closer to Stoicism than he would be willing to acknowledge. For the classical anti-hedonistic strategy used by the Stoics, as Diogenes Laertius tells us, is to argue that pleasure is not the primary attachment, but a by-product (*epigennēma*),[85] a term derived from the verb *epigignetai* used by Aristotle for the so-called supervenience relation (cf. *EN* 1174b33). It is thus conceivable that although Alexander purports to provide a faithful interpretation of Aristotle, his account would not persuade all of the Aristotelians, in particular those who are inclined to set up a close link between Aristotle and the hedonistic tradition. Theoretically considered, at least four elements in Alexander would be controversial: (1) The supervenience relation between

---

83   Cf. *EN* VII.1.1145a25–27; 12.1153a30–31; b25–32; 14.1154b25–28; X.2.1173a1–5; 5.1176a5–9; 7.1177a23–24.

84   *PE* 127.10–13.

85   DL 7.86: ἐπιγέννημα γάρ φασιν, εἰ ἄρα ἔστιν, ἡδονὴν εἶναι ὅταν αὐτὴ καθ' αὑτὴν ἡ φύσις ἐπιζητήσασα τὰ ἐναρμόζοντα τῇ συστάσει ἀπολάβῃ. ὃν τρόπον ἀφιλαρύνεται τὰ ζῷα καὶ θάλλει τὰ φυτά. Cf. the anti-hedonistic argument of Cleanthes in SVF III 155. For a more sophisticated interpretation of the Stoic understanding of pleasure as *epigennēma*, in particular in Seneca, see McVane in this volume.

pleasure and activity is evenly distributed in the sense that the supervenience of pleasure upon an excellent *energeia* does not enjoy any privilege in comparison with the supervenience of pleasure upon the *energeiai* that are bad or neutral. (2) Although good pleasure must derive from a good *energeia*, it is not conversely warranted that a good *energeia* must intrinsically entail a corresponding pleasure. (3) Pleasure and pain do not have any independent causal effect. (4) Since every concrete pleasure and pain obtains its evaluation respectively from the activities accompanied by them in opposed ways, the value of pleasure and pain as a whole is indeterminate.[86]

How would the other Aristotelians object to these theses? If Alexander accuses them of degenerating into Epicureanism, they could counter him by questioning whether his proposal dresses Aristotle up as a Stoic sage. No doubt, they must agree with Alexander that pleasure *as a whole* can be good or bad. But this does not mean that pleasure by its very nature is axiologically indeterminate. On the contrary, they would reply, one of Aristotle's primary concerns in his two accounts of pleasure is to defend the positive value of pleasure as such by appeal to the affinity between pleasure and good activity. Pleasure, in short, does not only necessarily supervene on a good activity, if there is no external hindrance, but also as its perfection causally *completes* this activity.[87] For this reason, pleasure is for them good, even if not all pleasures are good.

To understand why Alexander's interpretation is in tension with Aristotle's account, it may be useful to take a glimpse at the debate between Aristotle and Eudoxus over the argument from pleasure as an additional good. Eudoxus argues that pleasure is the ultimate good because if pleasure is *added* to (*prostithemenēn*) something, it makes this thing more valuable (*EN* x.2, 1172b23–34). A full explication of this argument and Aristotle's reply is beyond the scope of my survey. But if we pay attention to the subtle divergence between Aristotle and Eudoxus in their debate, we might better grasp why some Aristotelians would reject Alexander's extrinsic reading of pleasure. Aristotle's diagnosis of this argument is intriguing. He does not dismiss the claim that the addition of pleasure makes other things better, nor does he seem to be bothered by any hedonistic conclusion to be drawn from this premise. On the contrary, he complains that this argument is *not 'hedonistic' enough* in the sense that it cannot fulfil Eudoxus' initial purpose, namely to prove that

---

86   Although Alexander does not thus evaluate pleasure and pain as indifferent, his position is very close to this Stoic classification of pleasure and pain. Cf. Stobaeus ii. 5a; 7b.

87   *EN* 1174b22: τελειοῖ δὲ τὴν ἐνέργειαν ἡ ἡδονή, cf. 1174b24, b31–32, 1175a15, a17, a21, a28, a30, 1176a26–29.

pleasure is *the good* or *the best thing*. For the most we can draw from the ability of pleasure to increase any other thing's good is a moderate thesis: i.e., pleasure is *a* good thing (*EN* x.2, 1172b26–32). This diagnosis helps us better understand why Aristotle introduces supervenience to re-determine the relation between pleasure and activity. The intention of his proposal is actually to render their relation more intimate, which aims to show that pleasure, in the strict sense, is *the* good, by connecting and assimilating pleasure with perfect activity.[88]

To conclude then, I suggest that Alexander's approach in the *PE* is considerably determined by his intention to resist the hedonistic implication his opponents draw from Aristotle's account of pleasure. The main target of Alexander's anti-hedonistic arguments is those who adopted a hedonistic reading of Aristotle's accounts of pleasure. To refute them, Alexander is forced to underrate the normative structure implied in the supervenience between pleasure and good activity, so that it is understandable that he denies any intrinsic link between pleasure and goodness. The cost of his reading is that pleasure, as something that is neither good nor bad in its own right, is deprived of any causal effect or normative standing. A merit is that this proposal can well explain why pleasures differ in kind according to Aristotle (*EN* 1173b28). In addition, it allows the positive evaluation of some pains, so that the Peripatetic demand of moderate emotions is kept consistent with Aristotle's doctrines about pleasure and pain. Moreover, it leads him to take the problem of pain more seriously than any other commentators on Aristotle. For although the neutralization of pain can accommodate an influential pain-friendly tradition, i.e., a tradition in which pain was taken as constitutive of the path to happiness, it seems at odds with Aristotle's use of the premise that pain is something bad in many dialectical arguments. To address this *aporia*, Alexander attempts to classify different kinds of pains, trying to figure out a way to explain in what sense Aristotle can take pain as bad even if there are pains which are good or neutral.

---

88 Alexander does not mention Eudoxus explicitly in the whole text of the *Ethica Problemata*. From his frequent quotations of the argument from contraries (Pr. §6, §7, §17), however, it is clear that he is familiar with the Eudoxean arguments supporting hedonism (cf. Sharples 1990a, 31, n73). Unfortunately, he fails to notice the significance of the debate between Eudoxus and Aristotle over the argument from pleasure as an additional good. Otherwise he would have endeavored to distance his own concept of supervenience from Eudoxus' thesis in which pleasure functions as an additional good.

CHAPTER 11

On Grief and Pain[1]

David Konstan

In my book on *The Emotions of the Ancient Greeks*,[2] I included two chapters on emotions—if they are emotions—that Aristotle did not discuss in his analysis of the *pathê* in the second book of his *Rhetoric*: one of these was jealousy, and the other was grief, the topic I take up here. One of the reasons for this omission, I suggested, was that Aristotle regarded grief as a more elementary kind of response than the kinds of sentiments he included under the label *pathos*. The common Greek term for grief was *lupê*, which also designated physical pain. When Aristotle defines the emotions as 'those things through which, by undergoing change, people come to differ in their judgments and which are accompanied by pain and pleasure, for example, anger, pity, fear, and other such things and their opposites' (*Rhetoric* 2.1, 1378a20–23), the words for pain and pleasure are precisely *lupê* and *hêdonê*. Pleasure and pain are thus constituents of emotions, and not emotions as such.

What is more, the kinds of affects that Aristotle treats as examples of *pathê* typically involve moral evaluations of human behavior. Anger or *orgê* is a reaction to an insult, and more especially one on the part of those not in a position to belittle you; a complex assessment of status and intention is implied in this definition. Love and hatred are based on perceptions of qualities of character, pity and indignation are aroused by unmerited suffering or prosperity, gratitude is evoked by a favor that is selflessly bestowed, shame is a function in part of how others judge one and in part of one's own sense of virtue, and fear depends on an assessment of the hostile intentions of others as well as on their relative power. Even envy, the worst of the lot, is aroused by the belief that people of one's own status are faring better than oneself. Grief, however, is not elicited by the intentional behavior of another or by a perception of inequality

1 This article benefitted from a fellowship at the Swedish Collegium for Advanced Study during the period 1 September to 16 December 2016, and from a fellowship at the Paris Institute for Advanced Studies (France), with the financial support of the French State managed by the Agence Nationale de la Recherche, programme 'Investissements d'avenir', (ANR-11-LABX-0027-01 Labex RFIEA+), during the period 1 February to 30 June 2017. It was originally presented at a seminar on AITIA/AITIAI, held at the Centre de recherches sur la pensée antique (Centre Léon Robin) on 8 June 2017 at the Sorbonne, organized by Cristina Viano.
2 Konstan 2006.

or unfairness relative to one's own or another's fortune. It is simply a response to the loss of someone dear, something that irrational animals are capable of feeling as well when they are suddenly deprived of their young, for example. The feeling of grief is unprocessed, as it were; it strikes us without being mediated by judgment or assent, at a more primitive level than the kinds of sentiments that Aristotle collects under the heading *pathos*. It is the result, we may say, of a different kind of cause or causal process.

Of course, grief differs from corporeal pain: the death of a person we love is not the same as a physical blow. When Epicurus or the Stoics wished to identify a specifically physical pain, they used the words *algos* or *algêdôn*, as opposed to the more general *lupê*; in order to bridge the semantic range of *lupê*, modern scholars writing in English tend to translate it as 'distress' (more precisely characterized by Epicureans, for example, as *tarakhê*).[3]

But perhaps we should be wary of ascribing to the Greeks a distinction between mental and physical agony that may seem natural to us. The news that someone we love has died may not feel very different from bodily harm, and even today we speak of 'blows of fortune' and employ various other physical metaphors for psychic distress.[4]

In this respect, it is worth taking a closer look at how pleasure and pain are experienced in connection with the reactions that Aristotle identifies as *pathê*. We may take the case of anger as paradigmatic. Aristotle defines anger as 'a desire, accompanied by pain, for a perceived revenge, on account of a perceived slight on the part of people who are not fit to slight one or one's own' (*Rhetoric* 2.2, 1378a31–33).[5] In connection with this definition, I have observed:[6]

> Pain and pleasure themselves do not count, for Aristotle, as emotions. Rather, they are sensations or *aisthêseis*. A painful sensation may arise either as a result of direct perception, or else by way of *phantasia*, that is, through recollection or anticipation of something perceived. In

---

3   On the variety of terms for pain, see the chapter by Véronique Boudon-Millot in this volume, in the section, 'The vocabulary of pain and pleasure'.

4   On some of the dangers that may follow upon a casual equation of physical pain and psychological distress, see Iannetti et al. 2013, who note that 'Physical pain can be clearly distinguished from other states of distress. In recent years, however, the notion that social distress is experienced as physically painful has permeated the scientific literature and popular media. This conclusion is based on the overlap of brain regions that respond to nociceptive input and sociocultural distress. Here we challenge the assumption that underlies this conclusion—that physical pain can be easily inferred from a particular pattern of activated brain regions' (371).

5   On the translation, see Harris 1997.

6   Konstan 2006, 42.

Aristotle's own words: 'since feeling pleasure is in the perception of some experience [*pathos*], and *phantasia* is a weak kind of perception [*aisthê-sis*], some *phantasia* of what one remembers or expects always occurs in a person when he remembers or expects something.... Thus, it is necessary that all pleasures are either present in perception or arise in remembering things that have happened or in expecting things that will happen.

> *Rhetoric* 1.11, 1370a27–34

But it now seems to me that I was too casual in assuming a simple contrast between sensation and mental events. If pain, like pleasure, may arise in the recollection or anticipation of events, then it is hardly reducible to a direct physical ache. What is more, Aristotle does not specify in this passage the kind of event in question. In the case of anger, the pain must be of the sort that arises from a feeling of humiliation, of having been insulted or put down while lacking the ability to respond in kind. Hence, one must bide one's time and nourish the hope of exacting revenge, which consists in causing in the other a similar sense of disgrace or mortification (Aristotle uses the term *antipathein, Rhetoric* 2.4, 1382a14–15). One can derive some pleasure in the meantime from the expectation (*elpis*) of exacting a condign form of revenge. Now, neither the pain resulting from an insult nor the pleasure that accompanies an imagined revenge is a corporeal sensation; in fact, there is nothing that obviously distinguishes the quality of the pain associated with anger from that deriving from the loss of a dear one, except our awareness of the cause. With anger, I must be conscious of having been diminished by another person's words or behavior (such as the slap in the face that Meidias inflicted on Demosthenes), and judge that the relative statuses of myself and the offender are such that I can and should seek vengeance (if revenge is impossible, as Aristotle observes, then we cannot properly feel anger, or at least not very much: *Rhetoric* 2.2, 1370b13–15). If, as an orator, I wish to deflect anger, I can argue that the offense was unintentional or misunderstood, or show that the offender made, for example, similar remarks about himself or others where a deliberate insult was out of the question.

When it comes to grief, we do not typically find it necessary to judge the nature of our relationship to the deceased: we see or learn of her or his death and we feel it instantly as a deprivation. There are, perhaps, implicit assessments involved. I suppose that one way of alleviating sorrow at the death of someone close to us is to show that the other never really loved us and in fact attempted repeatedly to do us harm or was a thoroughly evil individual; thus, we are mourning not for the death of a *philos* but an *ekhthros*. I do not know of any consolation in classical antiquity that adopts this strategy, and for good

reason; the genre addresses our response to genuine loss, not our mispercep-
tion of the other's feelings or character. At a certain level, indeed, such evaluations may be irrelevant: if we feel grief at the death of a young child, for
example, it is not because we have formed a judgment of its character or affections; parental love is instinctive, we may say, and does not arise in the same
way as friendship, which according to Aristotle may emerge when another is
useful to us, or provides pleasure, or is virtuous. When Aristotle seeks to demonstrate that *philia* resides more in loving than in being loved, he offers the
following remarkable illustration:

> Some [mothers] give out their own children to be raised, and they love
> and know them, but they do not seek to be loved in return, if both [loving
> and being loved] are not possible; but it seems to them to suffice if they
> see them [i.e., their children] doing well, and they love them even if they,
> as a result of their ignorance, provide in return none of the things that
> are due a mother.
>
> *NE* 8.8, 1159a28–33

The second-century AD Greek commentator Aspasius observed of this passage
that the love in question seemed not to fit Aristotle's definition of *philia* earlier
in the same book of the *Nicomachean Ethics*, in which he specifies that friends
must 'be well-disposed toward one another and wish good things, not escaping
[the other's] notice, in regard to some one of the abovementioned kinds [i.e.,
usefulness, pleasure, or goodness]' (8.2, 1155b31–56a5). Aspasius noted that
'*philia* is in those who love mutually. But nevertheless the [love] of parents
for their children is a trace of *philia*. I say 'a trace', because sometimes sons do
not love in return. But it strongly resembles *philia*, because parents wish good
things for their sons for their sakes' (179.28–180.5 Heylbut, trans. Konstan).
At the very beginning of the eighth book of the *Nicomachean Ethics*, where
Aristotle introduces the topic of *philia*, he states that *philia* 'seems to inhere
by nature in a parent toward offspring, not only among human beings but also
among birds and most animals, and also in those of the same species toward
one another, and this above all in human beings' (8.1, 1155a16–22). The idea of
a natural *philia* suggests a form of attachment that is prior to or more elementary than the appreciation of another's qualities from which *philia* in the sense
of friendship arises, and the loss we experience at the death of those whom we
love in this manner is, I suggest, similarly unreflecting.

Of course, even in the case of such deprivations there are what we may call
cognitive considerations. For example, we may be mistaken as to the identity
of the dead person, and so be grieving falsely, as it were; as soon as we are set

straight, we cease to mourn. But we register the loss of a child in the same natural or instinctive way that we love the child in the first place. We do not reflect on whether it was good or bad; desert is beside the point, as is intentionality. The cause of this kind of pain is qualitatively different, I suggest, than the cause of the pain that is associated with anger and forms part of its definition. We may wonder whether the grief we feel upon the loss of a friend has more of the character of an emotion, since our affection for friends is based on appreciation of their qualities and is not simply an instinctive attachment. Here too, however, I would note that the death of a friend is not subject to the kind of moral and social appraisal that we employ in the case of the *pathê* that Aristotle discusses in the *Rhetoric*. Of course, we may believe that a friend has lost his life unjustly, whether by murder or neglect or some other means. In this case, we may well respond with pity or else with indignation or anger, since the death was undeserved and the injustice is an offense against both the victim and those who cared for him. But in that case, the emotion that is aroused is not grief per se but the pain associated with the relevant emotion: pain or *lupê* forms part of the definition of pity, indignation, and anger. The two kinds of pain, one resulting from the simple loss, the other from the perceived offense, may be difficult to distinguish experientially, and in a sense are mutually interdependent—we feel the injustice more intensely in proportion to the love we bear for the deceased—but they are not due to the same cause and can be discriminated logically. A good literary example is Sophocles' *Electra*, where Electra's suffering for the death of her father Agamemnon at the hands of her mother Clytemnestra and her lover, Aegisthus, is a product of both anger and grief.[7]

Ancient thinkers were concerned, however, that the natural and instinctive grief that human beings, like other animals, experience upon the loss of loved ones is often prolonged and exaggerated, as they regarded it, by beliefs concerning the nature of death, beliefs which non-rational creatures are incapable of holding. Socrates had led the way in affirming that death is not an evil, and Plato, the Epicureans, and the Stoics all followed suit. This counsel promoted equanimity in the face of one's own extinction, but there remained the pain we feel when we survive the deaths of others. Phaedo gave voice to the sentiment in Plato's dialogue by that name, when he spoke of the mixture of sadness and cheer he felt upon seeing Socrates conversing as usual when he was at the point of taking the hemlock (58E–59A):

---

7 Further discussion in Konstan 2016a.

No pity overcame me, as if I were present at the death of someone dear to me: for the man himself seemed happy, Echecrates, both in his demeanor and in what he said.... Thus no sense of pity overcame me, as would seem natural in the presence of grief, nor again pleasure as when we were philosophizing together as usual—for in fact there was such a discussion—but rather I felt some entirely strange emotion, an unusual mixture compounded of pleasure and pain at once.

Since Socrates is untroubled by his imminent death, Phaedo cannot feel sorrow on his behalf, but he nevertheless feels a proleptic pain at the thought that he will no longer have the company of his dear friend, or so I suppose; since he speaks also of pity, it is hard to be sure of the cause of Phaedo's grief, and perhaps he persists in believing that death is somehow an evil to be lamented.

Lucretius described the misery of a cow that has been deprived of its calf in moving lines in the *De rerum natura* (2.352–66):

for often a calf, slain in front of a temple of the gods, has fallen at the incense-bearing altars, pouring a warm river of blood from its breast; but its bereft mother, wandering through the green fields, recognizes [*novit*] the traces left by its cleft hooves in the ground, scans every place with its eyes, if perhaps she may detect somewhere her lost newborn, and she stops and fills the leafy woods with her cries, and again and again returns to the stable, transfixed with longing [*desiderio*] for the calf.... Nor can other kinds of calf in the flourishing meadows divert her mind and relieve her anxiety: that is how much she seeks what is her own and familiar to her (my translation).

The sorrow of the cow is the other side of the coin of its instinctive attachment to its offspring. It is of course independent of any beliefs the cow may have about death, since presumably she has none. Indeed, she does not even know that the calf has been slain; it is simply missing, and so she is searching for it. This is the elementary sense of loss or missing of a loved one that has not the moral or cognitive complexity of a *pathos*, as Aristotle understood the term. Although Epicurus believed that the fear of death was at the root of human anxiety and that we are naturally attracted to pleasure, he had no wish to disparage or eliminate such longing, painful as it is. Plutarch notes that that Epicurus wrote a consolatory letter to a certain Dositheus and Pyrson upon the death of Hegesianax, Dositheus' son and Pyrson's brother (*On Why it is Impossible to Live Pleasurably according to Epicureanism* 1101a–b1 = *Epistles* fr. 16 Arrighetti), and remarks that the Epicureans polemicize against those who eliminate grief [*lupai*], tears and groans at the death of dear ones, and they say that freedom from grief [*alupia*] that is carried to the point of insensitivity [*to apathes*] arises from another and greater vice, namely ruthlessness or uncontrolled vanity or insanity. It is therefore better to feel [*paskhein*] something and to grieve [*lupeisthai*] and even, by Zeus, for one's eyes to glisten and melt with tears, and all the other things which, when people suffer and write them, they are thought to be sensitive and loving sorts.

Plutarch treats this attitude as a sign of Epicurus' hypocrisy, but Epicurus had in mind the immediate sense of loss we inevitably experience at the absence of someone we love, which is independent of beliefs we may or may not hold concerning death. His view has nothing in common with the harshness of the remark attributed to Anaxagoras (and others) upon hearing that his son had died: 'I knew he was mortal when I fathered him' (Diogenes Laertius 2.31).

The distinction between the kind of grief that results from the loss of a person (or even an object) to which we are attached and that which is consequent upon false beliefs concerning death is abundantly clear in Stoic texts, above all those by Seneca. Non-rational animals, according to Seneca, experience a sense of longing (*desideria*) for a fellow creature that has died or disappeared, but although their sorrow is intense it is short lived. As Seneca writes: 'no animal has a lengthy sorrow for its offspring except man, who adheres to his grief and is stirred not to the extent that he feels it but to the extent that he has decided to be' (*Consolatio ad Marciam* 7.2). In the 99th epistle to Lucilius (99.18), Seneca again remarks that birds and wild animals love their young with a fierce passion, but it is quickly extinguished after they have died (99.24). In one respect, their response is similar to that of human beings: humans have a strong reaction to the death of a dear one: 'when the first news of a bitter death strikes us, when we hold the body that is about to pass from our embrace into the fire, a natural necessity forces out our tears'. Such tears are shed independently of our will or decision (99.19). Human beings, unlike other animals, remember the dead; Seneca affirms that to forget loved ones and bury the memory of them together with their bodies is inhuman. A good person, then, will keep their memory alive but will no longer grieve (*lugere*) for them.

I am inclined to believe that our initial and unpremeditated reaction to the loss of a loved one takes the form of what the Stoics called a *propatheia*, that is, a pre- or proto-emotion and what Seneca identifies in his treatise on anger as 'the initial preliminaries to emotions' (*principia proludentia adfectibus*, *On Anger* 2.2.6). Such responses, Seneca makes clear, are not emotions (*adfectus*) properly speaking, but rather 'motions that do not arise through our will', and consequently are irresistible and do not yield to reason. Some examples of such elementary reactions are, Seneca says, shivering or goose-pimples when one is sprinkled with cold water, aversion to certain kinds of touch (presumably slimy things and the like), the rising of one's hair at bad news, blushing at obscene language, and the vertigo produced by heights, but also our responses to theatrical spectacles and narratives of historical events, songs and martial trumpeting, horrible paintings, and the sight of punishments even when they are deserved, as well as contagious laughter and sadness. Such sadness, Seneca explains, is not genuine grief any more that a grimace we may make upon seeing a shipwreck in a play; so too, we do not experience genuine fear when we read a description of the Roman disaster in the battle of Cannae.

The list may seem odd, ranging as it does from goosebumps and dizziness to literary and theatrical representations, but what they all have in common is that they are evoked irrespective of our judgment or assent. Anger, by contrast, as a true emotion, 'does not venture anything on its own but only when the mind approves; for to accept the impression of an injury that has been sustained and desire vengeance for it—and to unite the two judgments, that one ought not to have been harmed and that one ought to be avenged—this is not characteristic of an impulse [*impetus*] that is aroused without our will [*voluntas*]. For the latter kind is simple, but the former is composite and contains several elements: one has discerned something, grown indignant, condemned it, and takes revenge: these things cannot occur unless the mind consents to those things by which it was affected' (2.1.4). Sages do not get angry because they do not consent to the idea that they have been harmed—the only true evil is the loss of one's virtue—and they do not judge that they ought to seek vengeance. When it comes to bereavement, however, even the strongest minds feel a sting simply when friends are absent, not to mention when they have died, as Seneca affirms in his *Consolation to Marcia* (7.1). It is entirely natural to miss our loved ones (*desiderium suorum*), so long as the emotion is moderate.[8]

There is good reason, I believe, to assume that animals too experience these 'initial preliminaries to emotions', although Seneca does not describe them as such, presumably because, since animals do not experience emotions in the strict sense of the word, in their case these elementary responses are not preliminary to anything else. As Seneca writes: 'We must affirm that wild animals, and all creatures apart from human beings, are without anger; for since anger is contrary to reason, it does not arise except where reason has a place.

---

8   I discuss Seneca's conception of emotion and pre-emotion in Konstan 2014b and Konstan 2016b ('Reason vs. Emotion').

Animals have violence, rabidity, ferocity, aggression, but do not have anger any more than they have licentiousness.... Dumb animals lack human emotions, but they do have certain impulses that are similar to emotions'. He continues: 'their onrushes and outbreaks are violent, but they do not have fears and worries, sadness and anger, but rather things that are similar to these' (*On Anger* 1.3.4–8). So too, in the *Consolation to Marcia* 5.1, Seneca remarks that animals do not experience sadness and fear, any more than stones do. It is worth noting that among the examples he provides of pre-emotions, Seneca mentions the way 'the ears of a soldier prick up at the sound of a trumpet, even when peace reigns and he is wearing the toga, and the noise of arms rouses army horses' (*On Anger* 2.2.6); here, then, the reaction of animals is evidently analogous to that of human beings.

The cause of initial grief, then, is reasonably clear: it derives from the perception or imagination (*species, phantasia*) of a loss, to which human beings, even the wisest, react naturally, just as animals do. Aristotle, Epicurus, and the Stoics all shared this view in one form or another. Humans alone, however, extend the period of mourning beyond what is natural or due. The reason, as Seneca explains in the *Consolation to Marcia*, is that opinion adds more than nature demands (*sed plus est quod opinio adicit quam quod natura imperauit*). The opinion to which Seneca refers clearly has to do with false beliefs concerning the nature of death as well as what is of fundamental value in life, which for the Stoics, as I have said, is virtue and virtue alone. This kind of second-order grief, if I may call it so, threatens to become habitual and so constitutes a disease—we may label it 'melancholy', with Freud—that it is the task of philosophy to cure. We may say, then, that erroneous beliefs, when added to the initial and instinctive response to loss that is perfectly natural and unobjectionable, are the cause of that excess of mourning that is properly described as pathological.

We have thus identified the causes of both kinds of grief, but a question remains: is the perverse kind of grief, in which the pre-emotional reaction is extended and amplified beyond all measure, a *pathos* in the sense that Aristotle or the Stoics employed the term? The Stoics, of course, differed from Aristotle in condemning all *pathê*, such as anger and pity, although they left room for certain approved kinds of sentiments which they labeled *eupatheiai*; for Aristotle, only envy was a *pathos* unworthy of a virtuous person. If grief for Aristotle was merely the pain or *lupê* that results from loss, instinctive in character and hence not susceptible to rational persuasion, then it is clear why he would not have regarded it as part of an orator's toolkit and so beyond the purview of a treatise on rhetoric. But if he had turned his attention to the more complex sentiment that arises from mistaken opinion superadded on to such a loss, might he then have included it among the *pathê*? In other words, is such grief an emotion?

The fact that prolonged grief arises from false rather than true belief does not tell against it as a *pathos*. Aristotle, as we have seen, defines anger as 'a desire, accompanied by pain, for a perceived revenge, on account of a perceived slight'. I believe that the emphasis on perception answers to the fact that we want to see the offender suffer when we take our revenge (cf. *antipathein*) rather than just do away with him or her, which suffices in the case of hatred, according to Aristotle (*Rhetoric* 2.4, 1382a1–14). But it also suggests that we interpret a gesture or remark as insulting, and our perception is open to correction; Aristotle proceeds to show how to alter such perceptions in his analysis of *praotês* or calming down. For the Stoics, in turn, all *pathê* result from incorrect beliefs. Like the *pathê* Aristotle discusses in the *Rhetoric*, prolonged or obsessive mourning is open to being assuaged by arguments; this is what the genre of the consolation is designed to do, after all, and various strategies for helping the bereaved to overcome their anguish were developed. Nevertheless, I think that there are fundamental differences between inveterate grief and the kind of sentiments that Aristotle included under the term *pathos*. In part, it is the very rootedness of such grief that distinguishes it from the occurrent emotions (to use the modern term) that Aristotle subsumes under this heading: *orgê* as a *pathos* differs from *orgilotês* or 'irascibility' as a state, that is, a *diathesis* or perhaps a *hexis*. Someone like Seneca's Marcia, who has been in mourning for her deceased child for three years, is unlikely to be persuaded to alter her thoughts or behavior by a courtroom speech. The emotions do indeed involve judgments, which presumably are subject to change if one's view of the situation proves to be unfounded: an insult, for example, may not have been intended or was misunderstood, or a person we are inclined to pity turns out to be a criminal and so deserves his fate. But Aristotle did not, I think, have in mind cases in which anger or pity had hardened into chronic or ingrained attitudes, and so become immune to ordinary techniques of persuasion. As Plutarch writes in his consolation to his wife, most mothers, if their children die, 'dissolve into empty [*kenon*], ungrateful grief [*penthos*], not out of goodwill [*eunoia*] (which is a good and reasoned [*eulogiston*] thing) but because a large admixture of empty opinion [*to pros kenên doxan*] in a small quantity of natural emotion [*tôi phusikôi pathei*] makes the act of grieving [*ta penthê*] wild, insane [*manika*], and difficult to sedate' (6, trans. D. A. Russell, slightly modified).

But there may also be another reason for the exclusion of grief, even of this more cognitive sort, from the list of *pathê* as Aristotle understood the term. In a recent paper, Olivier Renaut affirms, rightly in my view, that 'Aristote est sans doute, c'est vrai, le premier « théoricien » des « émotions ». Contrairement à Platon, Aristote nous indique plus exactement quels types de jugements sont susceptibles d'infléchir, de causer, ou d'être la conséquence de certaines affections émotives'. Renaut takes as exemplary the emotion of anger, and concludes: 'la colère reçoit une analyse inédite dans le corpus, pour promouvoir une rhétorique technicienne (elle demeure neutre du point de vue éthique et politique), plus soucieuse de la justesse de l'émotion, plus attentive aussi à la valeur du *logos* que sont susceptibles d'employer les rhéteurs, et que sont capables de recevoir et comprendre les auditeurs'. In response to Renaut, I suggested, as indicated above, that the other *pathê* analyzed by Aristotle have a similarly moral and social dimension. Thus hatred (*to misein*) is a response to perceived vice in others, just as affection is induced by the perception of another's virtue (although there are other causes of *philia*, specifically pleasure and utility). Shame, rivalry (*zêlos*), gratitude, and even fear are morally inflected reactions. Envy too, or *phthonos*, which Aristotle says is not characteristic of a decent of virtuous person (*epieikês*), has an ethical aspect, insofar as one judges that one's equals are prospering more than oneself. I then proposed, very tentatively, the hypothesis that Aristotle may have collected the various sentiments he did under the specific category of *pathê* in the *Rhetoric* precisely because all of them, and not just *orgê*, more or less involved a concern for justice and a responsiveness to the value of reason or *logos*.

In a way, this is to turn Renaut's argument on its head, as Karl Marx claimed to be doing with Hegel's metaphysics: instead of arguing that Aristotle's *pathê* have a moral aspect, I suggest that he identified as *pathê* just those responses that have an ethical character, as he understood or chose to represent them. It is true that Aristotle's list of *pathê* is remarkably similar to the kinds of affects that are today recognized as emotions. In this sense, he is indeed, as Renaut says, 'the first theoretician of the emotions'. But if so, it is not necessarily because there exists an abstract and transhistorical category that corresponds to what we call 'emotion'. It may rather be a kind of sublime coincidence that Aristotle, working from very different premises about the kinds of affects to include in his advice to orators, arrived at a selection that we now perceive as precisely corresponding to the modern notion of emotion.

It may also be the case that Aristotle's principle of selection was implicitly at work in the modern period, even though the passions were largely taken to be irrational in nature. At all events, it is fair to say that Aristotle's classification of the *pathê* influenced the development of subsequent taxonomies of the emotions by Cicero, Thomas Aquinas, Descartes, Hume, Adam Smith, and others, even when Aristotle's original principle of selection was no longer recognized or accepted. At all events, if, as Renaut puts it, 'Normativité technique et éthiques sont ... difficilement dissociables' in Aristotle's treatment, it is in part because Aristotle selected the responses that he wished to arouse or assuage by technical means precisely on the basis of their ethical dimension, as he saw it. Grief, even the pathological or inveterate kind, is not an ethical affect in this same way, and so, even though its causes may be ascribed to false beliefs that contaminate an initial natural response to loss, it remained outside the gamut of what Aristotle conceived of as *pathê*.

CHAPTER 12

Nero in Hell: Plutarch's *De Sera Numinis Vindicta*[1]

Marcus Folch

1   Introduction

This essay approaches pleasure and pain in antiquity through the lens of
Plutarch's *De Sera Numinis Vindicta* (henceforth DSNV), a short, often over-
looked dialogue in the *Moralia*. DSNV begins *in medias res*, as an Epicurean
(named Epicurus, appropriately enough) departs abruptly, leaving his interlocutors to defend divine providence (πρόνοια) in his absence.[2] Plutarch's
apology focuses on the topic that gives the dialogue its title—delays in divine
punishment, that is, retribution that occurs (if at all) long after a crime has
been committed—with an extended excursus on the doctrine of 'ancestral
fault' (προγονικὸν ἁμάρτημα), the notion that subsequent generations may pay
for the vices of their forbears.[3] The dialogue divides into two philosophical
speeches (the first concerning delays in divine punishment, the second inheritance of ancestral fault) and a myth, modeled on Plato's Er, in which one
Aridaeus—a degenerate, who squanders his inheritance and refrains from no
crime to recover it—falls, strikes his head, and is presumed dead. Tethered to
his body as though by the rode of an anchor, his soul wanders through the lowest strata of the heavens, witnessing the fates of those who lived immorally—
a harrowing vision that convinces Aridaeus to live a just and moderate life.

Recent literature on DSNV has sought principally to appraise the dialogue's
argumentative merits and adjudicate among its philosophical, literary, rhetorical, and religious characteristics.[4] My (loosely narratological) approach
emphasizes instead its engagement with classical Athenian literature, the clas-
sically trained readership it presupposes, and its careful positioning vis-à-vis

---

1   I wish to thank Professors W. V. Harris and J. Howley for reading, commenting on, and
    improving earlier drafts of this essay.
2   As Klaerr and Vernière (1974: 97–101) observe, the dramatis personae in DSNV are most prop-
    erly understood as idealized interlocutors. For discussion of providence in Plutarch, see
    Swain 1989.
3   For difficulties translating προγονικὸν ἁμάρτημα, see Gagné 2013: 54–55.
4   For general treatments of DSNV see Soury 1945: 167–169; Ziegler 1949: 212–213; Brenk 1973;
    Klaerr and Vernière 1974: 89–124; Torraca 1991; Saunders 1993; Helmig 2005: 323–326; Scholten
    2009: 102–111; Frazier 2010; Opsomer and Steel 2012: 50–59; Gagné 2013: 39–49.

DOI:10.1163/9789004379503_013

Roman imperial politics. Whatever one's assessment of Plutarch as a philosopher, stylist, rhetorical theorist, or religious thinker, DSNV is the product of the renewed Hellenism of the first and second centuries CE, and like much of Plutarch's corpus, it adapts generic models associated with fifth—and fourth-century Athenian literature to the radically different political realities of Greece under Rome. Particularly in its closing myth—which features Nero's tortured soul on the verge of being reborn into the body of a mysterious creature—DSNV participates directly in the contestation over the legacy of the Julio-Claudian dynasty that erupted shortly after (if not before) the emperor's demise. Approaching the dialogue with an awareness of its tailoring of classical literary forms to the Roman imperial context, I make three claims:

The first, which takes up the bulk of the next section, is that for Plutarch injustice that goes unpunished presents not only a metaphysical problem; it is also a problem of sentiment. As we shall observe, Plutarch consistently calls attention to the sensations of pleasure and pain, joy and despondency to which the injustices of human history give rise. At stake in DSNV is thus both a philosophical account of how the world may be recognized as good despite wrongdoings that appear to go unpunished, and the pleasure we enjoy and the pain we suffer when surveying the drama of human passions. In this respect, DSNV offers a case study in the history of pleasure and pain in antiquity, in which philosophy provides the resources to make sense of, and possibly even to find pleasure in (or despite), the most painful dimensions of human history.

My second claim, addressed in the third section ("'Viewing" history, reading text'), is hermeneutic: through a series of theatrical similes and metaphors which emphasize the ways we view the pleasures and punishments of others, Plutarch furnishes readers with the tools to decipher the dialogue. In other words, DSNV establishes the terms of its own interpretation. In doing so, it delineates the outlines of an ideal interpreter of the dialogue—one who perceives, even in the most extreme instances of human suffering, the rational order of the cosmos while at the same time apprehending the intertextual strategies DSNV brings to bear on the question of providence.

My third claim, discussed in the section 'Revisiting Nero', is that when approached from the interpretive parameters that the dialogue itself proposes and encourages its readers to adopt, DSNV is surprisingly subversive, inviting its audience to reinterpret its defense of providence as oblique criticism of the Roman emperor. A source of perennial controversy, the final scene of Aridaeus' journey—Nero's tortured soul on the verge of rebirth in the body of an unidentifiable creature—has seemed to many commentators to be discordant with the dialogue's otherwise philosophical and historically distanced claims.[5] Yet, I contend that Nero is not an aberration from the dialogue's argument but its central problem. Not only is Nero's life—the pleasures he enjoyed, the pains he inflicted—what makes a defense of providence necessary in the first place. A careful rereading of the dialogue, necessitated by the emperor's anomalous appearance, also suggests that Nero has been the implicit subject of philosophical exploration long before his soul emerges in the afterlife.

2 Overview of Plutarch's Argument

2.1 First Speech

The dialogue begins with a prefatory exchange, in which Plutarch's interlocutors summarize Epicurus' most disquieting claims. Patrocleas complains of feeling 'disturbed' (ἠγανάκτουν) when hearing Euripides' adage that 'Apollo lags' (μέλλει, 548d2), and he insists that god should be indolent in nothing— particularly when punishing the wicked, who are anything but idle in the pursuit of vice.[6] He also emphasizes the psychological states of those who perpetrate, suffer from, or witness others committing crimes: chastisement that immediately follows a crime comforts the injured and deters future misdeeds, but injustices that go unpunished leave the victim 'weak' (ἀσθενῆ), robbed of 'hopes' (ἐλπίσι), and 'downcast' (ταπεινόν); at the same time, justice delayed fortifies the criminal's resolve, giving him 'confidence and boldness' (θρασύτητι καὶ τόλμῃ) to commit further crime (548d10–e5). Olympichus adds that delinquency on the part of the divine is suggestive of a world without order; justice that is slow resembles 'the fortuitous (τῷ αὐτομάτῳ) rather than providence' (πρόνοιαν, 549d5–6). At stake in Epicurus' claims are both the affective responses (ἀσθενῆ, ταπεινόν, θρασύτητι, τόλμῃ) that history provokes and a metaphysical argument over the nature of the cosmos.[7] Such concerns, Plutarch concedes,

---

5 Cf. Saunders 1993: 74: 'whereas Plato [in the *Laws*] applied Platonic penology in an ambitious model penal code based on contemporary law, Plutarch draws back from showing how a revised Platonic penology could affect contemporary policy, in which he takes little direct interest (and it is noticeable too how many of his illustrations are drawn from the distant past)'.

6 Unattributed Stephanus page numbers are to DSNV. Translations of DSNV are based on de Lacy and Einarson's (1959) with slight modification.

7 It is notable, however, that there is nothing especially Epicurean in the arguments to which DSNV responds; Epicurus has merely triggered troubling recollections based on such canonical writers as Euripides, Thucydides, and Bias. The literary roots of the positions against which DSNV reacts should warn against interpreting the text as a volley in a philosophical in-game among second-century Platonists and their Epicurean critics. DSNV rather represents

touch on unknowable dimensions of reality. The appropriate posture, when one contemplates the divine, is circumspection (549e). We must trust that god knows the right time to apply punishment as medicine, but beyond that divine law is inscrutable (549f–550a). A defense of providence cannot aspire to scientific knowledge (550b); it aims instead for 'persuasiveness' (τῷ πιθανῷ) in the face of 'philosophical impasse' (ἀπορίαν), and ought to be received as such (550c11–12). What follows, then, is a philosophical foray beyond the limits of scientific and empirical reasoning, speculative arguments leveraging Platonic doctrines to delineate the contours of the most impenetrable dimensions of human existence.

The preliminary strategy of the first speech is to re-describe delays in divine punishment as the hallmark of god's benevolence. God, Plutarch insists, has fashioned reality as an image of himself to serve as a 'model' (παράδειγμα, 550d1) for human virtue. He has, for instance, implanted rhythm and harmony in the movements of planets and stars, so that we might gaze upon the heavens and 'become habituated to welcome and love all that moves in stateliness and order, and thereby come to hate discordant and errant passions' (550d9–e1). Humanity's normative relationship to the physical world is a species of 'mimesis' (μιμήσει, 550e3), a replicating of the goodness that inheres in 'nature' (φύσις, 550d4)—which includes history's recurrent patterns—within the psyche and its sentiments. Because knowledge of virtue may be derived by observing and mimicking nature, it is reasonable to infer that we ought to emulate the unhurried timing of divine retribution. Doing so allows the soul to rid itself of the 'animalistic' (θηριῶδες) and 'turbulent' (λάβρον, 550e8) passions that motivate our desire for revenge. Nature teaches us not to lash out in anger or permit madness to seize control of our psyches, but to remain dispassionate as we correct those who, despite their criminal activities, share our humanity (550e–551c). Adhering to such principles, Plato and Archytas refrained from beating miscreant slaves, stopping mid-blow and citing their own passions as the reason *not* to punish (Plato delivered his slave to Speusippus for a sound drubbing).[8] Plutarch's apology for delays in divine punishment thus resolves into a critique of the psychology of ὀργή, θυμός, and μανία—the conventional sentimental bases for seeking restitution in ancient penal thought—and it

---

a rejoinder to conventional readings of Greek literature and history, and its defense of provi-dence, as we shall see later, attempts to present an alternative reading of the same canonical sources.

8   Cf. Riginos 1976: 155–156. See Gellius (1.26), in which the philosopher who punishes a delin-quent slave is none other than the moralist from Chaeronea. I owe this reference to Joseph Howley.

participates in the ideology of anger control characteristic of Hellenistic and Roman philosophy.[9]

Long before the speech draws to a conclusion, however, Plutarch abandons its initial premise—the doctrine of 'imitate god.' For the remainder of the speech Plutarch and his interlocutors unpack the implications of Plato's medicinal penology. Because of its association with psychological pathology, punishment, as it is practiced in judicial institutions, has a singular goal and an intrinsic limitation; it seeks only 'to requite pain for pain' (ἀντιλυποῦν, 551c7–8).[10] God, by contrast, is unharmed by injustice, and therefore harbors no vindictive motives. Rather, he apprehends the passions that lead to crime and seeks to heal the criminal's sickened soul (551c). If the soul is predisposed to repentance and its evil eradicable, god grants it a period of time for reform (551c–d). Some god cures with a course of 'therapy' (θεραπευθέν, 551d6), but those whose vices are irremediable god 'amputates' (551d9) straightaway. Others commit crimes out of ignorance of the good rather than love of evil; these god patiently remediates (551e). God's medicinal approach to justice, which adapts punishment to the innate nobility of the criminal's soul and its potential to harm others or redeem itself, arises from privileged insight into the quality of human psyche. However large a portion of virtue a soul may have had prior to its incarnation, god recognizes that inhabiting a human body may retard the realization of one's potential goodness (551d). Upbringing and bad company lead to bad habits, shaping the soul's character profoundly but in many cases not indelibly (551e). However negligent it may appear, divine retribution allows souls to heal from the effects of embodiment.[11]

It might seem intuitive to interpret Plutarch as directing his interlocutors (and readers) to look to their own lives for demonstration that a criminal's soul may redeem itself over time, but his illustrations consist entirely of tyrants and would-be autocrats: Gelon, Hieron, Peisistratus, Lydiadas, Miltiades, Cimon, and Themistocles (551f–552b). The unifying thread connecting this pageantry of ruthless, cold-blooded murderers—drawn entirely from earlier periods of Greek history—is the violence with which they seized power, the ethical transformation they underwent, and the justice with which they ruled their subjects. As important is their civilizing function; all these latter-day Cecropses spread Hellenic culture. Such accomplishments demonstrate the seminal Platonic

---

9   Cf. σὺν ὀργῇ, 550e9; ὀργῆς, 551a1; ὀργήν, 551a9; θυμός, 551a6; θυμός, 550e10; θυμόν, 551a9; μανίας, 551a2. For the ideology of anger control, see Harris 2001: chs. 6 & 8. For ὀργή as motivation for penal action, see Allen 2000a: 137–38; cf. Allen 2000b: chs. 4–9.
10   For ὀργή as an object of medical speculation, see Allen 2000a: 141–42.
11   Cf. Becchi 2012: 43–44.

principle that 'great natures (μεγάλαι φύσεις) bring forth nothing trivial, and the vigor and enterprise in them is too keen to remain inert' (551b11–c1); they wander restless before attaining a determinate character, effecting great destruction but eventually greater virtue.[12]

Some villains have no such redeeming qualities—in which case, just as Egyptian law stays the execution of pregnant women under sentence of death until they have given birth, god postpones punishment for humanity's benefit (552d). The brutality of tyrants and the anger of rulers serve as purgatives, cleansing a people of moral vice (553a). God, Plutarch insists, 'does not destroy the rank and thorny root of a glorious race until it has borne its proper fruit' (553c4–7). Tyrannies are sometimes instances of the divine employing vices of some to cure others. At other times god may postpone punishment to design a penalty that is even more 'timely and fitting' (ἐν καιρῷ καὶ τρόπῳ τῷ προσήκοντι, 553d1). Divine retribution might therefore have aesthetic properties, part of a cosmic narrative with its own pacing, dramatic inversions, and unforeseen climaxes.[13]

If much of the first speech argues that we must model punishment and the management of the passions on the delayed pace of divine retribution, and that such delays are signs of god's benevolence, its final contention is that there are no delays. Taking up Hesiod's (*Op.* 266) maxim that the wicked plan is most evil for the one who devises it, Plutarch argues that, 'vice frames out of itself each instrument of its own punishment' (554a10–b1; cf. Gellius 4.5). From the moment of his first iniquity a tyrant's soul is afflicted with doubt, self-loathing, and fear (553f–556e). Such tortured passional states are just the beginning of a retribution that will follow the evildoer until death. A naïve spectator may misconstrue the wrongdoers' successes as fortune, but god recognizes the trappings of success as part of the punishment. From the perspective of the divine, for whom the interval of a human life is nothing, a man whose punishment arrives thirty years after his crime has been stretched on the rack in the evening rather than the morning, having spent the intervening period as though in prison, playing dice as a noose swings overhead (554d). Those who live long after committing injustice 'are not punished once they have grown old, but have grown old in punishment' (554c11–d1). Even the most prosperous moments in the lives of criminals may therefore be viewed as part of elaborate rituals of retribution, in which the vicious are tormented by delusions and memories of their misdeeds, all of which portend impending penalties (554f–555c). Once the madness by which one is convinced to violate

---

12   Cf. discussion of 'great natures' in *Demetr.* 1, *Cor.* 1.2–3, with Duff 1999: esp. 317–318.

13   We return to the aesthetic properties of punishment in the next section.

laws has abated, all that is left is remorse and the knowledge that ill-gotten gains are easily lost (555f–556e). Punishment, therefore, is virtually unnecessary; memory and the fleeting nature of the passions suffice as penalties.

2.2 Second Speech

The second speech, which, we are led to believe, addresses the most serious accusation against providence, responds to Timon's contention that inheritance of ancestral fault violates the basic principles of justice. Either the guilty party has already been punished, in which case justice demands that god not exact two payments for the same crime; or, because it is inadmissible to punish the innocent, once the culpable have died, god has missed the only opportunity legitimately to seek restitution (556f). Timon further observes that the vices of ancestors have furnished generals, tyrants, heroes, and gods with pretexts to despoil neighbors, depopulate cities, and plague the innocent sometimes centuries after the ancestors' wrongdoings—an especially troubling observation, in light of the claim of the first speech that one ought to emulate divine behavior (556f–557e).

Plutarch's reply is periphrastic, consisting of a preamble and a proper speech. Noting that many of the examples of inherited punishments that Timon has adduced are fictional 'anomalies' (ἀτοπίας, 557e8), Plutarch insists that divine restitution obeys the logic of ancestral 'reciprocity' (χάριν, 558c1). Because the 'family' or 'race' (γένει, 558c1) receives hereditary honors, it is also the appropriate site for retribution. It is thus inconsistent to denounce the gods for imposing penalties on children and heirs while simultaneously praising transmissible social privilege—of which, incidentally, Plutarch and Timon have both been recent beneficiaries (558a–b). The preamble has clear meta-dialogic relevance; the analogical structure of punishment and honor, Plutarch insists, should temper the vehement emotions that Timon (whose histrionic disposition recalls Plato's Thrasymachus) has exhibited in criticizing inherited ancestral fault (558b–c).[14] The effect is to delineate the appropriate emotive disposition for receptivity to the principal argument of the second speech—namely, that crime, like 'illness' (νόσημα, 558e2), is communicable within a γένος. Vice is comparable to such diseases as dropsy and phthisis; just as doctors order the children of parents who have died of either condition to sit with feet in water, until the corpses have been cremated, we should not be surprised if god treats descendants of evildoers with what appears to us as deferred punishment (558d). In such cases god is healing an infected family.

---

14   Cf. Klaerr and Vernière 1974: 97–98.

To explain the mechanism whereby vice is transferred from one generation to the next, Plutarch proposes a theory of somatic, political, and psychological inheritance. Certain 'forces' (δυνάμεις) have a capacity for 'contagion' (ἀφάς) and 'transmission' (διαδόσεις), covering great intervals of time and space and 'reaching one object by passing through another' (558e6–8). Disease and injustice are among such forces; plague traveled from Ethiopia to kill Pericles and attack Thucydides; guilt (and with it retribution) found its way to the children of sacrilegious Delphians and Sybarites (558e–f). Such forces revert from their 'farthest points' (τῶν ἐσχάτων) to their 'origins' (τὰ πρῶτα), effecting 'connections' (συνάψεις) between extremities (558f3–4). Although we do not know the precise cause that creates such linkages, nevertheless it 'silently achieves its proper effect' (τὸ οἰκεῖον, 558f5). Cities, Plutarch continues, provide one context in which such forces circulate. Although a city may change over time, it remains sufficiently identical to itself to warrant punishment postponed or displaced onto subsequent generations, provided that the 'association' (κοινωνία) by which it was created preserves its 'unity' (ἑνότητα, 559a7, cf. b–c).[15]

Another such context is the γένος. All members of a family spring from and remain attached to a 'single origin,' which reproduces a 'certain power and common quality pervading them all' (δύναμίν τινα καὶ κοινωνίαν διαπεφυκυῖαν ἀναφερούσης, 559d1–2). Unlike an 'artefact' (τι δημιούργημα πεποιημένον), descendants are created 'out of' (ἐξ) their ancestor, not 'by' (ὑπ') him, and thus contain within themselves a portion of what is his (559d4).[16] An ancestor's 'principal part inheres and is innate' (τὸ κυριώτατον ἐμπέφυκε καὶ πάρεστι μέρος) within his descendants; 'by it they live, are nourished, are governed, and think' (ζῶσιν αὐτῷ καὶ τρέφονται καὶ διοικοῦνται καὶ φρονοῦσι, 559e3–5).[17] Because an ancestor's principal part animates and guides the thoughts of the members of a γένος, descendants receive their ancestor's due when they inherit his punishments and honors.

It is, therefore, possible to imagine conditions in which god might cure descendants, as a doctor treats the body—by cauterization, scarring, and

---

15   Cf. Aristotle's (*Pol.* 1276b1–2) claim that, because a city is a 'partnership' (κοινωνία) of citizens in a 'constitution' (πολιτείας), it remains identical to itself as long as its constitution is unchanged.

16   Cf. Aristotle's (*Gen. Animal.* 730b9–31) claim that the semen of the father is the efficient and formal cause of the child, fashioning the material cause of the mother's menstrual blood as a carpenter sculpts inert material.

17   Inspiration for this claim appears to be a passage from the *Laws* in which Plato argues that the human race is 'coeval with all time' (συμφυὲς τοῦ παντὸς χρόνου); as such, it innately desires immortality—a desire that is satisfied through procreation and perpetuation, by which humanity remains 'one and the same in perpetuity' (ταὐτὸν καὶ ἓν ὂν ἀεί, 721c2–6).

bleeding, oftentimes applied to intermediaries and appendages even before symptoms of the disease appear (559d). Indeed, the soul is a more efficient vehicle for remediation than the body; medicine applied to one part of a body may heal another part of the same body, but treatment of one person will not cure another. By contrast, 'dispositions, afflictions, and corrections' (διαθέσεις καὶ κακώσεις καὶ ἐπανορθώσεις, 560a6) may be communicated from soul to soul. Because the soul is led by 'imagination' (φαντασίαις, 560a9), it feels confidence and terror when it perceives or envisions the others undergoing treatment. Heirs of a family's vicious profile may, as a result, be treated through punitive remedies applied within a γένος, while bystanders may learn to avoid vice by observing others undergoing torturous therapy.

Plutarch concedes that the argument of the second speech presupposes the immortality of the soul, which competes 'like an athlete' (ὥσπερ ἀθλητής, 561a2) and receives its deserts in the afterlife (560b–561a). To the living, who are bonded to the body and limited by the somatic knowledge it affords, the vicious may seem to go unpunished and the innocent to suffer without reward; but much depends on perspective; in the eternal sequence of reincarnation and transmigration of souls, all debts are paid in the end (561a). In the afterlife ancestral fault serves a new punitive function; it becomes an instrument of retribution turned against one's culpable ancestors. For the greatest punishment is not to suffer posthumous retribution but to witness one's children, friends, and family paying the price for one's crimes and suffering terrible calamities through no fault of their own (561b).

In the final section of the second speech, Plutarch anticipates a counter-argument, conventionally associated with Bion of Borysthenes: namely, punishing the children of wicked men is akin to administering medicine to a son or grandson for a father's or grandfather's illness (561c). Such objections, Plutarch insists, only support his case. While it may be true that treatment administered to the child of an ill father or grandfather will never cure his ailing family member, punishments visited on descendants 'provide a spectacle' (δείκνυνται, 561c8) and therefore have the second-order benefit of dissuading onlookers from committing like crimes. More significantly, Plutarch's critics miss the seminal point that what is transmitted along the γένος is not culpability but *potentiality*. Souls, like bodies, inherit congenital predispositions; members of a γένος may bear a 'family resemblance in vice' (κακίας δ'ὁμοιότητα συγγενικήν, 561f5). The propensity for evil is thus hereditary, and must be treated before it becomes 'evident in the passions' (πάθεσιν ἐμφανής, 562a2).

Once again, god's privileged insight into the nature of the soul is of crucial importance. Whereas an animal's 'congenital character' (τὸ συγγενὲς ἦθος) is evident at birth, humans are born into 'customs, doctrines, and laws'

(562b5–7). Social conventions allow the heir of a vicious nature to 'conceal' her or his predisposition, and to 'imitate' virtue (562b7–8). She or he may thereby ablate 'the genetic stain of vice' (ἐγγενῆ κηλῖδα τῆς κακίας), or temporarily escape detection by wrapping her or his depravity 'as though with a covering' (οἷον ἔλυτρόν τι, 562b9–10). God is not fooled by such concealments, nor does he make the mistake of believing that humans 'become' unjust the moment they 'appear' unjust (562c8). Thieves and tyrants possess vice from the outset; they merely act upon their thievish and lawless instincts when presented the occasion and power. God 'innately perceives' (αἰσθάνεσθαι πεφυκώς, 562d2) soul rather than body, and knows the nature and disposition of each individual. He need not wait for violence to reveal itself in the hands, impudence in the voice, and licentiousness in the sexual organs before inflicting punishment; and in such cases, god's purposes are not retaliatory but medicinal, aiming to remove vice, like epilepsy, before the seizure (562d). If the 'family trait' (τὸ συγγενές) bypasses a generation, god withholds punishment, reserving remediation solely for heirs, in whom the family's 'vicious resemblance' (τὴν ὁμοιότητα τῆς κακίας, 563a3–4) must necessarily reassert itself. What appears as inherited punishment is more properly understood as selective, prophylactic therapy, administered throughout the γένος before an ancestor's animating force has exhibited itself.

2.3   Myth

The eschatological myth provides a graphic and palimpsestic restatement of the claims of the first two speeches (cf. Hirsch-Luipold 2014: 172–174). Struck free of its body, Aridaeus' soul feels first like a pilot cast from the helm of a ship and submerged in an abyss (563e). Soon it rises to the fiery empyrean and gazes upon stars that appear magnified in size and at vast distances apart, emitting light along which his soul travels like a ship (563e–f). It joins a procession of disembodied souls as they are sorted according to virtue and purity, and eventually encounters a distant kinsman, who guides Aridaeus (rechristened Thespesius) on a tour of many 'spectacles' (θεαμάτων, 563f4). Of the latter, the first is a tripartite schema of posthumous remediation overseen by Adrasteia (563e–565e). Those whose crimes were punished while they were alive fall under Poine's purview, whose methods are comparatively swift and gentle. Any who require posthumous correction are given to Dike. Erinys, Adrasteia's third minister, 'disappears and incarcerates' (ἠφάνισε καὶ κατέδυσεν) incurables in a place called 'the nameless and unseen' (τὸ ἄρρητον καὶ ἀόρατον, 564f5–565a1). Dike's punishments, which Plutarch narrates in detail, involve a dynamic of dramatic unmasking and exhibition, as she 'exposes' (καταφανῆ, 565a10) the soul of each naked, so that he is 'seen' in every way. In this state Dike 'shows' (ἔδειξε) him to his virtuous parents and ancestors—if such they were; if they were wicked, he 'sees' them punished and 'is seen' by them (565b2–6). Such souls then undergo prolonged treatment, as each of their passions is removed through 'agonies and labors' (ἀλγηδόσι καὶ πόνοις, 565b7), whose magnitude exceeds the torments of the body as much as waking reality is more vivid than dreams. Some are cured after several rounds of therapy; but those from whom the passions cannot be eradicated, sink back into the world below, borne into bodies of living things by the force of their ignorance and the 'form of the love of pleasure' (φιληδονίας εἶδος, 565d7), impressed upon the soul by a lifetime of hedonism.

The second spectacle is the path by which Dionysos entered the underworld to retrieve Semele (565e–566a). There, Aridaeus observes souls seduced by the memory of bodily pleasure: enchanted by Bacchic revelry, the rational parts of their psyches dissolve, while the remaining, irrational portion puts on flesh and is drawn back into the process of birth.

The penultimate scene involves a series of oracles—of Night and Moon, the Sibyl, and Apollo (566a–e). His guide attempts 'to show' him the rarified light of Apollo's tripod at Delphi; 'although he desired to, [Aridaeus] did not see it' (προθυμούμενος...ἰδεῖν οὐκ εἶδεν, 566d3–5). Instead, he hears the voice of the Sibyl, foretelling his death, the eruption of Vesuvius, the (otherwise unattested) conflagration of Dicaearcheia, and the demise of the emperor Titus (566e). This sequence—which provides a *terminus post quem* for the dating of the dialogue—is one of only two instances in which Plutarch ruptures the myth's illusion of ahistoricity, alluding directly to known historical figures and events (the second is the appearance of Nero).[18]

In the final spectacle, souls undergo punishment before being reborn within the bodies of various animals—a scene notable for its macabre detail as well as its departure from Plato's strictly medicinal penology (566e–567f). Among the condemned Aridaeus sees his own father, crawling out from a pit, guilty of poisoning and robbing guests in their sleep, and forced to confess his crimes to his son (566e–f). As he 'gazes upon the torture' (ἐθεᾶτο... τὴν αἰκίαν, 567a6–7) of the condemned, Aridaeus discovers that those whose vices were evident and punished in life receive the mildest remediation, while men and women who 'cloaked themselves in a costume and reputation for virtue' (πρόσχημα

---

18   The contrast between Nero and Titus is pointed. Suetonius (*Vit. Tit.* 7.1–3) observes that Titus spent his youth in such violence and dissipation that he was expected to be a second Nero. Instead, he proved to be a virtuous leader, thereby demonstrating precisely the antipodal trajectory of moral development to the one *DSNV* illustrates with respect to Nero. I wish to thank the anonymous reader for calling attention to this cross-reference. For the date of *DSNV*, see Klaerr and Vernière 1974: 93.

καὶ δόξαν ἀρετῆς περιβαλόμενοι, 567a9–10) receive the harshest penalties; some are sentenced to writhe and twist inward like sea-scolopendras on a hook until they turn inside out; others are flayed, ulcerated, and exposed to the elements; others still coil like vipers in a nest, devouring one another. Demonic craftsmen then forge the souls anew, smelting them in the molten rivers that encircle the underworld (567b–d). Most pitiable are those who thought they had fulfilled their sentences, only to discover that their guilt had transferred to their descendants. Heirs of ancestral punishment rush upon their parents and grandparents, 'displaying the signs of their sufferings' (τὰ σημεῖα τῶν παθῶν ἐδείκνυεν, 567d–8), and dragging them back for further retribution; upon some great swarms of souls descend like bees and bats, enraged at the memory of all they had suffered through no fault of their own.[19] Aridaeus sees Nero's soul, twisted, cut, and fitted to new somatic forms, condemned first to the body of a serpent and later to that of a singing swamp creature. Immediately thereafter a terrifying and beautiful woman appears, intending to lead Aridaeus off to undergo remediation, but another interposes, and his soul is snapped away as though by a cord, a strong wind returning it to his body (568a).

3   'Viewing' History, Reading Text

There is more going on here than moralistic mythologizing appended to a collection of conventional arguments in favor of providence and inherited culpability. It often goes unnoticed that in tandem with its doctrinal defense of providence, DSNV presents its reader a meditation on the emotions of pain and pleasure that human suffering and vice engender. That history often appears governed by irrational passions and that humanity's most noble intentions seem to lead to greater forms of evil is itself a source of psychological distress. On the other hand, phenomena that provoke sentiments of despondency and grief, when viewed from another perspective—the right perspective—offer a distinct form of pleasure: consolation in the knowledge that evil will receive its just deserts. In this sense, philosophy—or at least the right kind of philosophy—is shown throughout DSNV to provide the resources to rewrite history's greatest injustices as part of a script that governs the cosmos, to see its criminal actors as inexorably directing themselves toward a just and aesthetically satisfying conclusion.

My use of theatrical metaphors is not accidental. Plutarch often represents history in dramatic terms, as though adhering to a plot whose structure and

---

19   The imagery in this passage recalls *Odyssey* 24.5.

conclusion may be inferred from theater, Platonic dialogues, and canonical Greek literature.[20] The claim, for instance, that vice immediately afflicts the perpetrator's soul is explained by way of analogy with Roman punitive rituals, in which participants reenacted mythological and historical events, often culminating in the execution of the convict protagonist:[21]

> Some people are no wiser than little children, who see criminals in the theater, frequently clad in tunics of cloth of gold and purple mantles, wearing chaplets and dancing Pyrrhic measures, and struck with awe and wonderment suppose them supremely happy, till the moment when before their eyes the criminals are stabbed and scourged and that gay and sumptuous apparel bursts into flames. (554b4–9)

Against the vantage of such a naïve spectator we may juxtapose Plutarch's account of the criminal's nascent self-awareness. When evil men perceive wickedness within themselves, their souls are moved from a state of 'pleasure' to one of 'terrors (φόβων), pains (λυπῶν), unpleasant memories (μνήμης ἀτερποῦς), misgivings for the future and mistrust of the present' (555f6–556a2). In a similar vein, Plutarch cites Euripides' *Ino* to argue that 'the thought that the soul of every wicked man resolves within itself and dwells upon is this: how it might escape the memory of its iniquities, drive out of itself the consciousness of guilt, regain its purity (καθαρά), and begin its life anew' (556a7–b1). The linguistic and conceptual framework within which divine punishment becomes interpretable evokes the *anagnôrisis, peripeteia,* and *katharsis* of an Aristotelian tragic plot.[22] The emphasis on sight, vision, spectacle is not limited to the first speech; even within the vast temporal frame of the second— which posits a sweeping theory of cosmological sympathy and circulation of powers and in which predispositions for vice inhere in the psychology of a γένος—spectatorship remains the principal axis along which the argument of *DSNV* advances. One who is predisposed to vice may conceal his nature behind a costume (πρόσχημα, ἔλυτρόν), and, like an actor, mime (μιμεῖται) the virtues

---

20 As we observe below, moreover, theatrical imagery serves an important meta-textual function, calling attention to the psychological state of those who interpret history and pointing to the manner in which *DSNV* asks to be read. For theatrical imagery in Plutarch, see de Lacy (1952: esp. 159–168), who argues that terminology for tragedy, drama, and theater are usually terms of censure; but his study omits *DSNV*.

21 Cf. Coleman 1990: 47.

22 Cf. the later claim that, just as performers 'on receiving applause in the theater suddenly give a sigh, as their appetite for glory subsides to become mere love of wealth' (556c11–d2), criminals are soon filled with remorse, discovering that wickedness is its own punishment.

of good men, but god's aesthetic perception penetrates the illusion and sees beyond the performance of social convention. The criminal's vicious family trait is visible (ἐμφανής) later in life, and those who seem from one perspective to inherit punishment, appear from another to undergo anticipatory treatment of a congenital disorder. Theatricalizing divine punishment reaffirms the philosophical point that it matters little whether one agrees that crime is its own penalty and that it is impossible to conceal vice; whatever onlookers or participants may believe, the criminal is part of a tragic plot, a villain fated to receive just deserts. The dramatic imagery also gestures back to the prompt from which the conversation began; the literary canon and the poet, whose claim that Apollo lags threw Plutarch's interlocutors into a state of despondency, are rewritten to affirm the providential nature of the cosmos.

The key observation here is that our hedonic response to human history is a kind of 'reading', an act of deciphering in which literary education and philosophical commitments are put on display.[23] A passage from the first speech is especially relevant in this respect:

> Just as one ignorant of agriculture, on seeing a piece of ground overgrown with dense thickets and weeds, overrun with wild animals and watercourses and covered with mud, would not find it to his liking, while to him who has learned to discriminate and judge (διαισθάνεσθαι καὶ κρίνειν) these very circumstances reveal the vigor, depth, and looseness of the soil, so great natures put forth at first many strange and villainous shoots, and we, at once impatient of their rough and thorny quality, fancy that we should clear them away and cut them short; whereas the better judge discerns even in this their good and noble strain, and waits for them to reach the maturity that lends support to reason and virtue and the season when their nature yields her proper fruit. (552c3–d3)

Comparing the villainous soul to a tangled field and the imperceptive attitude of the inexperienced to the knowing farmer, suggests that the capacity to identify immanent virtue may be cultivated. The effect is to call attention to the responsibility we bear when deciding whether to view an individual's life as symptomatic of divine dereliction. Our reading of history—and thus our hedonic response to its most painful dimensions—depends not (only) on the

---

23   I have chosen 'reading' as my primary analytical metaphor, because, although Plutarch prefers imagery of theatrical and dramatic display, his approach to the interpretation of history is essentially literary, emphasizing the use of written, canonical texts (dramatic and philosophical) to illuminate history's underlying plot structures.

providential nature of the cosmos per se, but on the literary and philosophical expertise to which we make recourse when assessing the figures that have caused history's most painful developments. At stake in Plutarch's theatrical apologetics are the narratives by which we make sense of human suffering and the positions that such narratives permit us to occupy. What this passage points to, then, is an idealized reader or—to adopt Plutarch's perceptual metaphorics—an ideal 'spectator' of history, one whose vantage is distinguished by its literary and philosophical competence.[24] The literary and philosophically competent reader perceives in history patterns that are more unambiguously visible in canonical Greek literature (such as tragedy) and especially Platonic philosophy.[25] Such competence, frequently represented in *DSNV* in visual and theatrical terms, appears as an implicit and normative viewpoint from which history's most violent dimensions ought to be focalized and narrated.

Philosophically and narratologically competent readings of history enable us to contextualize human suffering and injustice within a providential narrative, and thus to make sound judgments regarding the management of pleasure and pain. At the same time, the notion of an ideal reader of history also has metatextual relevance for the interpretation of *DSNV* itself. Consider the analogy with which Plutarch illustrates the claim that punishment begins at the moment the crime is committed:

> What is to keep us from denying that even prisoners under sentence of death are punished until their necks are severed, or that one who has drunk the hemlock and is walking about, waiting for his legs to become heavy, is punished until he is overtaken by the chill and rigor that immediately precede the loss of all sensation, if we account as punishment only the final moment of punishment and ignore the intervening sufferings, terrors, forebodings, and pangs of remorse to which every wicked

---

24 By 'competence' I mean to combine Culler's (1975: 144) notion of 'literary competence' as 'what an ideal reader must know implicitly in order to read and interpret works in ways which we consider acceptable, in accordance with the institution of literature'; and Rowe's (2010: 40–42) 'practiced reader' of philosophy, one who knows (how) to bring the arguments from one Platonic dialogue to bear in the interpretation of other Platonic dialogues. Rowe's comments pertain principally to the *Laws* but may be adapted to the Platonic corpus in general and its reception in Plutarch.

25 In this respect, the ideal reading of history delineated in *DSNV* resembles what Konstan (2004: 8) calls 'the radical and remarkably modern approach to literature that Plutarch inaugurates in [*How a Youth Should Listen to Poems*],' an approach that places responsibility for interpretation on the reader. As I argue below, in *DSNV* responsibility for one's 'reading' of history and of the dialogue itself is also deflected to the reader.

man, once he has done evil, is prey, as if we denied that a fish which has
swallowed the hook is caught until we see it set to broil or cut in pieces
by the cook? (554d10–f1)

In the most just world, penal law positions the convicted in a state of rational-
ized suffering, the severity of which is calibrated to the crime and designed,
inter alia, to restore dignity to the victim.[26] Yet, it would be mistaken to construe the *punitive* as coterminous with the *sentence*; for punishment begins
where pain begins—not in the slitting of the throat or deadening of the limbs,
but in the passions, premonitions, and fears that attend the criminal act. In this
respect, rituals of punishment may have no bearing whatsoever on whether
an individual is being punished. Indeed, Plutarch later argues that divine retribution may involve various forms of pleasure—'feasting, business, gifting,
receiving of gifts, and entertainment' (554d7–8). The point is that what we
mean when we designate a particular phenomenon as punitive—the object
description—is in need of critical reevaluation; for only once we are clear on
the definitional assumptions we bring to the question of punishment will we
be equipped to assess whether it is delayed.

   On one level, then, *DSNV* interrogates the notional borders of the punitive,
and the conclusion it leads to is that the labeling of an action or mental state as
penal depends on the presuppositions of the one who characterizes an event
as punishment.[27] But Plutarch's penology involves 'reading' on another level as
well—for, as every reader will have recognized, the image of an incarcer-
ated convict at 554d10–f1 alludes (by antithesis) to Plato's Socrates, awaiting
execution with equipoise (*Phaed.* 53b–c, 114d–115a). Of course, the intertextual background reinforces Plutarch's claim that punishment hinges on perspective; whether one experiences the same sentence as a terrifying punitive
ritual or, in Socratic fashion, as liberation depends on one's philosophical
commitments.[28] In this respect, our reading of history is intimately connected
to how we read texts. In other words, historical and textual interpretations
involve identical hermeneutic activities; the ideal reader will conduct parallel
modes of interpretation: she or he will construe history as a theater (or amphi-
theater) peopled by Platonic souls, who enact plots and perform scripts familiar from Greek tragedy and the Platonic dialogues; at the same time, she or he

---

26   Cf. Coleman 1990: 45–46.
27   E.g., Plutarch later argues that divine retribution may involve various forms of pleasure—
      'feasting, business, gifting, receiving of gifts, and entertainment' (554d7–8).
28   On bondage and liberation in the *Phaedo*, see most recently Kamen 2013: 85–97.

will decode *DSNV* in light of the literary and philosophical works to which it alludes.[29]

4   Revisiting Nero

In the example above, the mental state of the condemned inmate underscores the degree to which Plutarch's classicizing Platonism is both philosophical and literary—that is, constituted in doctrines that may be used to disclose providential intent in otherwise unjust historical events, and in works of literature to which texts may allude and in view of which one may interpret other literary works. Plutarch's philosophical apologetics may thus appear to be confirmed by the literature to which he points his readers. Yet, the myth with which the dialogue concludes complicates the careful coordination of philosophical and literary modes of readings developed in the first two speeches. On the one hand, the final scene of the myth challenges the reader to consider the applicability of the claims of the previous arguments to the emperor. In doing so, it involves the reader in an act of retrospective reinterpretation, in which the first two speeches are revised not (only) as historically distanced apologetics but (also) as indirect commentary on Nero. On the other hand, we are also invited to read the final scene in light of the literary works to which Plutarch alludes. Here too we discover Plutarch altering, even violating the interpretive expectations that the dialogue has built and encouraged readers to adopt. For the intertextual backdrop of the scene remains so pointedly polyvalent and palimpsestic as to render any definitive reading of Nero's incarnation inconclusive. The result is a change in the basic rules of interpretation that throws in doubt the meaning of the earlier speeches as we read them.[30] Such change, moreover, has political ramifications; as we shall observe below, the act of making sense of Nero within the interpretive parameters that *DSNV* has set up

---

29   Although Plutarch in 556b1–c4, 556d5–9 relies extensively on Platonic philosophy, it must be stressed that the perspective of the competent reader is literary as well; Plutarch's Plato is an author of literary figures, and his historical illustrations are drawn from the literary record.

30   The language of this sentence borrows from Winkler's (1985: 8) analysis of Book 11.5 of Apuleius' *Golden Ass*: 'In what is virtually a breach of contract between narrator and audience, Mithras summarizes Lucius's history in new terms and throws in doubt the meaning of the earlier books as we had read them.'

leaves the reader accountable for occupying critical or complicitous positions vis-à-vis first—and second-century imperial culture.[31]

The passage in which Nero appears is worth quoting at length:

> He [Aridaeus] was viewing the final spectacle of his vision, the souls returning to a second birth, as they were forcibly bent to fit all manner of living things and altered in shape by the framers of these, who with blows from certain tools were welding and hammering together one set of members, wrenching another apart, and polishing away and quite obliterating a third, to adapt them to new characters and lives, when among them appeared the soul of Nero, already in a sorry plight and pierced with incandescent rivets (διαπεπαρμένην ἥλοις διαπύροις). For his soul too the framers had made ready a form, that of Nicander's [or Pindar's][32] viper, in which it was to live on eating its way out of its pregnant mother, when suddenly (he said) a great light shot through and a voice came out of the light commanding them to transfer it to a milder kind of race and frame instead a vocal creature, frequenter of marshes and lakes (ᾠδικόν τι μηχανησαμένους περὶ ἕλη καὶ λίμνας ζῷον), as he had paid the penalty for his crimes, and a piece of kindness too was owing him from the gods, since he had granted freedom to the nation which among his subjects was noblest and most beloved of Heaven. Thus much he was a spectator (θεατής). (567e4–568a3)

Nero in hell is, for Plutarch, an argument—perhaps *the* argument—against Epicureanism and a sign of the inherent goodness of the cosmos. But the creature into which Nero is incarnated has baffled many a commentator.[33] The periphrastic expressions with which Plutarch describes Nero's new form— ἄλλο γένος ἡμερώτερον, ᾠδικόν τι … περὶ ἕλη καὶ λίμνας ζῷον—recall a passage from Aristotle's *Historia Animalium*: 'swans are among the web-footed animals, and live around lakes and marshes (βιοτεύουσι περὶ λίμνας καὶ ἕλη) … They are

---

31   It should be clear, therefore, that although I find generally convincing the conventional interpretation of the myth as, in Hirsch-Luipold's (2014: 174) expression, 'a form of narrative philosophizing' that continues the argument of the dialogue by other, more literary means, my argument is that the final scene revises the preceding arguments in unexpected and politically loaded terms.

32   The text in this section appears corrupt, and various commentators have sought to correct the reading of the MS (Πινδαρικῆς ἐχίδνης), on which see Klaerr and Vernière 1974: 224, whose emendation ('Ἰνδικῆς) is based on Herodotus 3.109. Cf. Nicander, *Ther.* 133–134.

33   For the contours of the debate over the identity of the *zôion*, see Wyttenbach 1821: 596; Ziegler 1949: 212; Frazer 1971: 216–217; Klaerr and Vernière 1974: 224–225; Sansone 1993: 185, n. 25; Saunders 1993: 90; Zadorojnyi 1997: 29; Brenk 1987; Taufer 2010: 216–219.

musical (ᾠδικοί) and sing especially at the end of their lives' (9.615a31–b2).[34] Such Aristotelian resonances have led some to identify the odic, lacustrine ζῷον as a swan, Apollo's bird—apt for the 'actor emperor' (Plin. *Pan.* 46.4), who assimilated himself iconographically to the god of the lyre (Suet. *Nero* 25.2–3, 49.3; Tac. *Ann.* 14.14.1–2).[35] The tradition of identifying the ζῷον as a swan may well be ancient; it is attested an unpublished scolium in the first edition of the *Moralia* edited by Massimo Planude, which reads: Νέρωνος ψυχή· ἐχίδνη, κύκνος.[36]

Other commentators—more cynical than cygneous—have noted that Plutarch's description recalls the chorus of *ranae ridibundae* in Aristophanes' *Frogs.* 'Children of the lake and stream' (λιμναῖα κρηνῶν τέκνα, *Ran.* 211), it proclaims itself, and is later referred to as an 'ode-loving race' (φιλῳδὸν γένος, *Ran.* 240). Such critics also call attention to the hierarchy of metempsychosis in Plato's *Timaeus*, which the final spectacle of Aridaeus' journey follows closely. According to the eponymous interlocutor of the Platonic dialogue, the souls of those who studied astronomy but made the mistake of believing in the objects of sight are reborn as birds; the souls of men without philosophy as four-footed animals (of whom the especially foolish ones become snakes and worms); and the least intelligent and most impure souls as 'aquatic creatures' (ἔνυδρον/α, *Tim.* 92b1, 7, cf. 42b–d, 90e–92c).[37] If περὶ ἕλη καὶ λίμνας ζῷον in Plutarch is synonymous with Plato's τὸ ἔνυδρον γένος, the text appears to suggest that Nero will be reincarnated at the lowest stratum of animate life.[38] To such Hellenic overtones may be adduced a Roman tradition, predating Plutarch and preserved in Phaedrus' satirical fables and Petronius' *Satyricon* (77.6), of associating Nero (and princes in general) with frogs.[39] Nero's physiology, moreover, seems to some authors to have a froggy appearance. Suetonius describes the emperor's voice as 'thin and hoarse' (*exiguae uocis et fuscae, Nero* 20.1; cf., Dio 62.20.2) and his skin 'splotched and rank, hair light blonde, face more cute than august, eyes blue and weak, neck fat, stomach bloated, legs very skinny' (*Nero* 51.1).[40]

---

34   Cf. κύκνος μελῳδός, Eur. *IT* 1104–1105.

35   For the identification of Nero with Apollo, see Clark 1929: 172–173; Champlin 2003: 112–144.

36   Torraca 1991: 119–120 n. 178.

37   For the connections between Nero's fate in *DSNV* and Plato's *Timaeus*, see Brenk 1987: 135–136.

38   There are reasons, however, to be skeptical of connecting *DSNV* and *Timaeus* along these lines; aquatic (ἔνυδρον) for Plato entails not only or perhaps not principally amphibians but animals that do not breathe air (esp. fish and crustaceans)—one notch above vegetables. Yet, Brenk (ibid.) observes, even if frogs are classified as four-footed animals, reincarnation as such leaves Nero little better off than as a serpent or a worm.

39   Cf. Brenk 1987: 132–135.

40   Cf. Champlin 2003: 25–26.

In death Nero's visage becomes ever more raniform, his eyes bulging and pro-
truding from the sockets (Suet. *Nero* 49.4). Frazer makes the (too?) ingenious
suggestion that the name of the eponymous heroine of the *Canace Parturiens*,
verses of which Nero is known to have sung (see Suet. *Nero* 21.3), might have
sounded to a Latin-speaking audience reminiscent of the description of the
sounds of 'noisy frogs' (χαναχοί...βάτραχοι) in Nicander's *Theriaca* (620–621),
upon which Plutarch is known to have written a commentary.[41] During Nero's
performance a Roman soldier is said to have asked what the emperor was
doing, and was told 'Giving birth'.[42] The juxtaposition of frogs, parturition, and
bilingual double-entendre in Plutarch's portrayal of Nero—who built a golden
palace on the site of a drained swamp—would have seemed especially ironic
to an ancient audience, who would have recognized Nero as an Aristophanic
frog, a soul without philosophy, and the butt of a Roman joke.

Is Nero a swan or a frog? The answer to that question affects our reading of
the dialogue as a whole. Commentators who identify Nero as a swan stress that
metempsychosis as Apollo's bird is in harmony with the Delphic and philosophical themes of the two speeches; such a reincarnation, in other words,
allows us to interpret *DSNV* as serious philosophy and religious apologetics.[43]
If, by contrast, Nero is a frog—if, in other words, not Aristotle, but Aristophanes,
Plato, and early Roman depictions of the emperor are the fundamental intertextual background—*DSNV* appears at the end as a comic lampoon on the
model of Seneca's *Apocolocyntosis*. Both identifications also have political ramifications. If Nero were reborn as a symbol of Apollo, his reincarnation would
appear without irony as a sign of indulgence; the emperor's benevolence to
Greece would allow him to become a more perfected embodiment of the god
he sought to emulate. According to this line of interpretation, Plutarch betrays
a deep ambivalence regarding the Roman emperor, and *DSNV* represents a
carefully circumscribed but nonetheless pro-Neronian response to Nero's rein.
Rebirth as a frog, conversely, would lend the dialogue the opposite political
valence, undermining Nero's Apollonian ambitions, theatrical aspirations, and
monumental building program.[44]

---

41   Frazer 1971: 217.

42   Cf. Champlin 2003: 105–106.

43   Thus Torraca (1991: 119–120 n. 178) contends that reincarnation in the body of a frog would
      lend the image '*inevitabilmente un colorito grottesco, non congruo né alla serietà teologica
      del discorso*.'

44   As Taufer (2010: 217) observes, frogs are traditionally represented as antithetical to Apollo
      and are explicitly excluded from the group of animals sacred to the god of Delphi; cf. *de
      Pyth. or.* 399f–400a.

It is not impossible to reconcile both identifications. Zadorojnyi is possibly right to suggest that '[t]he closeness of the phrase [ᾠδικόν ... περὶ ἕλη καὶ λίμνας ζῷον] to Aristotle's account of swans is but a ruse, for readers are expected to see through it to appreciate the irony'.[45]

Yet we should perhaps be cautious of that approach; for it is not Plutarch who determines the emperor's identity. As appealing as an unequivocal interpretation of the emperor's incarnation may seem, we cannot ignore either identification, not least because swan-frog ambiguity is part of the dialogue's intertextual backdrop.[46] Aristophanes' Charon speaks of the chorus as 'frog-swans' (βατράχων κύκνων, *Ran.* 207), and they profess to be servants of Apollo *and* Dionysus 'of the Marshes' (ἐν Λίμναισιν, *Ran.* 217–18, cf. 229–234).[47] The interpretive *aporia* commentators find themselves in thus appears to be a byproduct of the reading strategies *DSNV* makes available. It is telling in this respect that Plutarch portrays Nero's reincarnation as a spectacle, viewed through the eyes of a θεατής, while at the same time quoting almost verbatim a section of the *Phaedo* that warns against belief in objects of pleasurable spectation:

> [The greatest evil befalls us is] that the soul of every human being, when it undergoes extreme pleasure or pain, is compelled to think that that for which it suffered such feelings the most is the most distinct (ἐναργέστατόν) and true. But it is not so. And these things are mostly the things we see (τὰ ὁρατά), are they not ... And is the soul not bound by the body most when it experiences this sensation? ... Because each pleasure and pain nails the soul to the body, as though with a nail, and rivets it, and makes it somatic in form (σωματοειδῆ), believing that those things are true which the body says are true.
>
> *Phaed.* 83c5–d6; cf. 567e4–568a3 above

---

45   Zadorojnyi 1997: 29.

46   Cf. Taufer (2010: 219), who is right to warn that we cannot ignore either identification and to note there are other sonorous animals besides swans and frogs that inhabit swamps, lakes, and wetlands (midges come to mind); but conclusion that ᾠδικόν ζῷον should be read as having a '*valenza generica*' only solves the problem by refusing to acknowledge it.

47   Artemidorus gives a comparably polyvalent interpretation of oneiric frogs; dreams of frogs, he claims, symbolize 'charlatans' and 'altar-lurkers,' but they are positive visions for those whose livelihood is made 'from crowds' (*Oneirocritica* 2.15). Is Nero in this configuration the charlatan and altar-lurker or the one who makes a living from the *okloi*, and is he the only frog in his house, or do others share the shores of his swamp? I owe Dan-el Padilla Peralta for this cross-reference.

Is Plutarch suggesting that Nero is a 'somatoeidetic' soul bound to the body by pleasure, or that we ought not to believe what we see—that is, we ought to be skeptical of the spectacle of Nero's punishment? The works to which the dialogue alludes appear calculated to prompt a plurality of identifications and to leave tensions between interpretations unresolved. The more literature and philosophy one has under one's belt, the more one conducts the idealized reading DSNV calls for, the more indeterminate Nero's identity appears, and the more impossible it becomes to pin down Plutarch's posture vis-à-vis the emperor's legacy. The reader is thus left accountable for decoding the emperor's ultimate signification and for deciding which connections to draw between DSNV and the secondary texts to which it alludes. Depending on our interpretative choices, we—not Plutarch—are made to occupy politically significant positions vis-à-vis the Roman emperor.

The question remains of how to make *intra*-textual sense of Nero—that is, how an ideal reader of history might interpret Nero as illustrative of the Platonic principles of first two speeches. Rebirth as Nicander's serpent, who eats its way out of its mother's womb and, as female, will suffer the same fate, befits the emperor who murdered his mother (Tac. *Ann.* 14.8–9; Cassius Dio 62.14.)—a 'mirroring' penalty, exemplifying the principle that god's retribution is 'timely and in an appropriate manner' (553d1).[48] Nero's largess to Greece, moreover, might seem to demonstrate the claim that great natures do nothing minor (551b11–c1). Although Plutarch does not cast the emperor in such explicitly Platonic terms, other ancient authors do; thus Pausanias's reflections on Nero's liberation of Greece: 'When I thought of Nero's deed, it seemed to me that Plato, the son of Ariston, had spoken most correctly, when he said that the greatest and most daring injustices have been committed not by common men but by a noble soul corrupted by unusual education' (7.17.3). By the same token, recall Plutarch's insistence that god 'does not destroy the rank and thorny root of a glorious race until it has borne its proper fruit' (553c4–7), that members of a γένος may inherit a 'family resemblance in vice' (561f5), and that one's genetic character progressively becomes 'evident in the passions' (562a2). It is remarkable in this respect that ancient historians almost uniformly represent Nero's life as a progressive revelation of congenital character and innate propensity for vice. Cassius Dio attributes Nero's depravity to the 'character' (τρόπων) of his father and mother (61.2, 3). Suetonius traces a deeper genealogy: 'although Nero degenerated from the virtues of his ancestors, he inherited his vices of each of them as though transmitted by natural inheritance' (*Nero* 1.2). Suetonius also claims that 'little by little [Nero's] vices grew stronger

---

48   'Mirroring' is Saunders' (1993: 90 n. 84) expression.

and he disposed of joking and secrecy, and with no care for disguise, he burst forth into greater crimes' (*Nero* 27.1). What Nero saw in himself, he believed of others; he claimed that most men were thoroughly perverse, and 'hid and concealed their vices adroitly', while in those who confessed their obscenities he forgave other vices (*Nero* 29.1). Tacitus makes a comparison between Nero— the first emperor to borrow another man's eloquence—and his ancestors and predecessors a point of mockery (*Ann.* 13.3). He, too, assumes Nero concealed his character; the execution of Narcissus, for instance, was against Nero's will, 'with whose as-yet hidden vices (*abditis adhuc vitiis*) he was miraculously in conformity through his greed and prodigality' (Tac. *Ann.* 13.1); and, later, Nero's nature is said to have been restrained by Burrus' discipline and *mores*, and Seneca's manners and lessons in eloquence (Tac. *Ann.* 13.2; cf. Dio 61.7.5–6). Compare Plutarch's contention that upbringing and bad company lead to bad habits and character (551e); that vice occasionally skips members of a γένος (563a3–4); and that, whereas animals reveal their congenital nature at birth, among humans customs, laws, and conventions slow the emergence of one's intrinsic predisposition, temporarily suppressing a propensity for violence, impudence, and intemperance (562b).

My point here is more than just a claim about how Nero may be made retrospectively to demonstrate the arguments of the first two speeches or to underscore the degree to which Platonism provides the unmarked conceptual categories through which ancient authors interpreted the Roman emperors. It is rather that the philosophical sections of Plutarch's defense of providence are consonant with contemporary and more overtly condemnatory representations of Nero. Important in this respect is an early Latin biography (now lost) of Nero upon which Suetonius' account relies and which may have inspired Plutarch's treatment of the emperor in *DSNV* and his (also lost) life of Nero. As Sansone suggests,[49] the Roman biographer appears to have based the emperor's final hours on Plato's myth of Er. Plato's Ardiaeus invites obvious comparison to Nero; one committed patricide and fratricide, the other matricide, fratricide (by adoption), and possibly patricide; and both are singled out as having undergone exceptionally long sentences (Ardiaeus is bound hand and foot, carded over thorns, and cast back into the underworld, *Resp.* 615c–616a). Similar comparisons may be drawn between Nero and Plutarch's Aridaeus, who, like the Roman emperor, squandered his family fortune and committed injustices to recover it (cf. Suet. *Nero* 30–32). For a readership familiar with the lines along which ancient authors elaborated criticism of the emperor, Plutarch's mobilization of a Platonic framework would have

---

49   1993: 186–189.

activated Neronian associations long before Nero appears at the end—and, I believe, it was designed to activate such associations. For the reading strategies that *DSNV* has implicitly advocated directs readers to make the necessary connections—to read Aridaeus as Ardiaeus as Nero.

Such readers would find other phenomena in the text that permit readers to connect Plutarch's apology to (critical representations of) the emperor, namely:

1. Eschatological geography. Aridaeus' journey along the path by which Dionysos retrieved Semele would, I believe, have called to mind Nero's grand tour of Greece. The entrance Aridaeus bypasses was thought to exit near Lerna at the Alcyonian Lake, which Nero endeavored to measure and found bottomless (cf., Paus. 2.37.5–6). Its topography was reputedly reedy and swampy; in the same passage Pausanias refers to it as a 'marsh' (λίμνην). The image of the Roman emperor exploring an entrance to the underworld a year before his death became a common motif; Suetonius' (or his source's) description, for instance, of Nero's flight through a boggy landscape to Phaon's estate recalls both Plato's account of the underworld in the myth of Er and the Alcyonian Lake.[50] Plutarch appears to have picked up the same constellation of timely circumstances— evoking the emperor's tour of Greece in the geography of the (also Platonic) underworld, by representing Nero as a creature of lakes and streams (567f–568a), and by persistent reference to stagnate geography throughout the dialogue (552c–d, 553c).

2. Panhellenic (esp. Delphic) cult. The sequence that immediately follows the reference to Dionysos' path—Aridaeus' failed attempt to gaze on the light of Apollo's tripod, followed by prophesies foretelling the deaths of a Roman emperor and of Aridaeus (whose vices echo Nero's)—also takes on a new significance in light of Nero's Hellenic activities. On tour Nero visited (and plundered) the major Panhellenic sanctuaries, including Delphi—a visit at which Plutarch may well have been present—and participated in the Pythian games; there, he received a cryptic oracle forecasting his death and warning him to guard against the seventy third year (Suet. 40.3).[51] That the prophecy is apocryphal is immaterial; what matters is the suggestion—implicit in Plutarch and explicit in Suetonius and possibly their common source—that the oracle at Delphi (ambiguously) signaled Nero's death.

---

50   See Suet. *Nero* 48.3. with Sansone 1993: 187–188.
51   For Nero in Delphi, see Champlin 2003: 133.

3. Theatricality. As was suggested earlier, theatrical display, spectatorship, masking, and unmasking are recurring motifs in *DSNV*'s eschatological myth;[52] and, as we observed before, Plutarch consistently draws attention to the spectatorial dimensions of divine retribution, making theatricality a fulcrum in the interpretation of history and the dialogue. We have also noted Nero's association with tragedy and penchant for performance.[53] Nero sponsored and participated in nearly every athletic event and dramatic genre from which *DSNV*'s spectatorial metaphorics are drawn.[54] The implications of this concinnity are discussed below.

4. Nautical imagery. Ships and sailing figure prominently in Nero's biography: the emperor inaugurated the custom of holding naval battles (*naumachia*) in the theater (Suet. *Nero* 12.1; Dio 61.9.5). Nero's optimistic misinterpretation of the Delphic oracle is followed by a catastrophic shipwreck in which he lost items of great value (which, he claimed, fish would return to him; Suet. *Nero* 4.3). The murder of Agrippina made use of a ship rigged for the purpose (Tac. *Ann.* 14.3–5); her death occurred on a starry night, and her boat found a sea smooth for sailing as she was borne into Nero's trap (Tac. *Ann.* 14.5.1); after which Nero is said to have been plagued by dreams in which he was sailing and the helm was wrenched from his hands (Suet. *Nero* 46.1). Recall Aridaeus' psyche, unmoored but still bound to its body as though to an anchor, feeling like a pilot cast from a ship and submerged in the sea, and subsequently gazing upon radiant stars, along whose light his soul sails.

5. Medicine and pharmacy. Both loom large in *DSNV*, whose apology rests on the assumption that divine penology is remedial; dropsy, for instance, is, by analogy, representative of the vices inherited from ancestors (558e). Just as doctors administer medicine to epileptics to prevent seizure, god sometimes cures vicious members of a family before their natures appear (562d). Aridaeus's father is guilty of poisoning his guests (566f5). Compare the death of Nero's father from dropsy (Suet. *Nero* 5.2), and the poisoning of Britannicus (passed off as epilepsy; Suet. *Nero* 33.3) as well as of Junius Silanus (Tac. *Ann.* 13.1).

6. Resurrection. It is remarkable that Aridaeus (568a) and Nero—whose afterlife included the proliferation of false Neros and reports that Nero remained alive in the East—undergo (or were at least expected to

---

52 See, e.g., 564f5–565a1, 565a10, 565b2–9, 566d3–5, 567a6–7, 567a9–10, 567d7–9.

53 For Nero as a tragic figure in Plutarch, see *Quomodo Adul.* 56e–f, *Galba* 14.1–3 1058e–f with de Lacy 1952: 164.

54 Cf. Tac. *Ann.* 14.14, 20–21, 16.4; Suet. *Nero* 10–13, 20–26.

undergo) reincarnation, and subsequently lead lives vastly different from the depravity for which they are both reputed.[55]

7. *Animalia.* Curry (2014: 200–214) has highlighted a strategy of 'animalizing' Nero in Suetonius, and imputing on the emperor 'a generic notion of negative animality' (226; cf. Suet. *Nero* 6.4). Other ancient authors also associate Nero as various kinds of beasts (Tac. *Ann.* 14.12; Dio 61.2.4, 61.9.1). Given this background, might animal imagery in *DSNV*—great natures analogized to fields plagued with wild beasts, the souls of humans contrasted to the apprehensible nature of animals, and the emperor's initial transformation into a snake and later a generic *zôion*—also have been interpreted as directing readers' attention to Nero?

To be sure, many of the points of contact between *DSNV* and Nero's legacy are conventional in ancient representations of tyrants, and we should not rule out the likelihood that Plutarch has crafted his apology as a heuristic for interpreting numerous historical figures—it would be strange if he had not. Yet, the Neronian subtext is made clear in the end, and once that much is recognized, it is simply a matter of questioning how much of the dialogue has already taken aim at the Roman emperor.

5   Conclusion

My proposal, then, is that *DSNV* engages in a sophisticated act of doublespeak and authorial deflection, in which its philosophical defense of divine providence is rewritten as censure of the Roman emperor, and in which the reader is left liable for a politically seditious, retroactive reinterpreting of the dialogue.[56] Such a reading, I admit, must remain speculative, less a robust philosophical argument than a heuristic strategy tacitly authorized by the allusive network and overdetermined imagery Plutarch brings to bear on the question of *pronoia*. Yet, it is essential to read *DSNV* in the hermeneutic climate of the late Republic and early Empire, in which manipulation of mythology, spectacle, and religious symbolism had become familiar technologies of imperial control.[57] This appears to have been especially true of Nero, whose power

---

55   For the connection between the rebirth/return of Nero and *DSNV*, see Charlesworth 1950: 73; cf. Champlin 2003: 9–22.

56   For the concept of doublespeak, see Bartsch1994: chs. 4–5; cf. Ahl's (1984) concept of 'the art of safe criticism.'

57   See Champlin 2003: 68–83.

rested with non-elites and whose popularity is often attributed to his use of myth, sponsorship of games, and theater.[58] Nero's recourse to such strategies, as Champlin (2003: 96) has argued, presupposes performers and spectators receptive to his ploys:

> the Roman people were accustomed to seeing their rulers everywhere presented as figures of well-known myths, and they were accustomed to performances on stage that commented directly on their own contemporary concerns.

Potential for double meaning was not lost on literary artists, who discovered innovative means of subverting the apparent sense of their words through innuendo, which audiences and readers would have been primed to detect. The emperor's posthumous incarnation as a swan, a frog, a swan-frog might therefore be understood as provocation to reread Plutarch's Platonic philosophy as an exploration of why Nero and his γένος—understood narrowly as tyrants or expansively as a family (the Julio-Claudians?) or a city (Rome?), all of which Plutarch cites as targets of divine retribution—have not been more swiftly punishment—if, that is, his audience had not entertained such a reading already.[59]

If this proposal is right, *DSNV* shows Plutarch responding to Nero on Nero's own terms. Just as Nero expected his audiences to interpret his performances as implicitly concerned with his reign, *DSNV* Plutarch makes it possible for his readers to rethink philosophy as commentary on first—and second-century politics. For *DSNV* constructs a readership prepared to draw connections between the text's philosophical arguments and the Roman emperor—to see in Nero a teleological principle unifying the dialogue's 'jumble of disordered remarks'. Readers of *DSNV* will be equipped with the philosophical arguments to perceive within history a providential plot, to manage hedonic response, and to find some consolation—perhaps even pleasure—in knowing that justice will emerge victorious in the hereafter. In the meantime, they may savor the fantasy of an emperor in hell.

---

58   See Champlin 2003: 84–111.

59   Scholten (2009: 113–115), who also recognizes the centrality of a Roman readership in *DSNV*, sees Plutarch as offering philosophical exhortation, positioning Greek education as the solution to the moral defects of its imperial rulers.

Bibliography

Adam, J., and Adam, A. M. (eds.), *Platonis Protagoras* (Cambridge, 1893).

Ahl, F., "The Art of Safe Criticism in Greece and Rome", *AJPh* 105 (1984), 174–208.

Algra, K., "Chrysippus, Carneades, Cicero: the Ethical *divisiones* in Cicero's Lucullus", in B. Inwood and J. Mansfeld (eds.), *Assent and Argument: Studies in Cicero's Academic Books* (Leiden, 1997), 107–39.

Aliotta, G., Piomelli, D., Pollio, A., and Touwaide, A., *Le piante medicinali del "Corpus Hippocraticum"* (Milan, 2003).

Allen, D. S., "Envisaging the Body of the Condemned: The Power of Platonic Symbols", *CPh* 95 (2000), 133–50. (2000a)

Allen, D. S., *The World of Prometheus: The Politics of Punishing in Democratic Athens* (Princeton, 2000). (2000b)

Amadesi, S., Reni, C., Katare, R., Meloni, M., Oikawa, A., Beltrami, A. P., Avolio, E., Cesselli, D., Fortunato, O., Spinetti, G., Ascione, R., Cangiano, E., Valgimigli, M., Hunt, S. P., Emanueli, C., and Madeddu, P., "Role for Substance p-based Nociceptive Signaling in Progenitor Cell Activation and Angiogenesis during Ischemia in Mice and in Human Subjects", *Circulation* 125 (14) (2012), 1774–86, S1–19.

Amigues, S. (ed. and trans.), *Théophraste, Recherches sur les plantes*, Livre IX (Paris, 2006).

Amundsen, D. W., "Romanticizing the Ancient Medical Profession: the Characterization of the Physician in the Graeco-Roman Novel", *Bulletin of the History of Medicine* 48 (3) (1974), 320–37.

Annas, J., "Hedonism in *Protagoras*", in Annas (ed.), *Platonic Ethics Old and New* (Ithaca, NY, 1999), 167–71.

Annas, J., "Carneades' Classification of Ethical Theories", in A. M. Ioppolo and D. N. Sedley (eds.), *Pyrrhonists, Patricians, Platonizers: Hellenistic Philosophy in the Period 155–86 B.C.* (Naples, 2007), 187–223.

Asmis, E., "Seneca's "On the Happy Life" and Stoic Individualism", *Apeiron* 23 (1990), 219–55.

Asmis, E., "Epicurean Poetics", *PBACAPh* 7 (1991), 63–93. Reprinted in D. Obbink (ed.), *Philodemus and Poetry: Poetic Theory and Practice in Lucretius, Philodemus and Horace* (Oxford, 1995), 15–34; and in A. Laird (ed.), *Oxford Readings in Ancient Literary Criticism* (Oxford, 2006), 238–66.

Asmis, E., "Lucretius' Reception of Epicurus: *De rerum natura* as a Conversion Narrative", *Hermes* 144 (2017), 439–61.

Atherton, C., *The Stoics on Ambiguity* (Cambridge, 1993).

Aufderheide, J., *The Value of Pleasure in Plato's* Philebus *and Aristotle's* Ethics, unpublished PhD dissertation, St Andrews: https://research-repository.st-andrews.ac.uk/bitstream/10023/2105/6/JoachimAufderheidePhDThesis.pdf, 2011.

Bacon, F., *The Major Works, including New Atlantis and the Essays* (ed. B. Vickers, Oxford, 1996 [1625]).

Bailey, C. (ed. and trans.), *Lucretius. De rerum natura* (Oxford, 1947), 3 v.

Barnes, J., "Medicine, Experience and Logic", in J. Barnes, J. Brunschwig and M. Burnyeat (eds.), *Science and Speculation. Studies in Hellenistic Theory and Practice* (Cambridge, 1982), 24–68.

Barnes, J., "Roman Aristotle", in Barnes and Griffin 1997, 1–69.

Barnes, J., "An Introduction to Aspasius", in A. M. Alberti and R. W. Sharples (eds.), *Aspasius: The Earliest Extant Commentary on Aristotle's Ethics* (Berlin, 1999), 1–50.

Barnes, J., and Griffin, M. (eds.), *Philosophia Togata* II, *Plato and Aristotle at Rome* (Oxford, 1997).

Bartels, E. M., Swaddling, J., and Harrison, A. P., "An Ancient Greek Pain Remedy for Athletes", *Pain Practice* 6 (2006), 212–18.

Bartsch, S., *Actors in the Audience* (Cambridge, MA, 1994).

Baumbach, L., "Quacks Then as Now? An Examination of Medical Practice, Theory and Superstition in Plautus' 'Menaechmi'", *Acta Classica* 26 (1983), 99–104.

Becchi, F., "The Doctrine of the Passions: Plutarch, Posidonius, and Galen", in L. R. Lanzillotta and I. M. Gallarte (eds.), *Plutarch and the Religious and Philosophical Discourse of Late Antiquity* (Leiden, 2012), 43–54.

Beck, L. Y. (trans.), *Pedanius Dioscorides of Anazarbos, De materia medica* (Hildesheim, 2005).

Bees, R., *Die Oikeiosislehre der Stoa* (Würzburg, 2004).

Benedetti, F., Mayberg, H. S., Wager, T. D., Stohler, C. S., and Zubieta, J.-K., "Neurobiological Mechanisms of the Placebo Effect", *Journal of Neuroscience* 25 (2005), 10390–10402.

Bergk, T., *Griechische Literaturgeschichte* III (Leipzig, 1884).

Betjeman, J., *Summoned by Bells* (London, 1960).

Blank, D., "Socratics versus Sophists on Payment for Teaching", *Classical Antiquity* 4 (1985), 1–49.

Bobzien, S., "The Stoics on Fallacies of Equivocation", in D. Frede and B. Inwood (eds.), *Language and Learning: Philosophy of Language in the Hellenistic Age* (Cambridge, 2005), 239–73.

Bonelli, M. (ed.), *Aristotele e Alessandro di Afrodisia (Questioni etiche e Mantissa): Metodo e oggetto dell'etica peripatetica* (Naples, 2015).

Bonner, C., *Studies in Magical Amulets, Chiefly Graeco-Egyptian* (Ann Arbor, 1950).

Borgeaud, P., *The Cult of Pan in Ancient Greece* (trans. K. Atlass and J. Redfield, Chicago, 1988; original ed.: *Recherches sur le dieu Pan*, Rome, 1979).

Boudon-Millot, V., "Le chagrin selon le médecin Galien de Pergame: une maladie comme les autres ?", in S. Franchet d'Espèrey (ed.), *L'homme et ses passions, Actes du XVIIᵉ Congrès international de l'Association Guillaume Budé* (Paris, 2016), 303–20.

Bourke, J., *The Story of Pain* (Oxford, 2014).

Bradley, K. R., "The Chronology of Nero's Visit to Greece A.D. 66/67", *Latomus* 37 (1978), 61–72.

Brenk, F. E., "'A Most Strange Doctrine.' *Daimon* in Plutarch", *Classical Journal* 69 (1973), 1–11.

Brenk, F. E., "From Rex to Rana: Plutarch's Treatment of Nero", in *Il protagonismo nella storiografia classica* (Genoa, 1987), 121–42.

Brennan, T., "The Old Stoic Theory of Emotions", in Sihvola and Engberg-Pedersen 1998, 21–70.

Brennan, T., "Emotion and Peace of Mind", *Philosophical Books* 43 (2002), 169–220.

Brennan, T., "Moral Pyschology", in B. Inwood (ed.), *The Cambridge Companion to the Stoics* (Cambridge, 2003), 257–94.

Brink, C. O., "Οἰϰείωσις and Οἰϰειότης: Theophrastus and Zeno on Nature in Moral Theory", *Phronesis* 1 (1956), 123–45.

Broadie, S., *Ethics with Aristotle* (New York and Oxford, 1991).

Brunschwig, J., "Arguments without Winners or Losers", *Jahrbuch, Wissenschaftskolleg zu Berlin* (1984–85), 31–40.

Buonopane, A., "La terapia antalgica nella medicina romana: le *Compositiones* di Scribonio Largo", in M. F. Petraccia (ed.), *Dadi, fratture e vecchi belletti* (Genova, 2014), 119–37.

Burckhardt, J., *The Greeks and Greek Civilisation* (abbreviated trans. by Sheila Stern, London, 1998; original ed.: *Griechische Kulturgeschichte*, Berlin and Stuttgart, 1898–1902).

Burkert, W., *Homo Necans. The Anthropology of Ancient Greek Sacrificial Ritual and Myth* (Berkeley, 1972).

Burnyeat, M., "Gods and Heaps", in M. Schofield and M. C. Nussbaum (eds.), *Language and Logos. Studies in Ancient Greek Philosophy Presented to G. E. L. Owen* (Cambridge, 1982), 315–38.

Byl, S., "Le traitement de la douleur dans le *Corpus* hippocratique", in J. A. López Férez (ed.), *Tratados hipocráticos (Estudios acerca de su contenido, forma e influencia)* (Madrid, 1992), 203–13.

Capitani, U., "Celso, Scribonio Largo, Plinio il Vecchio e il loro atteggiamento nei confronti della medicina popolare", *Maia* 24 (1972), 120–40.

Carpenter, A. D., "Pleasure as Genesis in Plato's *Philebus*", *Ancient Philosophy* 31 (2011), 73–94.

Castelli, L., "Alexander of Aphrodisias: Methodological Issues and Argumentative Strategies between the Ethical Problems and the Commentary on the Topics", in Bonelli 2015, 19–42.

Caston, V., "Aristotle and Supervenience", *SJPh* 31 (1993), 107–35.

Caston, V., "Epiphenomenalisms, Ancient and Modern", *Philosophical Review* 106 (1997), 309–63.

Cavenaile, R., "L'anesthésie chirurgicale dans l'antiquité gréco-romaine", *Medicina nei secoli* 13 (2001), 25–46.

Champlin, E., *Nero* (Cambridge, MA, 2003).

Chaniotis, A., "Introduction", in Chaniotis (ed.), *Unveiling Emotions: Sources and Methods for the Study of Emotions in the Greek World* (Stuttgart, 2012), 11–36.

Charlesworth, M. P., "Nero: Some Aspects", *Journal of Roman Studies* 40 (1950), 69–76.

Cheng, W., *Pleasure and Pain in Context: Aristotle's Dialogue with his Predecessors and Contemporaries*, unpublished PhD dissertation, Humboldt-Universität zu Berlin, 2015.

Classen, C. J., "Poetry and Rhetoric in Lucretius", *TAPhA* 99 (1968), 77–118. Reprinted in C. J. Classen (ed.), *Probleme der Lukrezforschung* (Hildesheim, 1986), 331–72.

Claus, D., "Phaedra and the Socratic Paradox", *Yale Classical Studies* 22 (1972), 223–38.

Clay, D., *Lucretius and Epicurus* (Ithaca. NY, 1983).

Coleman, K. M., "Fatal Charades: Roman Executions Staged as Mythological Enactments", *Journal of Roman Studies* 80 (1990), 44–73.

Cooper, J., "Posidonius on Emotions", in Sihvola and Engberg-Pedersen 1998, 71–112.

Cooper, J., "The Emotional Life of the Wise", *SJPh* 43 (2005), 176–218.

Crawford, D. J., "The Opium Poppy: a Study in Ptolemaic Agriculture", in M. I. Finley (ed.), *Problèmes de la terre en Grèce ancienne* (Paris and The Hague, 1973), 223–51.

Crismani, D. (ed.), *Elio Promoto Alessandrino: Manuale della salute* (Alessandria, 2002).

Crombie, I. M., *An Examination of Plato's Doctrines* (London, 1962–3), 2 v.

Culler, J., *Structuralist Poetics: Structuralism, Linguistics, and the Study of Literature* (London, 1975).

Curry, S. A., "Nero *Quadripes*: Animalizing the Emperor in Suetonius's *Nero*", *Arethusa* 47 (2014), 197–230.

Csikszentmihalyi, M., *Beyond Boredom and Anxiety* (San Francisco, 1975).

Csikszentmihalyi, M., *Flow: The Psychology of Optimal Experience* (New York, 1990).

Csikszentmihalyi, M., *Finding Flow: The Psychology of Engagement with Everyday Life* (New York, 1997).

Csikszentmihalyi, M. and Csikszentmihalyi, I. S. (eds.), *Optimal Experience: Psychological Studies of Flow in Consciousness* (Cambridge, 1992).

Davidson, J., "On the Fish Missing from Homer", in J. Wilkins (ed.), *Food in European Literature* (Exeter, 1996), 57–64.

Davidson, J., *Courtesans and Fishcakes. The Consuming Passions of Classical Athens* (London, 1997).

Davidson, J., "Making a Spectacle of Her(self). The Courtesan and the Art of the Present", in M. Feldman and B. Gordon (eds.), *The Courtesans' Arts* (Oxford, 2006), 29–51.

Davidson, J., *The Greeks and Greek Love* (London, 2007).

Debru, A. (ed.), *Galen on Pharmacology* (Leiden, 1997).

de Lacy, P. H., "Biography and Tragedy in Plutarch", *AJPh* 73 (1952), 159–71.

de Lacy, P. H., and Einarson, B. (eds. and trans.), *Plutarch: Moralia* VII (Cambridge, MA, 1959).

Denyer, N. (ed.), *Plato: Protagoras* (Cambridge, 2008).

de Romilly, J., 'La condamnation du plaisir dans l'œuvre de Thucydide', *Wiener Studien* 79 (1966), 142–8.

de Romilly, J., "Cycles et cercles chez les auteurs grecs de l'époque classique", in J. Bingen, G. Cambier and G. Nachtergael (eds,), *Le monde grec. Hommages à Claire Préaux* (Brussels, 1975), 140–52.

Detienne, M., *The Gardens of Adonis: Spices in Greek Mythology* (trans. J. Lloyd, Brighton, 1977; original ed.: *Les Jardins d'Adonis*, Paris, 1972).

Detienne, M., *Dionysos à ciel ouvert* (Paris, 1986).

Dickinson, A., and Balleine, B., "Hedonics: the Cognitive-Emotional Interface", in Kringelbach and Berridge 2010, 74–84.

Dillon, S., "Women on the Columns of Trajan and Marcus Aurelius and the Visual Language of Roman Victory", in S. Dillon and K. Welch (eds.), *Representations of War in Ancient Rome* (Cambridge, 2006), 244–71.

Dimas, P., "Good and Pleasure in the Protagoras", *Ancient Philosophy* 28 (2008), 253–84.

Dirlmeier, F., *Nikomachische Ethik* (Berlin, 1964).

Dodds, E. R. (ed.), *Plato, Gorgias* (Oxford, 1959).

Dover, K. J., *Greek Popular Morality in the Time of Plato and Aristotle* (Oxford, 1974).

Dow, J., "Aristotle's Theory of the Emotions: Emotions as Pleasures and Pains", in Pakaluk and Pearson 2011, 47–74.

Duff, T., "Plutarch, Plato and 'Great Natures '", in A. Pérez Jiménez, J. García López and R. M. Aguilar (eds.), *Plutarco, Platón y Aristóteles: Actas del V Congreso Internacional de la I.P.S.* (Madrid, 1999), 313–32.

Dunbabin, K., *Mosaics of the Greek and Roman World* (Cambridge, 1999).

Dyson, H., *Prolepsis and Ennoia in the Early Stoa* (Berlin, 2009).

Dyson, M., "Knowledge and Hedonism in Plato's *Protagoras*", *Journal of Hellenic Studies* 96 (1976), 32–45.

Eliasson, E., "The Account of the Voluntariness of Virtue in the Anonymous Peripatetic Commentary on Nicomachean Ethics 2–5", *OSAPh* 44 (2013), 195–231.

Engberg-Pedersen, T., *The Stoic Theory of Oikeiosis: Moral Development and Social Interaction in Early Stoic Philosophy* (Aarhus, 1990).

Engeser, S. (ed.), *Advances in Flow Research* (Boston, 2012).

Engeser, S., and Schiepe-Tiska, A., "Historical Lines and an Overview of Current Research on Flow", in Engeser 2012, 1–22.

Englert, W. G., "Stoics and Epicureans on the Nature of Suicide", *PBACAPh* 10 (1994), 67–98.

Evans, M., "Can Epicureans be Friends?", *Ancient Philosophy* 24 (2004), 407–24.

Evans, M., "Plato's Anti–Hedonism", *PBACAPh* 23 (2008), 121–45.

Evenepoel, W., "The Stoic Seneca on *virtus, gaudium* and *voluptas*", *L'Antiquité Classique* 83 (2014), 45–78.

Fabbri, L., *Il papavero da oppio nella cultura e nella religione romana* (Florence, 2017).

Fabricius, C., *Galens Exzerpte aus älteren Pharmakologen* (Berlin, 1972).

Fagan, G., *The Lure of the Arena: Social Psychology and the Crowd at the Roman Games* (Cambridge, 2011).

Falcon, A., *Aristotelianism in the First Century BCE: Xenarchus of Seleucia* (Cambridge, 2012).

Fausti, D., and S. Hautala, 'Sulla farmacologia antica: bibliografia', *Lettre d'informations médecine antique et médiévale* 8 (2009), 1–38.

Feldman, F., "On the Intrinsic Value of Pleasures", *Ethics* 107 (3) (1997), 448–66.

Feldman, F., *Pleasure and the Good Life: Concerning the Nature, Varieties and Plausibility of Hedonism* (Oxford and New York, 2004).

Festugière, A.-J., *Le Plaisir (Eth. Nic. VII, 11–14; X, 1–5), Introduction, traduction et notes* (Paris, 1936).

Figal, G., "Plato's Anti-Hedonism", *PBACAPh* 23 (1) (2008), 187–204.

Fink, J. L. (ed.), *The Development of Dialectic from Plato to Aristotle* (Cambridge, 2012).

Finkelberg, M., "The Sources of *Iliad* 7", *Colby Quarterly* 38 (2002), 151–61.

Fletcher, E., "Plato on Pure Pleasure and the Best Life", *Phronesis* 59 (2014), 113–42.

Forschner, M., "Oikeiosis. Die stoische Theorie der Selbstaneignung", in B. Neumeyr et al. (eds.), *Stoizismus in der europäischen Philosophie, Literatur, Kunst und Politik* I (Berlin, 2008), 169–92.

Fortenbaugh, W. W., and White, S. A., *Lyco of Troas and Hieronymus of Rhodes: Text, Translation, and Discussion* (New Brunswick, 2004).

Fowler, D. P., "Lucretius and Politics", in Griffin and Barnes 1989, 121–50.

Fowler, D. P., *Lucretius on Atomic Motion. A commentary on De Rerum Natura Book Two, lines 1–332* (Oxford, 2002).

Frazer, R. M., "Nero the Singing Animal", *Arethusa* 4 (1971), 215–18.

Frazier, F., "Le *De Sera*, dialogue pythique: hasard et providence, philosophie et religion dans la pensée de Plutarque", in F. Frazier and D. F. Leão (eds.), *Tychè et pronoia: la marche du monde selon Plutarque* (Coimbra, 2010), 69–91.

Frede, D., "Disintegration and Restoration: Pleasure and Pain in Plato's *Philebus*", in R. Kraut (ed.), *The Cambridge Companion to Plato* (Cambridge, 1992), 425–63.

Frede, D. (trans.), *Philebus* (1993), included in J. M. Cooper (ed.), *Plato's Complete Works* (Indianapolis, 1997).

Frede, D. (ed. and trans.), *Platon, Philebos* (Göttingen, 1997).

Frede, D., "Pleasure and Pain in Aristotle's Ethics", in R. Kraut (ed.), *The Blackwell Guide to Aristotle's Nicomachean Ethics* (Malden, MA, and Oxford, 2006), 255–75.

Frede, D., "Nicomachean Ethics VII.11–12: Pleasure", in C. Natali (ed.), *Symposium Aristotelicum: Nicomachean Ethics VII* (Oxford and New York, 2009), 183–208.

Frede, M., "The Stoic Doctrine of the Affections of the Soul", in M. Schofield and G. Striker (eds.), *Norms and Nature: Studies in Hellenistic Ethics* (Cambridge, 1986), 93–110.

Frede, M., "Stoics and Skeptics on Clear and Distinct Impressions", in M. Frede (ed.), *Essays in Ancient Philosophy* (Minneapolis, 1987), 151–76.

Frede, M., "Introduction", in S. Lombardo and K. Bell (trans.), *Plato: Protagoras* (Indianapolis, 1992), vii–xxxiv.

Frier, B. W., "More is Worse: Observations on the Population of the Roman Empire", in W. Scheidel (ed.), *Debating Roman Demography* (Leiden, 2001), 139–59.

Furley, D. J., "Lucretius the Epicurean. On the History of Man", *Entretiens* [de la Fondation Hardt] *sur l'antiquité classique* 24 (1978), 1–37.

Gagné, R., *Ancestral Fault in Ancient Greece* (Cambridge, 2013).

Gale, M., *Myth and Poetry in Lucretius* (Cambridge, 1994).

Gantz, T., *Early Greek Myth* (Baltimore, 1993).

Garofalo, I. (ed.), *Anonymus Medicus [Anonymus Parisinus], De morbis acutis et chroniis* (Leiden, 1997).

Gauthier, R.-A., and Jolif, J. Y. (ed. and trans.), *Aristote, l'Éthique à Nicomaque* (Louvain and Paris, 1958).

Girard, C., "L'hellébore, panacée ou placébo?", in P. Potter, G. Maloney and J. Desautels (eds.), *La maladie et les maladies dans la collection hippocratique. Actes du VIe Colloque International Hippocratique* (n.p., 1990), 393–405.

Gosling, J. C. B., and Taylor, C. C. W., *The Greeks on Pleasure* (Oxford, 1982).

Gottschalk, H. B., "Aristotelian Philosophy in the Roman World", *ANRW* II, 36, 2 (1987), 1079–1174.

Gottschalk, H. B., "Continuity and Change in Aristotelianism", in R. Sorabji (ed.), *Aristotle and After* (London, 1997), 109–15.

Graver, M. R., *Stoicism and Emotion* (Chicago, 2007).

Green, C., Anderson, K. O., Baker, T. A., Campbell, L. C., Decker, S., Fillingim, R. B., Kaloukalani, D. A., Lasch, K. E., Myers, C., Tait, R. C., Todd, K. H., and Vallerand, A. H., "The Unequal Burden of Pain: Confronting Racial and Ethnic Disparities in Pain", *Pain Medicine* 4 (2003), 277–94.

Griffin, M., and Barnes J. (eds.), *Philosophia Togata* (Oxford, 1989).

Grimal, P., "La critique de l'aristotélisme dans le *De vita beata*", *Revue des études latines* 45 (1967), 396–419.

Grimal, P. (ed.), *L. Annaei Senecae, "De vita beata"* (Paris, 1969).

Grmek, M. D., and Gourevitch, D., "Les expériences pharmacologiques dans l'Antiquité", *Archives internationales d'histoire des sciences* 35 (1985), 3–27.

Grote, G., *Plato and the Other Companions of Sokrates* (London, 1865), 4 v.

Grube, G. M. A., "The Structural Unity of the Protagoras", *CQ* 27 (1933), 203–7.

Guthrie, W. K. C. (trans.), *Plato, Protagoras and Meno* (London, 1956).

Hackforth, R., "The Hedonism in Plato's *Protagoras*", *CQ* 22 (1928), 39–42.

Hackforth, R., *Plato's Examination of Pleasure: a Translation of the* Philebus *with Introduction and Commentary* (Cambridge, 1945).

Hadreas, P., "Aristotle's Simile of Pleasure at NE 1174b33", *Ancient Philosophy* 17 (1997), 371–4.

Hahm, D. E., "Critolaus and Late Hellenistic Peripatetic Philosophy", in A. M. Ioppolo and D. N. Sedley (eds.), *Pyrrhonists, Patricians, Platonizers: Hellenistic Philosophy in the Period 155–86 BC* (Naples, 2007), 47–101.

Hambruch, E., *Logische Regeln der platonischen Schule in der aristotelischen Topik* (Berlin, 1904).

Hamilton, R., Choes *and* Anthesteria: *Athenian Iconography and Ritual* (Ann Arbor, 1992).

Harari, Y. N., "Combat Flow: Military, Political, and Ethical Dimensions of Subjective Well-being in War", *Review of General Psychology* 12 (2008), 253–64.

Hardie, W. F. R., *Aristotle's Ethical Theory* (Oxford, 1968).

Harris, W. V., "Saving the φαινόμενα: A Note on Aristotle's Definition of Anger", *CQ* 47 (1997), 452–4.

Harris, W. V., *Restraining Rage: the Ideology of Anger Control in Classical Antiquity.* (Cambridge, MA, 2001).

Harris, W. V., "History, Empathy and Emotions", *Antike und Abendland* 56 (2010), 1–23.

Harris, W. V., "Popular Medicine in the Classical World", in Harris (ed.), *Popular Medicine in the Graeco-Roman World: Explorations* (Leiden, 2016), 1–64.

Harrison, J. E., "Mystica Vannus Iacchi", *Journal of Hellenic Studies* 23 (1903), 292–324.

Harte, V., "Commentary on Evans: Plato's Anti-Hedonism", *PBACAPh* 23 (2008), 147–53.

Harte, V., "The *Nicomachean Ethics* on Pleasure", in R. Polansky (ed.), *The Cambridge Companion to Aristotle's Nicomachean Ethics* (Cambridge, 2014), 288–318.

Hatzimichali, M., "The Texts of Plato and Aristotle in the First Century BC", in M. Schofield (ed.), *Aristotle, Plato and Pythagoreanism in the First Century BC* (Cambridge, 2013), 1–27.

Hayashi, T., *Bedeutung und Wandel des Triptolemos-bildes vom 6.-4. Jh. v. Chr.* (Würzburg, 1992).

Haynes, R. P., "The Theory of Pleasure of the Old Stoa", *AJPh* 83 (1962), 412–19.

Heinaman, R., "Pleasure as an Activity in the Nicomachean Ethics", in Pakaluk and Pearson, 2011, 7–46.

Heinricher, M. M., and Fields, H. L., "Central Nervous System Mechanisms of Pain Modulation", in McMahon 2013, 129–42.

Helmig, C., "A Jumble of Disordered Remarks? Structure and Argument of Plutarch's *De Sera Numinis Vindicta*", in M. Jufresa, F. Mestre, P. Gómez and P. Gilabert (eds.), *Plutarc a la Seva Època: Paideia i Societat* (Barcelona, 2005), 323–32.

Henriksén, C., *A Commentary on Martial, Epigrams Book 9* (Oxford, 2012).

Herman, G., *Morality and Behaviour in Democratic Athens* (Cambridge, 2006).

Heubeck, A., West, S., and Hainsworth, J. B., *A Commentary on Homer's Odyssey*, I [Books I–VIII] (Oxford, 1988).

Hirsch-Luipold, R., "Religion and Myth", in M. Beck (ed.), *A Companion to Plutarch* (Chichester, 2014), 163–76.

Horden, P., "Pain in Hippocratic Medicine", in J. R. Hinnells and R. Porter (eds.), *Religion, Health, and Suffering* (London, 1999), 295–315.

Iannetti, G. D., Salomons, T. V., Moayedi, M., Mourau, A., and Davis K. D., "Beyond Metaphor: Contrasting Mechanisms of Social and Physical Pain", *Trends in Cognitive Sciences* 17 (2013), 371–8.

Inwood, B., *Ethics and Human Action in Early Stoicism* (Oxford, 1985).

Inwood, B., "Seneca and Psychological Dualism", in J. Brunschwig and M. C. Nussbaum (eds.), *Passions & Perceptions: Studies in Hellenistic Philosophy of Mind* (Cambridge, 1993), 150–83.

Inwood, B., "The Will in Seneca the Younger", *CPh* 95 (2000), 44–60.

Inwood, B. (ed.), *Language and Learning: Philosophy of Language in the Hellenistic Age* (Cambridge, 2005).

Inwood, B., *Ethics after Aristotle* (Cambridge MA, 2014).

Irwin, T. H., "Euripides and Socrates", *CPh* 78 (1983), 183–97.

Irwin, T. H., *Plato's Ethics* (Oxford, 1995).

Irwin, T. H., *The Development of Ethics: A Historical and Critical Study* (Oxford, 2007).

Isager, S., and Pedersen P. (eds.), *The Salmakis Inscription and Hellenistic Halikarnassos* (Odense, 2004).

Israelowich, I., *Society, Medicine and Religion in the Sacred Tales of Aelius Aristides* (Leiden, 2012).

Jones, W. H. S. (ed.), *Hippocrates* volume II (London, 1923).

Jouanna, J., *Hippocrate* (Paris, 1992).

Jouanna, J., and Boudon, V., 'Remarques sur la place d'Hippocrate dans la pharmacologie de Galien', in Debru 1997, 213–34.

Jouanna-Bouchet, J. (ed. and trans.), *Scribonius Largus: Compositions médicales* (Paris, 2016).

Jünger, E., *On Pain* (trans. D. C. Durst, New York, 2008; original ed.: *Über den Schmerz*, Hamburg, 1934).

Kahn, C., "Socrates and Hedonism", in A. Havlíček and F. Karfík (eds.), *Plato's Protagoras: Proceedings of the Third Symposium Platonicum Pragense* (Prague, 2003), 165–74.

Kamen, D., "The Manumission of Socrates: a Rereading of Plato's *Phaedo*", *Classical Antiquity* 32 (2013), 78–100.

Kamtekar, R., "Good Feelings and Motivation: Comments on John Cooper 'The Emotional Life of the Wise'", *SJPh* 43 (2005), 219–29.

Kamtekar, R., *Plato's Moral Psychology* (Oxford, 2018).

Kawakita, Y., Sakai, S., and Otsuka, Y. (eds.), *History of Therapy: Proceedings of the 10th International Symposium on the Comparative History of Medicine—East and West* (Tokyo, 1990).

Kenny, A., *The Aristotelian Ethics: A Study of the Relationship between the Eudemian and Nicomachean Ethics of Aristotle* (Oxford, 1978).

Kim, J., "Supervenience as a Philosophical Concept", *Metaphilosophy* 21 (1991), 1–27.

King, D., *Experiencing Pain in Imperial Greek Culture* (Oxford, 2018).

King, H., *Hippocrates' Woman: Reading the Female Body in Ancient Greece* (London, 1998).

King, H., "Chronic Pain and the Creation of Narrative", in J. I. Porter (ed.), *Constructions of the Classical Body* (Ann Arbor, 1999), 269–86.

Klaerr, R., and Vernière, Y. (eds.), *Plutarque: Oeuvres morales* VII, 2 (Paris, 1974).

Kleingünther, A., *Protos Heuretes: Untersuchungen zur Geschichte einer Fragestellung. Philologus* suppl. 26 (Leipzig, 1933).

Klosko, G., "On the Analysis of *Protagoras* 351b–360e", *Phoenix* 34 (1980), 307–21.

Knörzer, K.-H., "Römerzeitliche Heilkräuter aus Novaesium (Neuß Rh.): Nachtrag", *Sudhoffs Archiv* 49 (1965), 416–22.

Konstan, D., "'The Birth of the Reader': Plutarch as Literary Critic", *Scholia* 13 (2004), 3–27.

Konstan, D., *The Emotions of the Ancient Greeks: Studies in Aristotle and Classical Literature* (Toronto, 2006).

Konstan, D., *Beauty: the Fortunes of an Ancient Greek Idea* (Oxford, 2014). (2014a).

Konstan, D., "Emotions", in S. Bartsch and A. Schiesaro (eds.), *The Cambridge Companion to Seneca* (Cambridge, 2014), 174–84. (2014b).

Konstan, D., "Understanding Grief in Greece and Rome", *Classical World* 110 (2016), 3–30. (2016a).

Konstan, D., "Reason versus Emotion in Seneca", in D. Cairns and D. Nelis (eds.), *Emotions in the Classical World: Methods, Approaches, and Directions* (Heidelberg, 2016), 231–43. (2016b).

Konstan, D., Clay, D., Glad, C. E., Thom, J. C., and Ware, J. (eds.), *Philodemus, On Frank Criticism* (Atlanta, 1998).

Kotsifou, C., "'Being Unable to Come to You and Weep with You': Grief and Condolence Letters on Papyrus', in A. Chaniotis (ed.), *Unveiling Emotions* (Stuttgart, 2012), 389–411.

Kovacs, D., "Shame, Pleasure, and Honor in Phaedra's Great Speech (Euripides, *Hippolytus* 375–87)", *AJPh* 101 (1980), 287–303.

Kovacs, D., "On Medea's Great Monologue (Eur. *Medea* 1021–80)", *CQ* 36 (1986), 343–52.

Kringelbach, M. L., and Berridge, K. C. (eds.), *Pleasures of the Brain* (Oxford and New York, 2010).

Lamb, Charles, *Essays* (New York, 1895 [original ed.: 1825]).

Landhäußer, A. and Keller, J., "Flow and Its Affective, Cognitive, and Performance-Related Consequences", in Engeser 2012, 65–85.

Lautner, P., Ἀέγει oder λήγει? Amelios und Sosikrates (?) über Timaios 37 A 6–7', *Hermes* 125 (1997), 294–308.

Lefebvre, D. 'Aristotle and the Hellenistic Peripatos: From Theophrastus to Critolaus', in A. Falcon (ed.), *Brill's Companion to the Reception of Aristotle in Antiquity* (Leiden, 2016), 11–34.

Leith, D., "How Popular Were the Medical Sects?", in Harris 2016, 231–50.

Leonhardt, J., *Ciceros Kritik der Philosophenschulen* (Munich, 1999).

Lewis, D. M., 'The Deme Ikarion', *Annual of the British School at Athens* 51 (1956), 172.

Lieberg, G., *Die Lehre von der Lust in den Ethiken des Aristoteles* (Munich, 1958).

Liolias, C. C., Graikou, K., Skaltsa, E., and Chinou, I., "Dittany of Crete: a Botanical and Ethnopharmacological Review", *Journal of Ethnopharmacology* 131 (2010), 229–41.

Lloyd, G. E. R., *Magic, Reason, and Experience: Studies in the Origin and Development of Greek Science* (Cambridge, 1979).

Lloyd, G. E. R., *Science, Folklore and Ideology* (Cambridge, 1983).

Lloyd, G. E. R., *Ambitions of Curiosity: Understanding the World in Ancient Greece and China* (Cambridge, 2002).

Lloyd-Jones, H., "Euripides, *Medea* 1056–80", *Würzburger Jahrbücher für die Altertumswissenschaft* 6a (1980), 51–9.

Lloyd-Jones, H., "The Pride of Halicarnassus"', *ZPE* 124 (1999), 1–14.

Lombardo, S., and Bell, K. (trans.), *Plato: Protagoras* (Indianapolis, 1992), reprinted with changes in J. M. Cooper (ed.), *Plato: Complete Works* (Indianapolis, 1997), 747–90.

Long, A. A., "Aristotle's Legacy to Stoic Ethics", *Bulletin of the Institute of Classical Studies* 15 (1968), 72–85.

Long, A. A., and Sedley, D. (eds.), *The Hellenistic Philosophers* (Cambridge, 1987), 2 v.

Loonen, A. J. M., and Ivanova, S. A., "Circuits Regulating Pleasure and Happiness: the Evolution of Reward-seeking and Misery-fleeing Behavioral Mechanisms in Vertebrates", *Frontiers in Neuroscience* 9 (2015), 394.

Luppe, W., "Die Ikarios-Sage im Mythographus Homericus", *ZPE* 112 (1996), 29–33.

Madigan, A., "Alexander of Aphrodisias: the Book of Ethical Problems", *ANRW* II, 36, 2 (Berlin and New York, 1987), 1260–79.

Majno, G., *The Healing Hand: Man and Wound in the Ancient World* (Cambridge, MA, 1975).

Malink, M., "The Beginnings of Formal Logic: Deduction in Aristotle's Topics vs. Prior Analytics", *Phronesis* 60 (2015), 267–309.

Mann, W.-R., "Rechtfertigung, I. Griechische Antike; Logik und Dialektik", in *Historisches Wörterbuch der Philosophie* VIII (Basel, 1992), 251–6.

Mann, W.-R., "These (Antike)", *Historisches Wörterbuch der Philosophie* X (Basel, 1998), 1175–7.

Mann, W.-R. rev. of T. Reinhardt, *Das Buch E der aristotelischen Topik*, *Archiv für Geschichte der Philosophie* 85 (2003), 91–8.

Mantovanelli, L. (ed. and trans.), *Scribonio Largo: Ricette mediche* (Padua, 2012).

Mastronarde, D. J. (ed.), *Euripides: Medea* (Cambridge, 2002).

Mattern, S. P., *The Prince of Medicine: Galen in the Roman Empire* (New York, 2013).

McMahon, S. B. (ed.), *Wall and Melzack's Textbook of Pain* (sixth ed., Philadelphia, 2013).

McNamara, L., "Conjurers, Purifiers, Vagabonds and Quacks? The Clinical Roles of the Folk and Hippocratic Healers of Classical Greece", *Journal of the Classical Association of Victoria* 16–17 (2003–4), 2–25.

Melzack, R., and Wall, P. D., *The Challenge of Pain* (second ed., London, 1996).

Mercken, H. P. F., "The Greek Commentators on Aristotle"'s Ethics", in Sorabji 1990, 407–43.

Merlan, P., *Studies in Epicurus and Aristotle* (Wiesbaden, 1960).

Merlin, M. D., "Archaeological Evidence for the Tradition of Psychoactive Plant Use in the Old World", *Economic Botany* 57 (3) (2003), 295–323.

Mette, H. J., "Zwei Akademiker heute: Krantor und Arkesilaos", *Lustrum* 26 (1984), 7–94.

Milanese, G., *Lucida carmina. Comunicazione e scrittura da Epicuro a Lucrezio* (Milan, 1989).

Mitsis, P., *Epicurus' Ethical Theory: the Pleasures of Invulnerability* (Ithaca, NY, 1988).

Mitsis. P., "Committing Philosophy to the Reader: Didactic Coercion and Reader Autonomy in *De Rerum Natura*", in J. S. Clay, P. Mitsis, and A. Schiesaro (eds.), *Mega nepios: il destinatario nell'epos didascalico* (Pisa, 1993), 111–28.

Moisan, M., "Les plantes narcotiques dans le Corpus hippocratique", in P. Potter, G. Maloney and J. Desautels (eds.), *La maladie et les maladies dans le Corpus hippocratique* (n.p., 1990), 381–92.

Moline, J., "Euripides, Socrates, and Virtue", *Hermes* 103 (1975), 46–67.

Monfort, M.-L., "*Quae quibus medicamenta danda*: études sur l'interprétation du fragment hippocratique *Peri Pharmakon*", in A. Thivel and A. Zucker (eds.), *Le Normal et le pathologique dans la Collection hippocratique* (Nice, 2002), 693–708.

Moraux, P., "La joute dialectique d'après le huitième livre des Topiques", in G. E. L. Owen (ed.), *Aristotle on Dialectic: The* Topics (Oxford, 1968), 277–311.

Moraux, P., *Der Aristotelismus bei den Griechen: Der Aristotelismus im I. und II. Jh. n.Chr.* (Berlin, 1984).

Moscoso, J., *Pain: a Cultural History* (trans. S. Thomas and P. House, London, 2012) (original ed.: *Historia cultural del dolor*, Madrid, 2011).

Moss, J., "Pleasure and Illusion in Plato", *Philosophy and Phenomenological Research* 72 (2006), 503–35.

Moss, J., *Aristotle on the Apparent Good* (Oxford, 2012).

Moss, J., "Hedonism and the Divided Soul in Plato's *Protagoras*", *Archiv für Geschichte der Philosophie* 96 (2014), 285–319.

Mossman, J. (ed.), *Euripides, Medea* (Oxford, 2011).

Müri, W., "Das Wort Dialektik bei Platon", *Museum Helveticum* 1 (1944), 152–68.

Nagy, G., *The Best of the Achaeans: Concepts of the Hero in Archaic Greek Poetry* (Baltimore, 1979).

Natali, C., "La scuola di Alessandro su piacere e sofferenza (Quaest. Eth. 5/4, 6, 7, 16)", in Bonelli 2015, 59–86.

North, H., *Sophrosyne: Self-Knowledge and Self-Restraint in Greek Literature* (Ithaca, NY, 1966).

Nunn, J. F., "The Origins of Anaesthesia", in R. S. Atkinson and T. B. Boulton (eds.), *The History of Anaesthesia* (London, 1989), 21–6.

Nussbaum, M., *The Fragility of Goodness* (Cambridge, 1986).

Nutton, V., "Therapeutic Methods and Methodist Therapeutics in the Roman Empire", in Kawakita et al. 1990, 1–35.

Nutton, V., *Ancient Medicine* (London, 2004; second ed., 2013).

Nutton, V. (ed.), *Galen, On Problematical Movements*, with an edition of the Arabic version by G. Bos (Cambridge, 2011).

Oakley, J. H., and Sinos, R. H., *The Wedding in Ancient Athens* (Madison, WI, 1993).

O'Brien, M. J., *The Socratic Paradoxes and the Greek Mind* (Chapel Hill, NC, 1967).

Ogden, D., *Drakōn. Dragon Myth and Serpent Cult in the Greek and Roman Worlds* (Oxford, 2013).

Oikonomopoulou, K., "Ancient Question-and-answer Literature and its Role in the Tradition of Dialogue", in S. Föllinger and G. M. Müller (eds.), *Der Dialog in der Antike* (Berlin, 2013), 37–63.

Opsomer, J., and Steel, C. (trans.), *Proclus: Ten Problems Concerning Providence* (London, 2012).

Otto, W. F., *Dionysus. Myth and Cult* (trans, R. B. Palmer, Bloomington, IN, 1965) (original ed.: *Dionysos: Mythos und Kultus*, fourth ed., Frankfurt, 1960).

Pakaluk, M., and Pearson, G. (eds.), *Moral Psychology and Human Action in Aristotle* (Oxford, 2011).

Parker, R., *Polytheism and Society at Athens* (Oxford, 2007).

Pembroke, S. G., "Oikeiosis", in A. A. Long (ed.), *Problems in Stoicism* (London, 1971), 114–49.

Petridou, G., and Thumiger, C. (eds.), *Homo Patiens—Approaches to the Patient in the Ancient World* (Leiden, 2016).

Pfeiffer, R., *History of Classical Scholarship from the Beginnings to the End of the Hellenistic Age* (Oxford, 1968).

Philippson, R., "Das 'Erste Naturgemäße'", *Philologus* 87 (1932), 447–66.

Pirenne-Delforge, V., *L'Aphrodite grecque*, Kernos Supplement 4 (Athens, 1994).

Platt, V., *Facing the Gods. Epiphany and Representation in Graeco-Roman Art, Literature and Religion* (Cambridge, 2011).

Pohlenz, M., *Grundfragen der stoischen Philosophie* (Göttingen, 1940).

Porter, A. J., "Compassion in Soranus' *Gynecology* and Caelius Aurelianus' *On Chronic Diseases*", in Petridou and Thumiger 2016, 285–303.

Potter, P. (ed.), *Hippocrates* volume 5 (Cambridge, MA, 1988).

Prince, S. (ed.), *Antisthenes of Athens: Texts, Translations, and Commentary* (Ann Arbor, 2015).

Prioreschi, P., Heaney. R. P., and Brehm E., "A Quantitative Assessment of Ancient Therapeutics: Poppy and Pain in the Hippocratic Corpus", *Medical Hypotheses* 51 (4) (1998), 325–31.

Prioreschi, P., *A History of Medicine* III (Omaha, 1998).

Puccetti, R., "The Sensation of Pleasure", *British Journal for the Philosophy of Science* 20 (1969), 239–45.

Raaflaub, K., "War and the City: the Brutality of War and its Impact on the Community", in P. Meineck and D. Konstan (eds.), *Combat Trauma and the Ancient Greeks* (New York, 2014), 15–46.

Rademaker, A., *Sophrosyne and the Rhetoric of Self-Restraint* (Leiden, 2005).

Ramoutsaki, I. A., Askitopoulou, H., and Konsolaki, E., "Pain Relief and Sedation in Roman Byzantine Texts: *Mandragoras officinarum*, *Hyoscyamos niger* and *Atropa belladonna*", in J. C. Diz, A. Franco, D. R. Bacon, J. Rupreht and J. Alvarez (eds.), *The History of Anesthesia*: Proceedings of the Fifth International Symposium on the History of Anesthesia (Amsterdam, etc., 2002) = *International Congress Series* 1242 (2002), 43–50.

Rapp, C., "Nichomachean Ethics VII 13–14 (1154a21): Pleasure and Eudaimonia", in C. Natali (ed.), *Aristotle's Nicomachean Ethics: Book VII* (Oxford, 2009), 209–35.

Rather, L. J., "The 'Six Things Non-Natural': A Note on the Origins and Fate of a Doctrine and a Phrase", *Clio Medica* 3 (1968), 337–47.

Raven, J. E., *Plants and Plant Lore in Ancient Greece* (Oxford, 2000).

Reeve, M., "Euripides, *Medea* 1021–80", *CQ* 22 (1972), 51–61.

Reinhardt, T., *Das Buch E der aristotelischen Topik. Untersuchungen zur Echtheitsfrage* (Göttingen, 2000).

Renaut, O., "Les *pathè*/émotions chez Aristote: une catégorie nouvelle? A propos de *Rh.* II". Unpublished paper.

Rey, R., *The History of Pain* (trans. L. E. Wallce, J. A. Cadden and S. W. Cadden, Cambridge, MA, 1995) (original ed.: *Histoire de la douleur*, Paris, 1993).

Ricken, F., *Der Lustbegriff in der Nikomachischen Ethik des Aristoteles* (Göttingen, 1976).

Ricken, F., "Wert und Wesen der Lust", in O. Höffe (ed.), *Aristoteles: Die Nikomachische Ethik* (Berlin, 1995), 207–28.

Rickert, G., "Akrasia and Euripides' *Medea*", *Harvard Studies in Classical Philology* 91 (1987), 91–117.

Riddle, J. M., "Folk Tradition and Folk Medicine. Recognitions of Drugs in Classical Antiquity", in J. Scarborough (ed.), *Folklore and Folk Medicines* (Madison, WI, 1987), 33–61; reprinted in Riddle 2002.

Riddle, J. M., *Quid Pro Quo: Studies in the History of Drugs* (Brookfield, VT, 2002).

Riginos, A. S., *Platonica: A Collection and Study of Anecdotes Dealing with the Life and Writings of Plato* (Columbia Studies in the Classical Tradition 3) (Leiden, 1976).

Rist, J. M., *Stoic Philosophy* (Cambridge, 1969).

Rist, J. M., "Pleasure: 360–300 B.C.", *Phoenix* 28 (1974), 167–79.

Robertson, M., "Two *pelikai* by the Pan Painter", *Greek Vases in the J. Paul Getty Museum* 3 (1986), 71–90.

Robinson, W., "Epiphenomenalism", *Stanford Encyclopedia of Philosophy* (Fall 2015 Edition), <http://plato.stanford.edu/archives/fall2015/entries/epiphenomenalism/>.

Roby, C., "Galen on the Patient's Role in Pain Diagnosis: Sensation, Consensus, and Metaphor", in Petridou and Thumiger 2016, 304–22.

Romano, I. B., "The Archaic Statue of Dionysos from Ikarion", *Hesperia* 51 (1982), 398–409.

Rorty, A., "The Place of Pleasure in Aristotle's Ethics", *Mind* 83 (1974), 481–93.

Rowe, C. J. (trans.), *Aristotle. Nicomachean Ethics* (Oxford, 2002).

Rowe, C. J., "Hedonism in the Protagoras again: Protagoras 351bff", in A. Havlíček and F. Karfík, (eds.), *Plato's Protagoras, Proceedings from the Third Symposium Platonicum Pragense* (Prague, 2003), 133–47.

Rowe, C. J., "The Relationship of the *Laws* to Other Dialogues: a Proposal", in C. Bobonich (ed.), *Plato's Laws: A Critical Guide* (Cambridge, 2010), 29–50.

Rudebusch, G., *Socrates, Pleasure, and Value* (Oxford, 2002).

Russell, D., "Virtue and Happiness in the Lyceum and Beyond", *OSAPh* 38 (2010), 143–85.

Ryle, G., *Dilemmas* (Cambridge, 1954).

Ryle, G., "Dialectic in the Academy", in R. Bambrough (ed.), *New Essays on Plato and Aristotle* (London, 1965), 39–68.

Ryle, G., "Dialectic in the Academy", in G. E. L. Owen (ed.), *Aristotle on Dialectic: The Topics* (Oxford, 1968), 69–79.

Salazar, C. F., *The Treatment of War Wounds in Graeco-Roman Antiquity* (Leiden, 2000).

Salim, E., *Four Puzzles on Aristotelian Pleasures and Pains*, unpublished PhD dissertation, University of Arizona, 2012.

Samama, É., *Les médecins dans le monde grec: sources épigraphiques sur la naissance d'un corps médical* (Geneva, 2003).

Sansone, D., "Nero's Final Hours", *Illinois Classical Studies* 18 (1993), 179–89.

Saunders, T. J., "Plutarch's *De Sera Numinis Vindicta* in the Tradition of Greek Penology", *Studi economico-giuridici* 54 (1993), 63–94.

Sauvé-Meyer, S., "Pleasure, Pain, and "Anticipation" in Plato's *Laws*, Book I", in R. Patterson, V. Karasmanis and A. Herman (eds.), *Presocratics and Plato: Festschrift at Delphi in Honor of Charles Kahn* (Las Vegas, 2012), 349–66.

Scarborough, J., "The Pharmacy of Methodist Medicine: the Evidence of Soranus' *Gynecology*", in P. Mudry and J. Pigeaud (eds.), *Les Écoles médicales à Rome* (Geneva, 1991), 203–16.

Scarborough, J., "The Opium Poppy in Hellenistic and Roman Medicine", in R. Porter and M. Teich (eds.), *Drugs and Narcotics in History* (Cambridge, 1995), 4–23.

Scholten, H., "Göttliche Vorsehung und die Bedeutung des Griechentums in Plutarchs *De Sera Numinis Vindicta*", *Antike und Abendland* 55 (2009), 99–117.

Schöne, H., "Hippokrates ΠΕΡΙ ΦΑΡΜΑΚΩΝ", *Rheinisches Museum für Philologie* 73 (1920), 434–48.

Schüler, J., "The Dark Side of the Moon", in Engeser 2012, 123–37.

Scott, K., "Plutarch and the Ruler Cult", *TAPhA* 60 (1929), 117–35.

Scullin, S. E., *Hippocratic Pain*, unpublished PhD dissertation, University of Pennsylvania, 2012.

Sedley, D., "Philosophical Allegiance in the Greco-Roman World", in Griffin and Barnes 1989, 97–119.

Sedley, D., "Plato's *auctoritas* and the Rebirth of the Commentary Tradition", in Barnes and Griffin 1997, 110–29.

Segal, C. P., "Shame and Purity in Euripides' *Hippolytus*", *Hermes* 98 (1970), 117–69.

Segvic, H., "No One Errs Willingly: The Meaning of Socratic Intellectualism", *OSAPh* 19 (2000), 1–45. Reprinted in her collected papers, M. F. Burnyeat (ed.), *From Protagoras to Aristotle* (Princeton, 2008), 47–88.

Seidensticker, B., "Euripides, *Medea* 1056–80 An Interpolation?", in M. Griffith and D. Mastronarde (eds.), *Cabinet of the Muses* (Atlanta, 1990), 89–102.

Sharples, R. W., "Ambiguity and Opposition: Alexander of Aphrodisias, Ethical Problems 11", *Bulletin of the Institute of Classical Studies* 32 (1985), 109–16.

Sharples, R. W., "Alexander of Aphrodisias: Scholasticism and Innovation", *ANRW* II, 36, 2 (1987), 1176–1243.

Sharples, R. W., *Alexander of Aphrodisias. Ethical Problems* (Ithaca, 1990). (1990a).

Sharples, R. W., "The School of Alexander?", in Sorabji 1990, 83–111. (1990b).

Sharples, R. W., *Alexander Aphrodisiensis, Supplement to On the Soul* (Ithaca, NY, 2004).

Sharples, R. W., *Alexander Aphrodisiensis, De anima libri mantissa* (Berlin, 2008).

Shaw, J. C., *Plato's Anti-hedonism and the Protagoras* (Cambridge, 2015).

Shields, C., "Perfecting Pleasures: The Metaphysics of Pleasure in Nicomachean Ethics X", in J. Miller (ed.), *Aristotle's Nicomachean Ethics: A Critical Guide* (Cambridge, 2011), 191–210.

Shields, C. (ed. and trans.), *Aristotle. De Anima* (Oxford, 2016).

Sidgwick, H., *The Methods of Ethics* (seventh ed., London, 1907).

Sihvola, J., and Engberg-Pedersen, T. (eds.), *The Emotions in Hellenistic Philosophy* (Dordrecht, 1998).

Smarczyk, B., *Untersuchungen zur Religionspolitik und politischen Propaganda Athens im Delisch-Attischen Seebund* (Munich, 1990).

Snell, B., "Das früheste Zeugnis über Sokrates", *Philologus* 97 (1948), 125–34.

Solmsen, F., "'Bad Shame' and Related Problems in Phaedra's Speech (Eur. *Hipp.* 380–388)", *Hermes* 101 (1973), 420–5.

Sorabji, R. (ed.), *Aristotle Transformed: the Ancient Commentators and their Influence* (London, 1990).

Sorabji, R., *Emotion and Peace of Mind: From Stoic Agitation to Christian Temptation* (Oxford, 2000).

Sourvinou-Inwood, C., "Something to do with Athens", in R. Osborne and S. Hornblower (eds.), *Ritual, Finance, Politics: Athenian Democratic Accounts Presented to David Lewis* (Oxford, 1994), 269–90.

Soury, G., "Le Problème de la Providence et le *De Sera Numinis Vindicta* de Plutarque", *Revue des études grecques* 58 (1945), 163–79.

Stannard, J., "Medicinal Plants and Folk Remedies in Pliny, *Historia Naturalis*", *History and Philosophy of the Life Sciences* 4 (1982), 3–23.

Steier, A., "Mandragoras", in *RE* XIV, 1 (1928), cols. 1028–37.

Striker, G., *Essays on Hellenistic Epistemology and Ethics* (Cambridge, 1996).

Strohl, M. S., "Pleasure as Perfection: Nicomachean Ethics X.4–5", *OSAPh* 41 (2011), 257–87.

Sullivan, J. P., "The Hedonism in Plato's *Protagoras*", *Phronesis* 6 (1961), 10–28.

Swain, S., "Plutarch: Chance, Providence, and History", *AJPh* 110 (1989), 272–302.

Szaif, J., *Gut des Menschen: Untersuchungen zur Problematik und Entwicklung der Glücksethik bei Aristoteles und in der Tradition des Peripatos* (Berlin, 2012).

Taub, L., "Problematising the *Problems*: the *Problemata* in Relation to Other Question-and-Answer Texts", in R. Mayhew (ed.), *The Aristotelian Problemata Physica: Philosophical and Scientific Investigations* (Leiden, 2015), 413–36.

Taufer, M., *Il mito di Tespesio nel De Sera Numinis Vindicta di Plutarco* (Naples, 2010).

Taylor, A. E., *Plato: the Man and His Work* (London, 1926).

Taylor, C. C. W. (ed. and trans.), *Plato: Protagoras* (Oxford, 1976; second ed., 1991).

Taylor, C. C. W., *Pleasure, Mind, and Soul. Selected Papers in Ancient Philosophy* (Oxford, 2008).

Tecusan, M. (ed.), *The Fragments of the Methodists* (Leiden, 2004).

Tell, H., *Plato's Counterfeit Sophists* (Cambridge, MA, 2011).

Thraede, K., "Das Lob des Erfinders: Bemerkungen zur Analyse der Heuremata-Kataloge", *Rheinisches Museum für Philologie* 105 (1962), 158–86.

Thumiger, C., *A History of the Mind and Mental Health in Classical Greek Thought* (Cambridge, 2017).

Torraca, L., "Linguaggio del reale e linguaggio dell'immaginario nel *De Sera Numinis Vindicta*", in G. D'Ippolito and I. Gallo (eds.), *Strutture formali dei Moralia di Plutarco* (Naples, 1991), 91–120.

Totelin, L. M. V., "A Recipe for Headache: Translating and Interpreting Ancient Greek and Roman Remedies", in A. Imhausen and T. Pommerening (eds.), *Writings of Early Scholars in the Ancient Near East, Egypt, Rome, and Greece* (Berlin, 2011), 219–37.

Trapp, M. B., *Philosophy in the Roman Empire: Ethics, Politics and Society* (Aldershot, 2007).

Usener, H. (ed.), *Epicurea* (Leipzig, 1887).

Vallance, J. T., *The Lost Theory of Asclepiades of Bithynia* (Oxford, 1990).

van den Berg, M., and Dircksen, M., "Mandrake from Antiquity to Harry Potter", *Akroterion* 53 (2008), 67–79.

van der Eijk, P. J., "Galen's Use of the Concept of 'Qualified Experience' in his Dietetic and Pharmacological Works", in Debru 1997, 35–57.

van Riel, G., "Does a Perfect Activity Necessarily Yield Pleasure? An Evaluation of the Relation between Pleasure and Activity in Aristotle, Nicomachean Ethics VII and X", *International Journal of Philosophical Studies* 7 (1999), 211–24.

van Riel, G., *Pleasure and the Good Life: Plato, Aristotle, and the Neoplatonists* (Leiden, 2000).

Vernant, J.-P., "One, Two, Three: Eros", in D. Halperin, J. J. Winkler and F. Zeitlin (eds.), *Before Sexuality* (Princeton, 1990), 465–78.

Vlastos, G., "Introduction" to B. Jowett (trans.), *Plato's Protagoras* (revised by M. Ostwald, Indianapolis, 1956).

Vlastos, G., "Socrates on Acrasia", *Phoenix* 23 (= *Studies Presented to G. M. A. Grube on the Occasion of His Seventieth Birthday*) (1969), 71–88.

Vogt, K. M., "Anger, Present Injustice and Future Revenge", in K. Volk and G. D. Williams (eds.), *Seeing Seneca Whole: Perspectives on Philosophy, Poetry and Politics* (Columbia Studies in the Classical Tradition 28) (Leiden, 2006), 57–74.

Vogt, K. M., "Why Pleasure Gains Fifth Rank: Against the Anti-Hedonist Reading of the *Philebus*", in J. Dillon and L. Brisson (eds.), *Plato's Philebus* (St. Augustin, 2010), 250–5.

Vogt, K. M., "I Shall Do What I Did: Stoic Views on Action", in R. Salles, P. Destrée and M. Zingano (eds.), *What is Up to Us? Studies on Agency and Responsibility in Ancient Philosophy* (Sankt Augustin, 2014), 107–20.

Vogt, K. M., "Taking the Same Things Seriously and not Seriously: a Stoic Proposal on Value and the Good", in D. R. Gordon and D. B. Suits (eds.), *Epictetus: His Continuing Influence and Contemporary Relevance* (Rochester, 2014), 55–75.

Vogt, K. M. rev. of Pakaluk and Pearson 2011, *Mind* 123 (2014), 1221–7.

Vogt, K. M., "Imagining Good Future States: Hope and Truth in Plato's *Philebus*", in J. Wilkins (ed.), *Selfhood and the Soul: Essays on Ancient Thought and Literature in Honour of Christopher Gill* (Oxford, 2017), 33–48.

Volk, K., *The Poetics of Latin Didactic* (Oxford, 2002).

Von Staden, H., *Herophilus: the Art of Medicine in Early Alexandria* (Cambridge, 1989).

Wager, T. D., and Fields, H. L., 'Placebo Analgesia', in McMahon 2013, 362–77.

Wallace-Hadrill, A., *Rome's Cultural Revolution* (Cambridge, 2008).

Warner, J. H., "From Specificity to Universalism in Medical Therapeutics: Transformation in the Nineteenth-century United States", in Kawakita et al. 1990, 193–223.

Warren, J., "Aristotle on Speusippus on Eudoxus on Pleasure", *OSAPh* 36 (2009), 249–81.

Warren, J., *The Pleasures of Reason in Plato, Aristotle, and the Hellenistic Hedonists* (Cambridge, 2014).

Warren, J., "The Bloom of Youth", *Apeiron* 48 (2016), 327–45.

Wehrli, F., *Hieronymos von Rhodos, Kritolaos und seine Schüler* (Basel, 1959).

Wehrli, F., *Lykon: Texte und Kommentar* (Basel, 1968).

Wehrli, F., Wöhrle, G., and Zhmud, L., "Der Peripatos bis zum Beginn der römischen Kaiserzeit", in H. Flashar (ed.), *Die Philosophie der Antike* III (second ed., Basel, 2004), 493–639.

White, S. A., "Happiness in the Hellenistic Lyceum", *Apeiron* 35 (2002), 69–94.

White, S. A., "Lyco and Hieronymus on the Good life", in W. W. Fortenbaugh and S. A. White (ed. and trans.), *Lyco of Troas and Hieronymus of Rhodes* (New Brunswick, 2004), 389–409.

White, S. A., "Stoic Selection: Objects, Actions, and Agents", in A. W. Nightingale and D. Sedley (eds.), *Ancient Models of Mind: Studies in Human and Divine Rationality* (Cambridge, 2010), 110–29.

Whitehead, D., "Competitive Outlay and Community Profit: *philotimia* in Democratic Athens", *Classica et Mediaevalia*, 34 (1983), 55–74.

Whitehead, D., *The Demes of Attica* (Princeton, 1986).

Whitehead, D., "Cardinal Virtues: the language of Public Approbation in Democratic Athens", *Classica et Mediaevalia* 44 (1993), 37–75.

Willer, L., "Iatromagie: Magie und Medizin im griechisch-römischen Ägypten", in A. Jördens (ed.), *Ägyptische Magie und Umwelt* (Wiesbaden, 2015), 281–301.

Winkler, J. J., *Auctor & Actor: A Narratological Reading of Apuleius's Golden Ass* (Berkeley, 1985).

Wolf, U., *Aristoteles' Nikomachische Ethik* (Darmstadt, 2002).

Wolfsdorf, D., "The Ridiculousness of Being Overcome by Pleasure: *Protagoras* 352B1–358D4", *OSAPh* 31 (2006), 113–36.

Wolfsdorf, D., "Hesiod, Prodicus, and the Socratics on Work and Pleasure", *OSAPh* 35 (2008), 1–18.

Wolfsdorf, D., "Epicurus on Εὐφροσύνη and Ἐνέργεια (DL 10.136)", *Apeiron* 42 (2009), 221–57.

Wolfsdorf, D., *Pleasure in Ancient Greek Philosophy* (Cambridge, 2013).

Wycherley, R. E., "The Garden of Epicurus", *Phoenix* 13 (2) (1959), 73–7.

Wyttenbach, D. A., *Animadversiones in Plutarchi Opera Moralia* II (Leipzig, 1821).

Zadorojnyi, A. V., "Nero's Transformation Again: Plutarch, *De Sera Numinis Vindicta* 567f–568a", *Pegasus* 40 (1997), 28–9.

Zanchin, G., "The Headache Remedies of the *Pseudo-Apuleius*: a Modern Reappraisal", in D. Michaelides (ed.), *Medicine and Healing in the Ancient Mediterranean* (Oxford, 2014), 164–6.

Zeyl, D. J., "Socrates and Hedonism: 'Protagoras' 351b–358d", *Phronesis* 25 (1980), 250–69.

Ziegler, K., *Plutarchos von Chaironeia* (Stuttgart, 1949).

Zohary, D., Hopf, M., and Weiss, E., *Domestication of Plants in the Old World* (fourth ed., Oxford, 2012).

Index

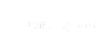

Printed in the United States
By Bookmasters